ADVANCES IN

Pharmacology and Chemotherapy

VOLUME 7

ADVISORY BOARD

ADVANCES IN

Pharmacology and Chemotherapy

EDITED BY

Silvio Garattini
Istituto di Ricerche Farmacologiche "Mario Negri" Milano, Italy

A. Goldin
National Cancer Institute Bethesda, Maryland

F. Hawking
National Institute for Medical Research London, England

I. J. Kopin
National Institute of Mental Health Bethesda, Maryland

VOLUME 7

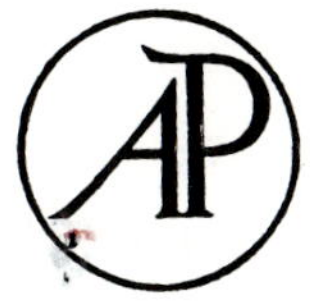

ACADEMIC PRESS New York and London, 1969

ACADEMIC PRESS, INC.
111 Fifth Avenue, New York, New York 10003

United Kingdom Edition published by
ACADEMIC PRESS, INC. (LONDON) LTD.
Berkeley Square House, London W1X 6BA

LIBRARY OF CONGRESS CATALOG CARD NUMBER: 61-18298

PRINTED IN THE UNITED STATES OF AMERICA

CONTRIBUTORS TO THIS VOLUME

Numbers in parentheses indicate the pages on which the authors' contributions begin.

BETTY J. ABBOTT (117), *Cancer Chemotherapy National Service Center, National Cancer Institute, National Institutes of Health, U.S. Public Health Service, Bethesda, Maryland*

RUBIN BRESSLER (91), *Departments of Medicine and Physiology and Pharmacology, Duke University Medical Center, Durham, North Carolina*

STANLEY G. BROWNE (211), *Leprosy Study Centre, London, England*

H. O. J. COLLIER (333), *Department of Pharmacological Research, Division of Medical and Scientific Affairs, Parke-Davis and Company, Hounslow, Middlesex, England*

CARL-GUSTAF HAMMAR (53), *Department of Toxicology, Swedish Medical Research Council, Karolinska Institutet, Stockholm, Sweden*

JONATHAN L. HARTWELL (117), *Cancer Chemotherapy National Service Center, National Cancer Institute, National Institutes of Health, U.S. Public Health Service, Bethesda, Maryland*

BO HOLMSTEDT (53), *Department of Toxicology, Swedish Medical Research Council, Karolinska Institutet, Stockholm, Sweden*

ERNEST JAWETZ (253), *Departments of Microbiology, Medicine, and Pediatrics, University of California Medical Center, San Francisco, California*

JOHN STEPHEN KIZER (91), *Departments of Medicine and Physiology and Pharmacology, Duke University Medical Center, Durham, North Carolina*

JAN-ERIK LINDGREN (53), *Department of Toxicology, Swedish Medical Research Council, Karolinska Institutet, Stockholm, Sweden*

JAMES A. MCFADZEAN (309), *The Research Laboratories, May & Baker Ltd., Dagenham, Essex, England*

H. R. PERKINS (283), *National Institute for Medical Research, London, England*

RICHARD THAM (53), *Department of Toxicology, Swedish Medical Research Council, Karolinska Institutet, Stockholm, Sweden*

ELLIOT S. VESELL* (1), *Section on Pharmacogenetics, Laboratory of Chemical Pharmacology, National Heart Institute, National Institutes of Health, Bethesda, Maryland*

*Present address: Department of Pharmacology, Milton S. Hershey Medical Center, Pennsylvania State University College of Medicine, Hershey, Pennsylvania

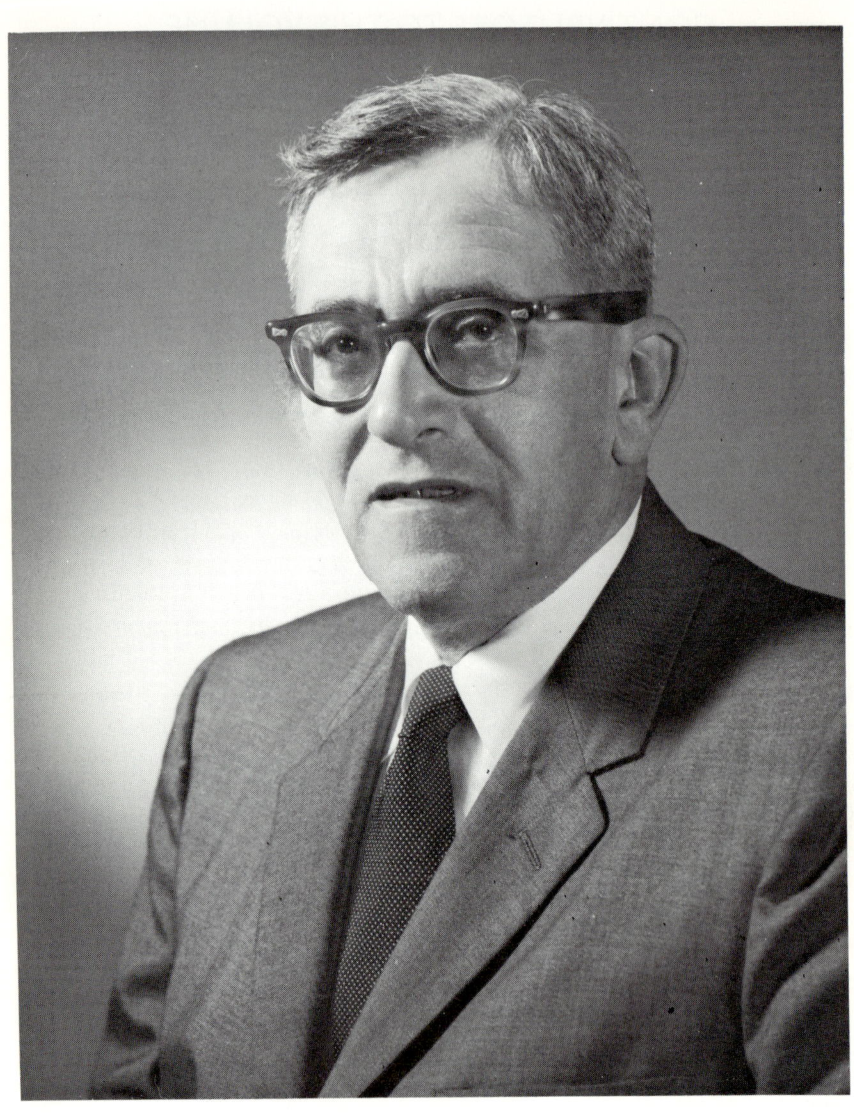

ROBERT J. SCHNITZER

FOREWORD

We would like to congratulate Dr. Robert J. Schnitzer on his seventy-fifth birthday.

Dr. Schnitzer was born in Berlin on May 16, 1894. He studied at the University in Berlin, and received his M.D. degree in 1919. From 1919 to 1928 he worked as a bacteriologist at the Institut Robert Koch in Berlin, and soon became involved in chemotherapy studies which have remained his major life interest. From 1928 to 1938 he was head of the Chemotherapy Laboratory, Farbwerke Hoechst, Hoechst/Main; from 1939 to 1941 he worked at the Connaught Laboratories, University of Toronto, and from 1941 to 1960 he was Director of the Chemotherapy Department of Hoffman La Roche, Inc., Nutley, New Jersey.

Dr. Schnitzer was the first to institute extensive routine screening tests of new compounds on many different infections—metazoal, protozoal, fungal, bacterial, viral—and on experimental neoplasms. This led to numerous discoveries: the action of quinoline compounds on *Trypanosoma congolense* and *T. vivax* (a step toward the discovery of Antrycide); the production of sulfisoxazole (Gantrisin) and sulfadimethoxine (Madribon); and, perhaps the greatest of all, the contribution to the discovery of isoniazid, the most active and widely used compound for the treatment of tuberculosis. He has also made many other important contributions to the practical and theoretical aspects of chemotherapy, including the relationship of immunological phenomena and drug resistance.

Since 1960 Dr. Schnitzer has served as a Consulting Editor to Academic Press, and has been instrumental in initiating and organizing the treatise "Experimental Chemotherapy," and other works, particularly the *Advances in Chemotherapy*, of which the present volume is an amalgamation and continuation.

Dr. Schnitzer, who is still as active as ever, is now Professorial Lecturer at the Mount Sinai School of Medicine, New York. We congratulate him on his achievements to date and wish him many more fruitful years.

SILVIO GARATTINI
ABRAHAM GOLDIN
FRANK HAWKING
IRWIN J. KOPIN

PREFACE

An observer of the developments in the fields of pharmacology and chemotherapy during the last decade could not fail to notice that the artificial separation of the two areas of experimental research in drug action cannot be maintained any longer. As the study of mechanism of drug action gained in depth, the correlation of active compounds with the biochemically and genetically defined properties of the target cells moved into the foreground of quantitative evaluation. Interpretations beyond the cellular level by the specific functions of subcellular structures and their enzymes seem to offer general concepts which may include organ, neoplastic, and microbial cells. Moreover, interactions of the response of host cells with pathological and pathogenic cells are characteristic for many therapeutic and toxic effects regardless of the etiological factors involved.

These considerations among others induced the editors and publisher of *Advances in Pharmacology* and *Advances in Chemotherapy* to combine these serial publications in the hope that the wider scope of the new work will offer to a larger audience a more complete insight into the interdigitations of chemical and biological action and open the way to new experimental approaches.

This volume, entitled *Advances in Pharmacology and Chemotherapy*, contains articles on pharmacological topics in a strict sense, namely, the contributions by Vesell, Hammar *et al.*, Kizer and Bressler, and Collier, whereas the articles by Hartwell and Abbott, Browne, Jawetz, Perkins, and McFadzean are devoted to topics of chemotherapy.

We cannot conclude the Preface without announcing with deep regret that Dr. Parkhurst A. Shore has completed his term of editorship of the Advances. Unfortunately, the burden of his academic commitments makes it impossible for him to continue his editorial work. The success of the first six volumes of *Advances in Pharmacology* was due to a great extent to his dedication to the difficult task as editor, his foresight, and his understanding of the essential events in pharmacology. We thank him for a job well done.

August, 1969

Silvio Garattini
Abraham Goldin
Frank Hawking
Irwin J. Kopin

CONTENTS

Antineoplastic Principles in Plants: Recent Developments in the Field

Jonathan L. Hartwell and Betty J. Abbott

The Evaluation of Present Antileprosy Compounds

Stanley G. Browne

Chemotherapy of Chlamydial Infections

Ernest Jawetz

Composition of Bacterial Cell Walls in Relation to Antibiotic Action

H. R. PERKINS

Advances in the Chemotherapy of Viral Diseases

JAMES A. MCFADZEAN

A Pharmacological Analysis of Aspirin

H. O. J. COLLIER

ADVANCES IN

Pharmacology and Chemotherapy

VOLUME 7

Recent Progress in Pharmacogenetics

Elliot S. Vesell*

Section on Pharmacogenetics
Laboratory of Chemical Pharmacology,
National Heart Institute, National Institutes of Health,
Bethesda, Maryland

I. History

In 1957 A. Motulsky and A. Vogel independently coined the term pharmacogenetics and laid the conceptual foundations for this new field (Motulsky, 1957; Vogel, 1959; Kalow, 1962). These two geneticists used the word to draw attention to several hereditary conditions then recently discovered through unusual responses elicited by the administration of various drugs. The examples available in 1957 were acatalasia, suxamethonium sensitivity, slow inactivation of isoniazid, inability to taste phenylthiourea, to smell hydrocyanic acid, and a self-limited hemolytic anemia occurring after ingestion of various drugs

* Current address: Department of Pharmacology, Milton S. Hershey Medical Center, Pennsylvania State University College of Medicine, Hershey, Pennsylvania.

caused by glucose-6-phosphate dehydrogenase deficiency. Increasing exposure of large numbers of individuals to various therapeutic agents and development of sensitive techniques for measuring activities of drug-metabolizing enzymes enabled the elucidation of these entities. Much recent work reviewed below has been devoted to these genetically transmitted conditions but few new examples have been described.

Widespread use of drugs constitutes a notable change in our environment. The possibility that this widespread dissemination of drugs might reveal additional hereditary disorders characterized by abnormal responses to potent commonly used therapeutic agents was anticipated in 1957. However, these expectations have not been realized over the past 12 years. Only rare and isolated examples have been reported: Sporadic cases of sensitivity to dicoumarol (Solomon, 1968) and Dilantin (Kutt *et al.*, 1964a) and of resistance to warfarin (O'Reilly *et al.*, 1964, 1968) have been published.

Clearly, adverse reactions to drugs are common; few new therapeutic agents lack side effects, either on the skin, gastrointestinal tract, blood, central nervous system, cardiovascular system, endocrine organs or genitourinary tract. However, the hereditary nature of these untoward responses remains to be established. Perhaps in the future some cases of blood dyscrasias after chloramphenicol, antibody formation to penicillin and other drugs, extrapyramidal symptoms after prochlorperazine, or a syndrome resembling disseminated lupus erythematosus appearing after hydralazine administration will be shown to be familial and their mode of inheritance elucidated.

II. Definitions

The term pharmacogenetics was employed originally to refer to hereditary disorders revealed solely by the use of drugs. Use of pharmacogenetics in this sense appears to be too restrictive. It excludes from consideration several hereditary diseases previously well described but only relatively recently discovered to be exacerbated by the administration of drugs: (1) diabetes mellitus precipitated by adrenocortical steroids, (2) acute gouty attacks after thiazide diuretics, and (3) porphyria worsened by barbiturates.

At the other extreme, pharmacogenetics has been defined to include conditions in which drug responses are modified by hereditary factors. This definition lacks specificity.

Experience during the 12 years since the introduction of the term pharmacogenetics has led to some disagreement over what limits should be imposed on the term and over how significant pharmacogenetic conditions and concepts will prove to be in the future. In this review the term pharmacogenetics will be applied to clinically significant consequences of hereditary variations in the handling of drugs. This article deals mainly with an increasing body of data on the defects in man enumerated above and only tangentially with the very large literature concerning experimental animals reviewed extensively and well earlier (Kalow, 1962; Meier, 1963).

III. Types of Response to Drugs

Search for hereditary variations affecting the way the body handles drugs has until recently turned up almost exclusively traits inherited as single factors; that is, traits produced by point mutations at a single genetic locus and transmitted either as Mendelian dominants or recessives.

Investigation of the responsiveness of the general population to a drug in terms of the amount of a drug required to produce a given effect may take the form of a continuous unimodal distribution curve or of a discontinuous polymodal curve (Fig. 1). Until recently, studies of drug responses that yield a

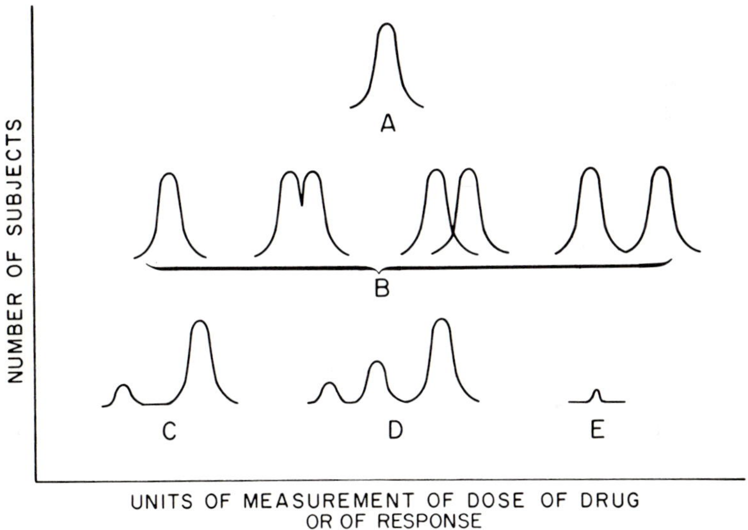

FIG. 1. Types of frequency distribution for the responsiveness of individuals to various drugs. Modified from Kalow (1962).

normal or continuous distribution curve have been almost entirely ignored in pharmacogenetic investigations. To construct unimodal, Gaussian distribution curves large populations are required. Furthermore, genotypes are hard to deduce from such curves. In contrast, discontinuous, bimodal, or trimodal curves of response obtained from disorders transmitted as Mendelian dominants or recessives are more easily analyzed because each discrete curve generally corresponds to a different genotype. In other words, the mutant genes and their corresponding phenotypes segregate both in pedigrees and in the distribution curves. Figure 1 compares the normal or Gaussian distribution curve obtained for graded metrical characters, typically under polygenic control (curve A), with the discontinuous multimodal curves for traits transmitted as Mendelian recessives and dominants. Curve E, though unimodal and continuous, actually indicates a response by individuals possessing a genetically transmitted polymorphic trait, a response which normal individuals do not exhibit. Such examples include hemolysis in some individuals with glucose-6-phosphate dehydrogenase deficiency after administration of antimalarials, or acute arthritic attacks in certain individuals with the gene for gout after receiving thiazide diuretics, or abnormal blood glucose tolerance curves in individuals with diabetes mellitus after receiving steroids.

Figure 1 includes under group B a unimodal curve, although all other examples under category B are multimodal. Because it may actually conceal genetic heterogeneity, this unimodal curve is included in group B. For example, Fig. 2 reveals that the total acid phosphatase activities in the general popula-

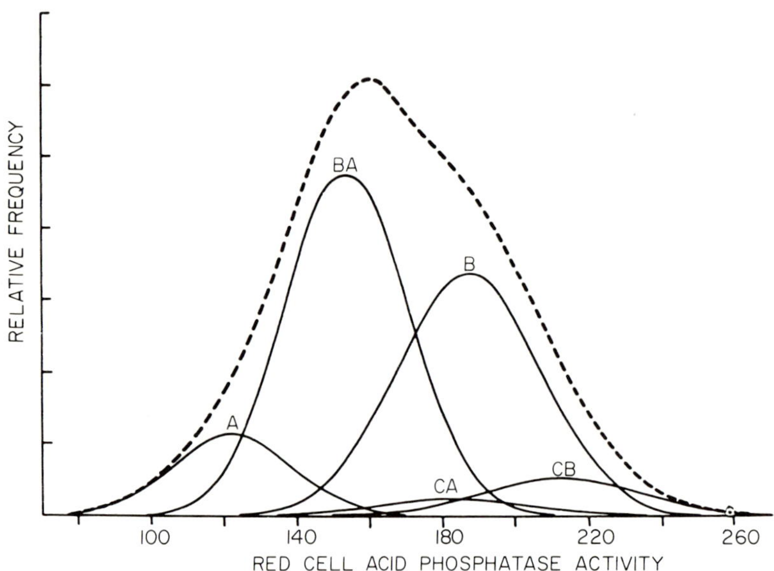

FIG. 2. Distribution of erythrocyte acid phosphatases in the general population (broken line) and in the separate phenotypes. The curves are reconstructed from data of Hopkinson *et al.* (1964) and are reproduced from Harris (1968).

tion superficially resemble a continuous unimodal curve, but in actuality this single curve is composed of five discrete curves representing five distinct phenotypes and genotypes (Hopkinson *et al.*, 1964). The frequency of each of these five curves was determined in an English population by separating the total acid phosphatase activity of erythrocytes into isozymes by starch gel electrophoresis; relatively different electrophoretic mobilities and different distributions of total activity among the isozymes permit classification of individuals into one of the five phenotypes (Hopkinson *et al.*, 1964).

Motulsky (1964) reported genetic investigations of variations in the half-life of dicoumarol in human plasma. An approximately continuous distribution was observed (Fig. 3). Analysis of family data by the method of Fisher (1954)

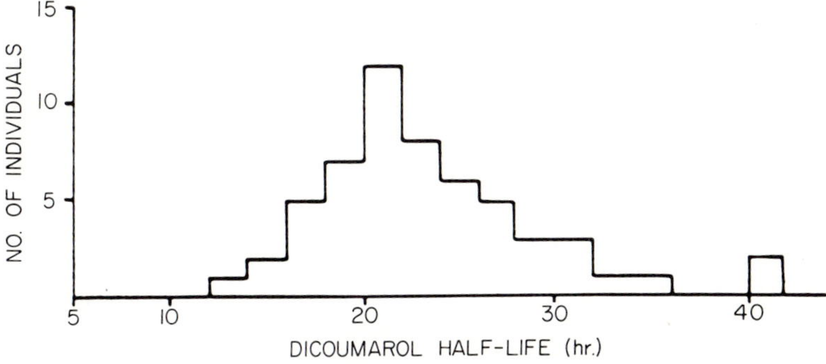

FIG. 3. Dicoumarol half-life in plasma in random subjects after a single oral dose of 2 mg/kg. (Reproduced from Motulsky, 1964.)

showed sib-sib correlations in the absence of sib-parent correlations. Attempts to fit the data to a single gene mechanism failed. To Motulsky these results suggested the operation of multiple recessive genes in controlling values for dicoumarol half-life in plasma. Such an interpretation is subject to the objection that young sibs may share a more similar environment than do parent and child. Thus sib-sib correlations in the absence of sib-parent correlations could result from the influence of environmental as well as genetic factors.

IV. Genetic Control of Drug Elimination from Human Plasma

Large differences in rates of elimination of phenylbutazone (Burns *et al.*, 1953), antipyrine (Brodie and Axelrod, 1950), and dicoumarol (Weiner *et al.*, 1950) from human plasma have been reported, but the basis for these differences was not established. Numerous environmental factors, such as exposure to inducing agents, degree of health or illness, and hormonal and nutritional status are known to alter the rates at which humans metabolize certain drugs. Several drugs such as phenylbutazone enhance their own metabolism (Conney,

1967). In mice, responsiveness to a drug such as hexobarbital differs according to age, sex, litter, painful stimuli, ambient temperature, degree of crowding, time of day of drug administration, and type of bedding (Vesell, 1968). Such experiments would imply that a large component in the causation of individual variations in human drug metabolism would be environmental.

Resistance to warfarin has been described in patients who metabolize the drug rapidly, with half-lives in plasma of 5.5 to 6.9 hours compared to normal values of 44 ± 10 hours (Lewis *et al.*, 1967). Abnormal plasma binding, anomalous apparent volume of distribution, and excretion of unchanged drug in the urine were eliminated as possible explanations; however, a history of prior drug administration was not provided and therefore a rapid rate of metabolism could arise from enzyme induction as well as from genetic factors.

To determine quantitatively the relative contributions of environmental and genetic factors to large variations among human subjects in drug metabolism, a study of identical and fraternal twins was performed. If individual variations in drug half-life were primarily due to environmental factors with a negligible effect of heredity, then intrapair differences would be of similar magnitude for monozygotic and dizygotic twins. However, if genetic factors played a significant role, then intrapair variations should be much smaller in identical than in fraternal twins. We anticipated a predominantly environmental influence.

Normal adult, Caucasian volunteers not receiving drugs at the time of, or for several weeks preceding, the study were typed for 30 blood groups to document the nature of their twinship. Each twin received a single oral dose of phenylbutazone (6 mg/kg); 2 months later a single oral dose of antipyrine (18 mg/kg) was given; 2 months later a single oral dose of dicoumarol (4 mg/kg) was administered. The half-lives of these three drugs determined in each individual are given in Table I (Vesell and Page, 1968a,b,c). Blood specimens were drawn at regular intervals after drug ingestion and the values for the concentration of drug in plasma plotted as shown in Figs. 4, 5, and 6. These curves illustrate for each of the three drugs tested typical examples of rates of elimination from plasma of identical twins and of fraternal twins. Half-lives of the three drugs, determined from these curves, appear in Table I.

The results clearly indicate that the major mechanisms for individual differences in rates of elimination of phenylbutazone, antipyrine, and dicoumarol are genetic rather than environmental. The contribution of heredity to the plasma half-life of these three drugs was estimated from the formula (Osborne and DeGeorge, 1959):

$$\frac{\text{Variance within pairs of fraternal twins} - \text{variance within pairs of identical twins}}{\text{variance within pairs of fraternal twins}}$$

Theoretically values derived from this formula could range from 0, indicating negligible contribution of heredity, to 1, indicating strong hereditary influence.

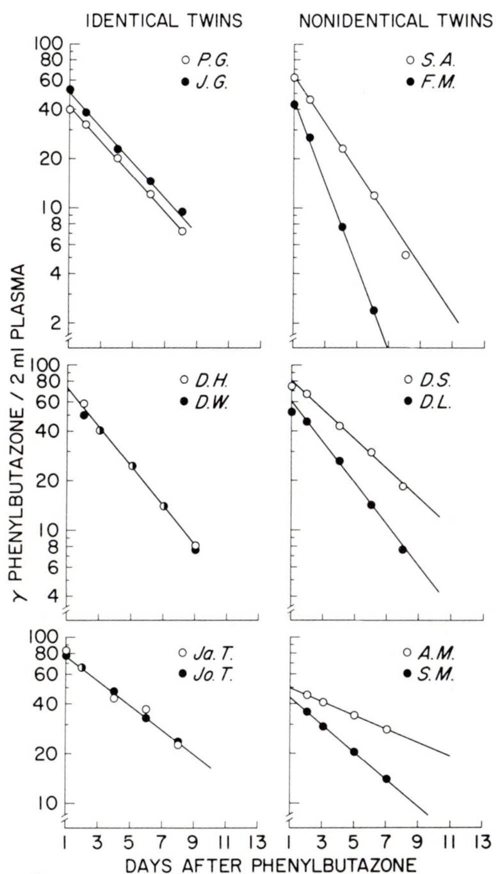

FIG. 4. Decline of phenylbutazone in the plasma of 3 sets of identical twins (left) and 3 sets of fraternal twins (right). The log of the phenylbutazone concentration in 2 ml of plasma is shown at intervals after a single oral dose (6 mg/kg). (Reproduced from Vesell and Page, 1968a.)

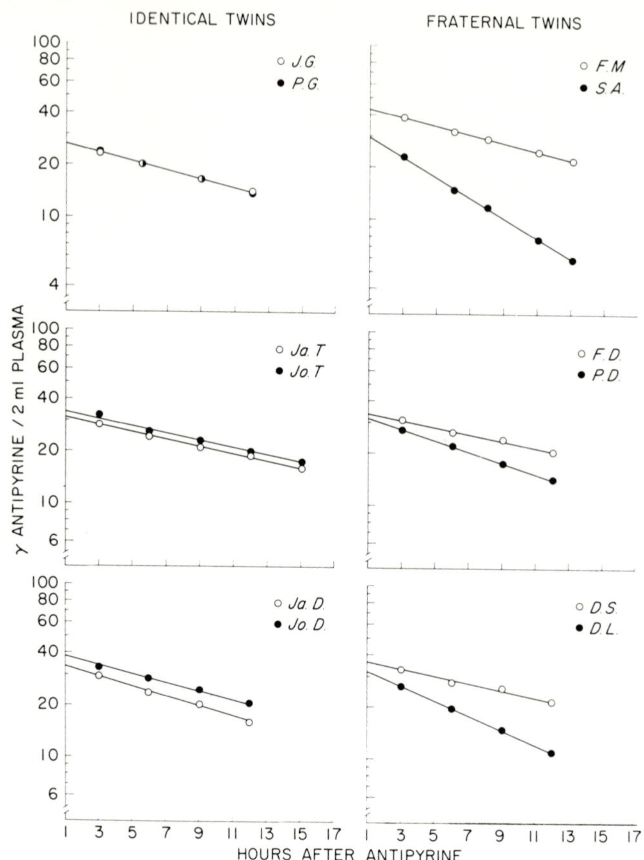

FIG. 5. Decline of antipyrine in the plasma of 3 sets of identical twins (left) and 3 sets of fraternal twins (right). The log of the antipyrine concentration in 2 ml of plasma is shown at intervals after a single oral dose (18 mg/kg). (Reproduced from Vesell and Page, 1968b.)

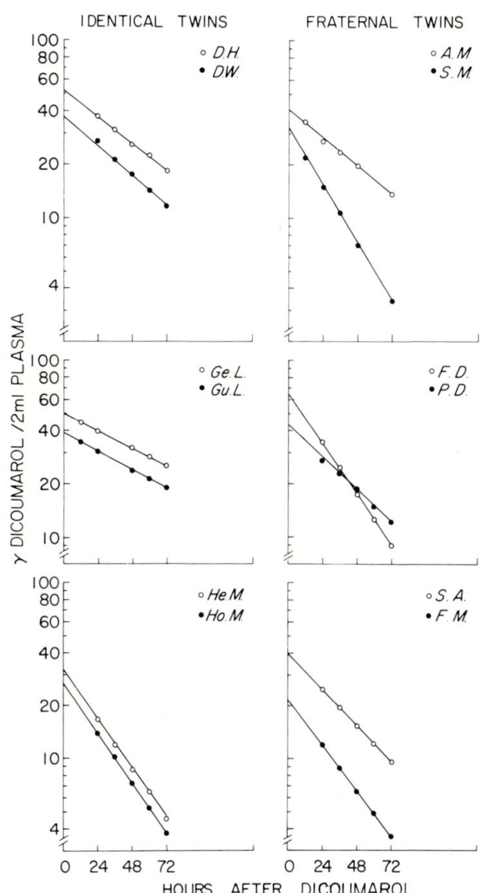

FIG. 6. Decline of dicoumarol in the plasma of 3 sets of identical twins (left) and 3 sets of fraternal twins (right). The log of the dicoumarol concentration in 2 ml of plasma is shown at intervals after a single oral dose (2 mg/kg). (Reproduced from Vesell and Page, 1968c.)

For phenylbutazone, antipyrine, and dicoumarol, values for the contribution of heredity were 0.99, 0.98, and 0.97, respectively.

Since phenylbutazone and dicoumarol are 98% bound to plasma proteins, variation in the elimination of these drugs from plasma might possibly involve binding of the drugs to albumin. However, antipyrine is not appreciably bound to plasma proteins. Therefore, it seems reasonable to conclude that for antipyrine, and possibly also for phenylbutazone and dicoumarol, variation in plasma half-life is due to differences in the metabolism rather than in distribution of drug. Appreciable variations do exist among humans in rates of metabolism of these drugs. Ranges in half-lives for phenylbutazone, antipyrine, and dicoumarol were 3-fold, 3-fold, and 10-fold, respectively, among the 28 individuals in the twin study (Table I).

These results have both clinical and theoretical implications. Toxicity may develop primarily in subjects in whom the half-life of drugs is long, whereas those with short drug half-lives may not attain sufficient or sufficiently sustained levels to derive therapeutic benefit.

Furthermore, half-lives of drugs such as Dilantin, phenylbutazone, and dicoumarol are dose-dependent; their rates of metabolism decrease as their dosage increases (Weiner *et al.*, 1950; Dayton *et al.*, 1967). Table II shows this dose-dependence of dicoumarol half-lives in normal individuals receiving a single dose of 2 mg/kg, a single dose of 4 mg/kg at a later date, and finally 2 mg/kg on each of 6 days. The dicoumarol half-lives were progressively prolonged. Although the mechanism for dose-dependent drug half-lives is not clear, it probably involves inhibition of metabolism by the drug itself (Dayton *et al.*, 1967). Regardless of the explanation, several important clinical implications relate both to wide individual variations in dicoumarol metabolism (10-fold in the 28 twins shown in Table I), and to the dose-dependence of dicoumarol half-life (Table II). The combination of large, genetically controlled variations in half-life and dose-dependence of half-life suggests the advisability of determining the half-lives of drugs in plasma before chronic therapy. Although the dose-dependence of drug half-life might be interpreted at first glance to argue against determination of individual rates of drug metabolism prior to long-term therapy, because of changing values of the half-life with each new dose, determination of half-life becomes of clinical importance precisely for this reason.

Patients who slowly metabolize drugs such as dicoumarol or phenylbutazone will be particularly susceptible to toxicity on chronic therapy. For example, with respect to the two individuals at the extremes of the data shown in Table I who have dicoumarol half-lives of 7 and 74 hours, no change in the half-life of the rapid metabolizer will occur after several daily doses. In contrast, the drug will accumulate on repeated administration to a patient with a drug half-life of 74 hours. The extent of variability of dicoumarol half-life will rise from 10-fold

TABLE I

Dicoumarol, Antipyrine, and Phenylbutazone Half-Lives with Smoking and Coffee History in 28 Twins[a]

Twin	Age, sex	Half-life			Smoking (Pack/day)	Coffee (Cups/day)
		Dicoumarol Hours	Antipyrine Hours	Phenylbutazone Days		
			Identical twins[b]			
HoM	48, M	25.0	11.3	1.9	0.5	2
HoM	48, M	25.0	11.3	2.1	1	3
DT	43, F	55.5	10.3	2.8	0	5–6
VW	43, F	55.5	9.6	2.9	2	8–10
JG	22, M	36.0	11.5	2.8	1	1–2
PG	22, M	34.0	11.5	2.8	1	1–2
JaT	44, M	74.0	14.9	4.0	0	6
JaT	44, M	72.0	14.9	4.0	0	2–3
CJ	55, F	41.0	6.9	3.2	0	2
FJ	55, F	42.5	7.1	2.9	0	2
Gel	45, M	72.0	12.3	3.9	0	4
Gul	45, M	69.0	12.8	4.1	0	4
DH	26, F	46.0	11.0	2.6	0	0–1
DW	26, F	44.0	11.0	2.6	0	3–4
			Fraternal twins[b]			
AM	21, F	45.0	15.1	7.3	1 5	2
SM	21, M	22.0	6.3	3.6	0	0
DL	36, F	46.5	7.2	2.3	0	2–3
DS	36, F	51.0	15.0	3.3	2	3–4
SA	33, F	34.5	5.1	2.1	1	2
FM	33, F	27.5	12.5	1.2	0.5	2
JaH	24, F	7.0	12.0	2.6	0	10–15
JeH	24, F	19.0	6.0	2.3	1.5	10
FD	48, M	24.5	14.7	2.8	0	1
PD	48, M	38.0	9.3	3.5	1.5	8
LD	21, F	67.0	8.2	2.9	1	6
LW	21, F	72.0	6.9	3.0	1	2–3
EK	31, F	40.5	7.7	1.9	0	0
RK	31, M	35.0	7.3	2.1	1	0

[a] From Vesell and Page (1968c).

[b] The difference between identical and fraternal twins in intrapair variance is significant: $P < 0.005$ ($F = 36.0$, $N_1 = N_2 = 7$).

TABLE II

Relationship of Dicoumarol Half-Life to Dose in 5 Unrelated Normal Adults[a]

Volunteer	Age, sex	Half-life (hr)[b] after dose of dicoumarol		
		2 mg/kg	4 mg/kg	2 mg/kg daily × 6
EV	34, M	25.0	42.5	80
JP	27, M	24.6	41.0	84
HC	53, F	30.5	68.0	144
FG	34, M	18.2	38.5	
HB	28, M	23.8	51.5	

[a] From Vesell and Page, (1968c).

[b] Mean half-life on 2 mg/kg dose = 24.4 hr; on 4 mg/kg dose = 48.3. Ratio of half-lives on these two dosages = 0.505.

after a single dose to 20- and even 30-fold after successive daily doses.

The increased liability to toxicity in individuals slowly metabolizing a drug whose half-life is dose-dependent raises the possibility that high drug-metabolizing activity may have conferred certain advantages during evolution. Such an advantage would occur in environments where individuals chronically ingest as food or drugs appreciable amounts of those alkaloids whose metabolism may be dose-dependent and whose accumulation in high levels within the body is toxic. Thus, natural selection in certain environments may have favored and possibly continues to favor individuals with high levels of drug-metabolizing enzymes.

These conclusions are based on the genetic control of the metabolism of certain drugs and the reproducibility of individual half-lives (Weiner *et al.*, 1950; Brodie and Axelrod, 1950; Burns *et al.*, 1953; Vesell and Page, 1968a,b,c). The genetic control of the rates for the elimination from plasma of phenylbutazone, antipyrine, and dicoumarol suggests that other drugs metabolized in the body may be under similar genetic regulation. If such proves to be the case, the application of pharmacogenetic concepts extends considerably beyond these few disorders with generally low incidence arising from single point mutations. The clinical significance of such conditions is limited mainly to avoidance of certain drugs in individuals of a particular genotype.

Rates of elimination of certain drugs from plasma can provide important therapeutic information to permit tailoring of dosage to individual requirements, thereby lessening instances of toxicity on the one hand, and of undertreatment on the other. Simple, direct, inexpensive, and accurate spectrophotometric procedures are available for the assay of phenylbutazone (Burns *et al.*, 1953), antipyrine (Brodie *et al.*, 1949), dicoumarol (Axelrod *et al.*,

1949), and many other drugs; new methods are being developed for an increasingly large number of drugs. Therefore, it appears feasible to estimate the half-lives of many drugs for routine clinical purposes.

Such a course would be greatly facilitated if correlations between various groups of drugs in rates of removal from plasma could be established. A search for such correlations was made by various statistical approaches in the 28 individuals whose half-lives for phenylbutazone, antipyrine, and dicoumarol are shown in Table I. The results show that although there is no correlation between rates of elimination from plasma of phenylbutazone and antipyrine and between those of dicoumarol and antipyrine, there appears to be a tendency toward correlation between rates of removal for phenylbutazone and dicoumarol. Figure 7 shows this correlation as estimated by the method of Bartlett

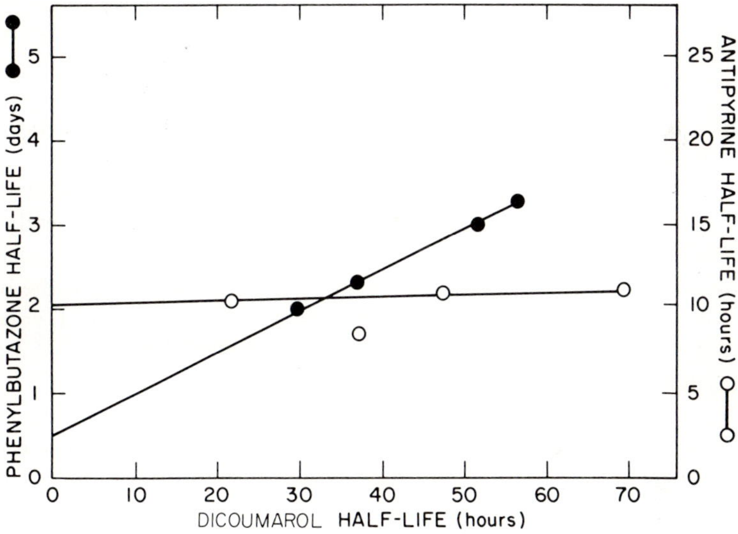

FIG. 7. Relationship between half-lives of dicoumarol and phenylbutazone and between half-lives of dicoumarol and antipyrine in various individuals according to the method of Bartlett (1949). (Reproduced from Vesell and Page, 1968c.)

(1949). The tendency toward correlation between rates of phenylbutazone and dicoumarol metabolism in an individual may be related to the fact that both drugs are avidly and almost entirely bound to plasma proteins. Alternatively, both drugs may be degraded by similar enzymatic steps. Whatever the explanation, the existence of such a correlation raises the possibility that within an individual the rates of metabolism of other drugs may also be correlated. Recent work by Hammer *et al.* (1969) demonstrates correlation of the rates of metabolism of desmethylimipramine, nortriptyline, and oxyphenylbutazone. The close correlation between the rates of metabolism of these three drugs is strikingly illustrated in Fig. 8 which shows that an individual metabolizing one drug slowly metabolizes the other two drugs slowly and that conversely, a rapid metabolizer transforms all three compounds at fast rates. Solomon (1968) also reported an individual who metabolizes both Dilantin and dicoumarol at abnormally slow rates.

Several environmental factors can alter rates of dicoumarol metabolism, including the size of the dose, the extent and rapidity of gastrointestinal

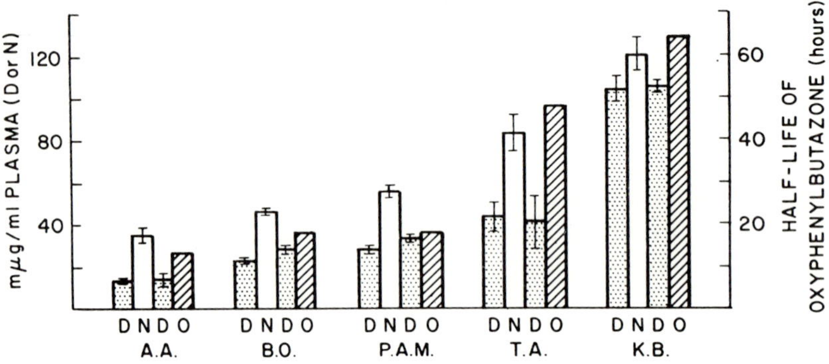

FIG. 8. Steady plasma levels (mean ± S.D.) of desmethylimipramine (D) (25 mg t.i.d.) and nortriptyline (N) (25 mg t.i.d.) and half-life of oxyphenylbutazone (O) in 5 hospitalized psychiatric female patients. The drugs were given separately in consecutive order, as shown in the figure. (Reproduced from Hammer *et al.*, 1969.)

absorption, and prior ingestion of substances capable of inducing drug-metabolizing enzymes located in liver microsomes (Weiner *et al.*, 1950; Dayton *et al.*, 1967; O'Reilly *et al.*, 1968; Conney, 1967). Various compounds induce hepatic microsomal drug-metabolizing enzymes, thereby shortening the plasma half-life of many therapeutic agents (Conney, 1967). In addition to phenobarbital and Dilantin, several substances in animals, such as 3,4-benzpyrene, 3-methylcholanthrene, nicotine (Wenzel and Broadie, 1966), and caffeine (Mitoma *et al.*, 1968), to which many individuals expose themselves, can also accelerate drug metabolism. Benzpyrene hydroxylase was enhanced in the placenta of smokers (Welch *et al.*, 1968). Therefore, a history of cigarette smoking and coffee ingestion was recorded in the 28 twins (Table I). No correlation with the rate of dicoumarol metabolism was detected; in a set of identical twins with closely similar dicoumarol half-lives, one individual did not smoke, whereas the other consumed two packs a day. Similar discordant examples occurred for both smoking and coffee consumption. To determine whether a relationship exists between these agents and levels of drug-metabolizing enzymes in humans will require much further work. Only two of the seven sets of identical twins lived in the same household; therefore, the close resemblance between identical twins in phenylbutazone half-lives, in antipyrine half-lives, and in dicoumarol half-lives cannot be attributed to those environmental factors, such as exposure to the same inducing agents, operating on individuals sharing the same home and meals.

Although the studies summarized in Table I clearly indicate the genetic control of rates of phenylbutazone, antipyrine, and dicoumarol elimination from human plasma, they elucidate neither the precise location of this control, which probably resides in the hepatic microsomal drug-metabolizing enzyme system, nor the precise mode of inheritance, which may be surmised to be polygenic like many other metrical traits.

Measurement of plasma levels of drugs represents a balance between rates of absorption, redistribution within tissues and binding, biotransformation, and excretion. Several of these processes involve several proteins subject to independent variation and control. Therefore, rates of drug elimination from plasma reveal only pale reflections of the actual sites at which genetic variations operate. Experimental animals offer an obvious advantage in permitting direct study of the enzymes themselves.

Recent therapeutic applications of various compounds capable of shortening either their own duration of action or that of other drugs administered simultaneously (Yaffee *et al.*, 1966; Crigler and Gold, 1969) raise the question of the magnitude of individual differences in responsiveness to such inducing agents. It might be assumed that subjects achieving comparable blood levels of an inducing agent would have their drug-metabolizing enzyme activity elevated to similar extents. However, very recent work (Vesell and Page, 1969) reveals that for the inducing agent most commonly employed therapeutically in man, phenobarbital, large, genetically determined differences exist in the inductive response. These individual variations were independent of absolute blood levels of phenobarbital. Antipyrine half-lives were determined in 4 sets of identical and 4 sets of fraternal twins before and after 2 weeks of sodium phenobarbital administered in a daily dose of 2 mg/kg. Intrapair differences in induction of antipyrine hydroxylase as reflected by the shortening of the plasma antipyrine half-life after phenobarbital were significantly less in identical than in fraternal twins (Vesell and Page, 1969). From these data, the contribution of heredity to the reduction in plasma antipyrine half-life and hence to the induction of drug-metabolizing enzymes produced by phenobarbital was calculated to be 99%.

Phenobarbital administration in these 16 twins decreased variations in antipyrine half-life from 2.8-fold before phenobarbital to 1.8-fold after 2 weeks on the drug (Vesell and Page, 1969). After phenobarbital the standard deviation of the mean antipyrine half-life decreased by more than 2-fold. Diminished size of individual differences in drug metabolism after phenobarbital suggests that possibly where extensive individual variations in the metabolism of a drug pose therapeutic problems, relatively innocuous inducing agents could be administered to minimize such individual differences.

V. Genetic Conditions, Probably Transmitted as Single Factors, Altering the Way the Body Acts on Drugs

As pointed out by Brodie and Hogben (1957) there are two facets to the problem of the biochemical and physical aspects of drug action: the influence of drugs on the body and the influence of the body on drugs. Six genetic conditions in the latter group and six that illustrate the former category will be reviewed. Although previous reviewers of pharmacogenetics have not employed this classification, it may prove a useful one in considering the consequences of the defects, in approaching their therapy, in searching for new, genetically determined variations in response to drugs, and finally, in analyzing variations in response to new drugs, in cases of drug toxicity and in drug trials.

A. Acatalasia

Acatalasia was discovered by the Japanese otorhinolaryngologist Takahara in 1946 when he operated on an 11-year-old Japanese girl with a friable granulating tumor in the right nasal cavity and maxillary sinus (Wyngaarden and Howell, 1966). After excising the necrotic areas, he used hydrogen peroxide to sterilize the wound. Takahara noted that the usual bubbles of oxygen, liberated by the action of catalase on hydrogen peroxide, did not occur. He also observed that the color of the tissue darkened, turning black, presumably through oxidative denaturation of hemoglobin by the drug. Takahara suspected that silver nitrate had been mistakenly applied; he washed the wound with saline and opened a new bottle of hydrogen peroxide. On reapplication, he observed the same events. Takahara postulated that his patient lacked the enzyme catalase and in a series of classic studies established that this was indeed the case and that the defect was transmitted as an autosomal recessive trait (Takahara, 1952, 1954; Takahara *et al.*, 1952, 1959; Takahara and Doi, 1958). Takahara reported that his initial patient lacked catalase activity in her oral mucosa and erythrocytes, that three of her five siblings also lacked the enzyme, and that her parents were second cousins.

The initial term "acatalasemia" suggesting restriction of the defect to blood has been dropped in favor of "acatalasia" because the enzyme has been shown to be deficient in such tissues as mucous membrane, skin, liver, muscle, and bone marrow. However, neither is acatalasia an entirely accurate designation since trace levels of catalase activity occur in certain patients for whom the term "severe hypocatalasia" seems more appropriate (Wyngaarden and Howell, 1966). "Intermediate hypocatalasia" would then refer to heterozygotes who generally exhibit values of catalase activity between those of the homozygous recessives and normal individuals. It should be emphasized that in certain Japanese kindred heterozygotes do not exhibit intermediate levels of catalase activity but rather values that overlap with the normal range; these kindred have been adduced as evidence that there are at least two forms of acatalasia in Japanese (Hamilton and Neel, 1963).

Takahara and Doi (1958) and Takahara *et al.* (1959) conducted an intensive search for individuals with acatalasia and by 1959 reported 38 cases in 17 families scattered throughout Japan in a fashion to suggest considerable geographic variation in the Japanese population, with "pockets" where this normally rare gene might occur in frequencies as high as 12%. In other regions of Japan the gene was present in much lower frequencies of approximately 0.3%.

The disease assumed mild, moderate, or severe expressions (Takahara *et al.*, 1960). Ulcers of the dental alveoli characterized the mild form; alveolar gangrene and atrophy developed in moderate types; and recession of alveolar bone with exposure of the necks of teeth, resulting eventually in their loss, was typical of the severe form.

Distribution of catalase activity in 66 members of five affected families was trimodal, revealing the existence of three phenotypes designated acatalasemic, hypocatalasemic, and normal by Nishimura and associates (1959). Males and females were equally affected.

In 1959 Yata reported in a Korean the first case of a non-Japanese subject with acatalasia. In 1961 Aebi and associates screened 73,661 blood samples from Swiss Army recruits and discovered 3 individuals with acatalasia. These three were in excellent health and exhibited none of the dental abnormalities; that is, the oral ulcers now called Takahara's disease, characteristic of the Japanese cases. Also in this connection, the Swiss cases, unlike the Japanese cases, exhibited some residual catalase activity, possibly protecting them against the hydrogen peroxide formed by certain microorganisms. Oral ulcers may occur as a result of peroxide-forming microorganisms.

Table III, from Aebi (1967a), provides a classification of varieties of acatalasia reported from several countries. Differences in frequency, enzyme activities, and clinical manifestations suggest that there are at least several different forms of the disease. Genetic heterogeneity is also suggested by different properties of the catalase molecule isolated from individuals with different forms of the disease (Shibata *et al.*, 1967).

Catalase molecules in normals and patients with Swiss acatalasia initially appeared identical with respect to enzymatic and antigenic properties (Micheli and Aebi, 1965; Aebi *et al.*, 1964). More recently, Aebi (1967a,b) reported that

TABLE III

CASES OF ACATALASIA AND RELATED ANOMALIES REPORTED IN LITERATURE UNTIL 1965[a]

Type (year of detection)	Origin (No. of families)	Number of homozygotes (Hom) and heterozygotes (Het)	Residual catalase activity percentage (normal = 100)	Remarks
I (1947)	Japan (31) Korea (1)	Hom: 66 Het: > 100	Hom: 0–3.2 Het: 37–56	Incomplete recessive inheritance; oral gangrene (Takahara's disease) in ~50% of homozygotes; activity: trimodal distribution curve (no overlap)
II (1959)	Japan (1) family 13 MI	Hom: 1 (male) Het: —	Hom: 3.2 Het: ~100	Complete recessive inheritance (involvement of modifier or suppressor genes?)
IIIa (1962)	Japan (1) kindred 29 OHH	Hom: 3 (Het: 17)	Hom: 0 (?) Het: > 56	Overlap between heterozygous carrier and normals (dual allelic control?)
IIIb (1961)	Switzerland (3) families V. B. and G.	Hom: 11 (Het: ~30)	Hom: 0.1–1.3 Het: 15-85	Synthesis of two different types of catalase in heterozygotes (normal catalase + unstable variant), all homozygotes in good state of health
IV (1963)	Israel (1) Iranian born	Hom: 1 (male) Het: 15	Hom: 8 Het: 49–67	Combination with deficiency of G-6-PD; intolerance to fungicide
V (1963)	United States (1) Scandinavian and British extraction	Hom: 0 Het: 6	All: ~100	Allocatalasia: synthesis of a variant catalase; activity and stability as normal catalase

[a] From Aebi (1967a).

the catalase from Swiss cases is not identical to the catalase from normal individuals. Further purification of catalase permitted detection of electrophoretic differences between the catalases of normal and deficient individuals. Differences in pH and heat stabilities were established. Normal catalase was demonstrated to differ from catalase of deficient subjects in sensitivity toward the inhibitors aminotriazole and azide. These observations by Aebi (1967b) led him to conclude that in Swiss families acatalasia was a structural, rather than a controller, gene mutation.

In human erythrocytes catalase appears in multiple molecular forms or isozymes (Price and Greenfield, 1954; Holmes and Masters, 1965; Nishimura *et al.*, 1964; Thorup *et al.*, 1964; Baur, 1963). These catalase isozymes all possess activity and exhibit molecular weights of approximately 250,000. The problem has been further complicated by the description of a minor component of catalase which, though reacting with rabbit antihuman catalase serum, lacks enzyme activity (Shibata *et al.*, 1967). This minor component occurs in erythrocytes of heterozygotes and acatalasics, although in the heterozygotes examined, the catalase activity was only half that of normal persons, and in the Japanese homozygotes studied it was entirely absent. The minor inactive component has a molecular weight of approximately 60,000 (Shibata *et al.*, 1967). If this minor component is a subunit or precursor of catalase, and other data suggest that bovine liver catalase is composed of three or four identical chains (Schroeder *et al.*, 1964; Tanford and Lovrien, 1962), then several interpretations of the molecular events responsible for acatalasia arise. The minor inactive component may be structurally different in acatalasics from normocatalasics. Such a structural abnormality might render the subunits unable to assemble into the polymeric form of the "apocatalase" molecule. Alternatively, the precursor subunits in acatalasics are entirely normal, but there exists a defect in a hypothetical "coupling" enzyme postulated to be required to join the subunits prior to addition of the prosthetic group (Shibata *et al.*, 1967).

B. Slow Acetylation of Isoniazid

Isoniazid (1-isonicotinylhydrazine) was first synthesized in 1912 by Meyer and Mally but not until 1952 was its bacteriostatic effect on *Mycobacterium tuberculosis* established in mice (Grunberg *et al.*, 1952) and man (Robitzek *et al.*, 1952). Bönicke and Reif (1953), Hughes (1953), and Hughes *et al.* (1954, 1955) described large variations in the metabolism of isoniazid in man. In studies of the excretory products of isoniazid Hughes, Schmidt, and Biehl (1955) observed that all the drug appeared in the urine either as acetyl isoniazid, isonicotinic acid, unchanged isoniazid, or small amounts of other derivatives. An inverse relationship occurred between the amount of free and acetylated urinary products, but each subject maintained his pattern of excretion during long-term therapy.

Consideration of the clinical consequences of the isoniazid polymorphism might lead to the expectation that rapid inactivators with lower plasma values for the drug than slow inactivators would respond less favorably to treatment. Harris (1961b) reported that in 775 patients with pulmonary tuberculosis on standardized isoniazid regimens cavity closure and sputum conversion were generally noted earlier in slow than in rapid inactivators but that the results after 6 months of treatment were no different in slow than in rapid phenotypes. However, responses are worse in rapid than in slow inactivator patients with tuberculosis when isoniazid is administered only once a week (Evans, 1968). Neither resistance to tubercle bacilli (Harris, 1961b) nor reversion (Gow and Evans, 1964) apparently develops more commonly in individuals of any particular acetylase genotype.

Polyneuritis does occur more frequently in slow inactivators; Hughes *et al.* (1954) reported that polyneuritis during isoniazid therapy occurred in four of five slow inactivators, but only in two of ten rapid inactivators. These conclusions are confirmed by the study in Madras of Devadatta *et al.* (1960). The administration of pyridoxine simultaneously with isoniazid prevents development of peripheral neuritis (Carlson *et al.*, 1956). The neuritis associated with isoniazid administration arises from pyridoxine deficiency which develops due to inactivation of pyridoxine and removal of the coenzyme from tissues through chemical interaction of the hydrazine group of isoniazid with the carbonyl group of pyridoxine to form a hydrazone. Also, isoniazid is believed to compete with pyridoxal phosphate for the enzyme apotryptophanase (Ross, 1958; Robson and Sullivan, 1963).

Hereditary differences in rates of isoniazid acetylation have clinical implications in that slow inactivators tend to develop polyneuritis on long-term therapy more than do rapid inactivators. Rapid acetylation is inherited as an autosomal dominant trait; slow acetylation is inherited as an autosomal recessive. The half-life of the drug in the plasma of rapid inactivators ranges from 45 to 80 minutes and of slow inactivators from 140 to 200 minutes (Kalow, 1962). Although rapid acetylators may excrete unchanged only 3% of a dose, whereas slow acetylators may excrete 30% (Hughes *et al.*, 1954; Peters, 1959, 1960a,b), differences between rapid and slow inactivation of isoniazid are unrelated to intestinal absorption, protein binding, renal glomerular clearance, or renal tubular reabsorption (Jenne *et al.*, 1961). The basis for differences between rapid and slow inactivators of isoniazid is that slow inactivators have reduced acetyl transferase (Evans and White, 1964; Peters *et al.*, 1965a,b), the liver supernatant enzyme mainly responsible for the metabolism of isoniazid, as well as such other monosubstituted hydrazines as phenelzine, hydralazine, and sulfamethazine (Evans, 1965). It should be emphasized that acetylation of other compounds such as *p*-aminosalicylic acid and sulfanilamide is monomorphic and probably accomplished by an acetylase different from that which acetylates isoniazid.

White and Evans (1968) compared the acetylation of sulfamethazine and sulfamethoxypyridazine. The latter drug was acetylated much less than sulfamethazine. Rapid inactivators acetylated a greater percentage of sulfamethoxypyridazine than did slow inactivators. However, serum concentrations of free sulfamethoxypyridazine in individuals of different acetylator phenotype were not significantly affected by the action of the polymorphism, presumably because of the operation of several other factors affecting elimination of the drug from plasma. Finally, White and Evans (1968) suggested the possibility that genetic factors beyond that of the acetylation polymorphism might cause differences among individuals, all of the same acetylator phenotype, in the amount of acetylated sulfamethazine excreted in urine. Environmental conditions for performance of the sulfamethazine test were carefully standardized and reproducibility of the percentage of urinary sulfamethazine acetylated in the same subject was high.

Many genetic studies of the isoniazid polymorphism have been performed. A twin study showed that the content of free isoniazid in 24-hour samples of urine was remarkably similar in identical twins, whereas much larger intrapair differences occurred in fraternal twins (Bönicke and Lisboa, 1957). Bimodal distributions of the percentage of a dose of isoniazid excreted unchanged in urine also suggested the existence of genetically distinct modes of handling the drug (Biehl, 1956, 1957). This concept was further supported by large differences between Caucasian and Japanese subjects in the frequency of rapid inactivators (Harris *et al.*, 1958), and by a study of 20 families showing that slow inactivation of isoniazid was probably recessive to rapid inactivation (Knight *et al.*, 1959). Evans *et al.* (1960) investigated plasma isoniazid concentrations 6 hours after an oral dose of 9.7 mg/kg in 267 members of 53 Caucasian families and observed a bimodal distribution permitting categorization of individuals as either rapid or slow inactivators. The mean concentration of isoniazid in plasma 6 hours after the oral dose was lower in heterozygotes than in rapid inactivators homozygous for the dominant gene; these observations established a dosage effect for the trait (Evans *et al.*, 1960). The genotype for isoniazid acetylation can be directly determined with a sensitive microbiologic assay (Sunahara, 1961). Table IV shows the differing frequencies for deficiency of isoniazid acetylase gathered by Motulsky (1964) from the work of various investigators (Armstrong and Peart, 1960; Harris, 1961a; Sunahara, 1961; Evans, 1962; Mitchell *et al.*, 1960; Devadatta *et al.*, 1960; Gangadharam and Selkon, 1961; Schmiedel, 1961; Szeinberg *et al.*, 1963). Deficiency is lowest in Eskimos and only slightly more common in Far Eastern populations. It is common in Negroes and European populations, where 70 to 80% of the individuals possess the gene either in homozygous or heterozygous state (Table IV).

Such polymorphisms as the rapid and slow acetylation of isoniazid are presumably perpetuated by natural selection; that is, the gene for slow inactivation may possess advantages in certain environments. Understanding of these hypothetical advantages will have to await better understanding of the action of the enzyme *in vivo*. Little information on naturally occurring hydrazine compounds is available. Peters, Miller, and Brown (1965b) measured dimethylaminobenzaldehyde-reacting substances in urine of individuals not receiving drugs and reported below 0.8 mg total hydrazine equivalents per 12 hours, a value suggesting that perhaps the body does not encounter many naturally occurring hydrazines. White and Evans (1967a,b) reported that neither hexosamine nor tryptophan metabolites are natural substrates for the acetylation polymorphism.

As previously mentioned, polymorphic acetylation occurs for the substrates isoniazid, sulfamethazine, sulfamaprine, phenelzine, and hydralazine, whereas acetylation of *p*-aminosalicylic acid, *p*-aminobenzoic acid, and sulfanilamide is monomorphic (Evans, 1965). These data suggest that acetylation proceeds by at least two enzymatically distinct pathways. Polymorphically acetylated drugs are generally all rapidly or slowly inactivated in a given individual; this observation implies that metabolism of compounds acetylated polymorphically may proceed by a single acetylase.

The human acetylase that transfers an acetyl group from acetyl coenzyme A to isoniazid has been studied *in vitro* by Evans (1962), Evans and White (1964), Jenne (1965), and Weber *et al.* (1968). Weber *et al.* (1968) purified the enzyme 300- to 500-fold from the 100,000 gm liver homogenate supernatant which contains all the acetyltransferase activity and described a Ping-Pong mechanism of action. Of particular interest were their kinetic data from rabbits that were rapid and slow inactivators of isoniazid; these studies suggested that the acetylase from slow inactivators differed structurally from the enzyme for rapid inactivators.

Since phenelzine is polymorphically acetylated, its side effects were observed in rapid and slow acetylators. Evans *et al.* (1965) reported that severe side effects of phenelzine, including blurred vision and psychosis, occurred predominantly in slow acetylators. Decreased toxicity in rapid as opposed to slow acetylators of a polymorphically acetylated drug may explain why toxic effects of the hydrazine drug phtivazid occurred infrequently in those patients who excreted the acetylated form in high concentrations (Smirnov and Kozulitzina, 1962). Finally, incidence of peripheral neuropathy and a syndrome resembling systemic lupus erythematosus is higher in slow than in rapid acetylators of hydralazine (Perry *et al.*, 1967).

TABLE IV

ISONIAZID INACTIVATION IN DIFFERENT POPULATIONS[a]

Population	No. studied	Percent slow inactivators (q^2)	Gene frequency (q)
Asiatic origin			
Eskimos[b]	226	0.05	0.22
Japanese[c]	30	0.10	0.32
Japanese[d]	1808	0.115	0.34
Ainu[d]	86	0.128	0.36
Korean[d]	65	0.108	0.33
Ryukyuan[d]	124	0.145	0.38
Chinese[e]	85	0.15	0.39
Thais[d]	108	0.278	0.53
American Indians[f]	15	0.21	0.46
Hindu Indians[g]	143	0.58	0.76
Hindu Indians[h]	299	0.60	0.77
African origin			
American Negro[c]	95	0.42	0.65
American Negro[f]	31	0.48	0.69
Sudanese Negro[e]	102	0.65	0.80
European origin			
United States whites[c]	112	0.47	0.69
German[i]	524	0.44	0.66
United States Scandinavian[c]	70	0.67	0.82
United States Italians[c]	14	0.64	0.80
United States Greek[c]	10	0.60	0.77
"Spanish Americans"[c] (Salt Lake City)[j]	23	0.60	0.77
"Spanish Americans"[f] (Denver)[j]	131	0.30	0.55
Jewish groups			
United States Askenazi[c]	11	0.55	0.75
Israeli Askenazi[k]	100	0.67	0.82
Israeli non-Askenazi[k]	179	0.69	0.83
Israeli Baghdad Jews[k]	60	0.75	0.87

[a] From Motulsky (1964).
[b] Armstrong and Peart (1960).
[c] Harris (1961a).
[d] Sunahara (1961).
[e] Evans (1962).
[f] Mitchell *et al.* (1960).
[g] Devadatta *et al.* (1960).
[h] Gangadharam and Selkon (1961).
[i] Schmiedel (1961).
[j] Variable degrees of Indian admixture in these "Spanish-American" populations probably explain the differences in gene frequency.
[k] Szeinberg *et al.* (1963).

C. Suxamethonium Sensitivity or Atypical Pseudocholinesterase

In 1952 several patients were reported to be abnormally sensitive to the muscle relaxant suxamethonium (Bourne *et al.*, 1952; Evans *et al.*, 1952). This drug, also called succinylcholine, Suxethonium, Scoline, and Anectine, was described in 1906 by Hunt and Taveau, and found 43 years later to be a muscle relaxant by Bovet *et al.* (1949). It is most commonly employed during general anesthesia, but also used in electroconvulsive therapy and in treatment of tetanus. The principal advantage of the drug is its short action; the usual dosage of 30 to 100 mg produces muscle paralysis and apnea only for approximately 2 minutes. However, in the atypical patients reported in 1952, the duration was 2 to 3 hours. The short duration of action in normal cases is due to rapid hydrolysis of suxamethonium by plasma pseudocholinesterase (Bovet-Nitti, 1949), which removes the choline radicals one at a time, with formation of the relatively inactive intermediate succinylmonocholine (Lehmann and Silk, 1953; Whittaker and Wijesundera, 1952). Effective treatment in prolonged apnea in patients with atypical pseudocholinesterase consists of transfusion of normal plasma or of a highly purified preparation of the human enzyme (Goedde *et al.*, 1968).

The initial reports of abnormally prolonged apnea in 1952 demonstrated low serum pseudocholinesterase activity. As more of these rare cases were published (Forbat *et al.*, 1953) it became clear that such abnormal individuals were otherwise healthy, and therefore had low pseudocholinesterase not because of liver disease, poisoning by organophosphorus compounds, malnutrition, or severe anemia, all of which can diminish plasma pseudocholinesterase activity (Lehmann and Ryan, 1956), but rather because of an inherited defect (Forbat *et al.*, 1953). Lehmann and Ryan (1956) investigated the families of five unrelated suxamethonium-sensitive probands and suggested that the disorder was inherited as an autosomal recessive trait. However, the three phenotypes could not be adequately separated simply by measurement of plasma pseudocholinesterase activity because there was considerable overlap.

Kalow and his associates are responsible for elucidating the nature of the enzymatic abnormality. They demonstrated that it was caused not simply by decreased amounts of the normal pseudocholinesterase but rather by the presence of an enzyme with kinetic properties markedly different from those of the usual enzyme (Kalow and Genest, 1957; Kalow and Staron, 1957; Kalow and Davies, 1959; Davies *et al.*, 1960).

Suxamethonium and other substrates have much lower avidity for the abnormal enzyme. At concentrations of suxamethonium present during anesthesia, the abnormal enzyme exhibits no detectable effect on the drug in contrast to the marked hydrolytic activity of the normal enzyme (Davies *et al.*, 1960). Kalow and Davies (1959) also demonstrated that the atypical enzyme was more resistant to many pseudocholinesterase inhibitors. At first it was thought that for differential inhibition the molecule must possess a positively charged nitrogen molecule, but fluoride (Harris and Whittaker, 1961) and organophosphorus compounds were later shown to inhibit differentially. Because of the importance of a positive charge on many inhibitors, it was suggested that the positively charged portion of the inhibitor combined with the anionic site of the enzyme and that only the anionic site on the atypical enzyme was defective either in accessibility or magnitude of charge (Kalow and Davies, 1959). Wilson (1954) had previously described two sites on cholinesterase molecules, an anionic site which accommodated the positively charged choline radical of the substrate and an esteratic site into which the acid portion of the substrate was positioned during hydrolysis. Recent work of Clark *et al.* (1968) demonstrated that the pK of the atypical enzyme is lower than that of the usual enzyme, that choline alters the pK of the usual but not of the atypical enzyme, and that choline has a lower affinity for the atypical enzyme. These observations support the conclusion that the anionic site of the atypical enzyme is altered. Stimulation by choline of the dephosphorylation step of the usual enzyme, but not of the atypical enzyme, and the difference in rates of dephosphorylation by sodium fluoride imply that the esteratic site must also be altered in the atypical enzyme (Clark *et al.*, 1968). It is not necessary to postulate two distinct point mutations on the atypical pseudocholinesterase to accommodate these concepts. Such a postulate would be in conflict with genetic dogma and previous experience with the hemoglobin molecule and several other proteins, where genetic variants exhibit a single amino acid substitution resulting from a single point mutation. Alteration of a single residue in the structure of the atypical pseudocholinesterase could modify both the anionic and esteratic sites.

Better understanding of the enzyme permitted development of tests to distinguish the three phenotypes which could not be satisfactorily separated simply by measuring plasma pseudocholinesterase activity. Dibucaine (cinchocaine), a differential inhibitor of normal and atypical pseudocholinesterase, was utilized by Kalow and Genest (1957) to separate the three phenotypes. They designated the percentage inhibition of pseudocholinesterase activity produced by 10^{-5} M dibucaine the "dibucaine number" or "DN." The normal enzyme is inhibited approximately 80%, whereas atypical pseudocholinesterase is inhibited only 20%. Heterozygotes exhibit dibucaine numbers between 52 and 69; the degree of inhibition is independent of enzyme concentration (Kalow and Genest, 1957).

Additional genetic variants were discovered by the use of sodium fluoride as an inhibitor (Harris and Whittaker, 1962a). Recently tetracaine, unlike other substances previously studied, has been shown to be hydrolyzed faster by atypical than by normal pseudocholinesterase and an even better separation of phenotypes has been achieved with the procaine-tetracaine ratio than with the DN (Foldes, 1968).

Family studies suggested the inheritance of various types of atypical pseudocholinesterase through allelic codominant genes at a single locus (Kalow and Staron, 1957; Harris *et al.*, 1960; Bush, 1961). Four alleles have been identified with the resulting ten genotypes shown in Table V (from Motulsky, 1964). Although penetrance is complete, the genes seem to vary in expression (Lehmann and Liddell, 1964). The frequency of homozygous affected individuals is 0.019 to 0.017, or approximately 1 in 2800, and of heterozygotes 3.8% in various populations (Kalow and Gunn, 1959; Kattamis *et al.*, 1962).

A series of four families are discussed by Lehmann and Liddell (1964) in which the dibucaine values do not conform to the pattern of autosomal inheritance. These individuals are believed to be heterozygous for a rare, so-called silent gene. A few rare individuals with complete absence of serum and liver pseudocholinesterase activity have been reported (Hodgkin *et al.*, 1965). All four normally occurring isozymes of serum pseudocholinesterase were absent; immunodiffusion and immunoelectrophoretic studies indicated the lack of antigenically cross-reacting material (Hodgkin *et al.*, 1965). Heterozygotes for the silent gene exhibit serum cholinesterase activity approximately two thirds of normal, and overlap considerably with normal values (Hodgkin *et al.*, 1965; Harris *et al.*, 1963). Motulsky (1964) states that such silent mutations may affect the controlling element of the gene, thereby causing complete failure of protein production, although he also acknowledges that the possibility of a single structural mutation affecting both the active site and the antigenic determinants cannot be eliminated. Goedde and Altland (1968) studied five individuals who were homozygous recessive for the silent gene. Residual enzymatic activity and antigenic determinants occurred in three subjects who revealed a single band on the starch gel at the C-4 position when their sera were concentrated 6-fold. In the remaining two cases, results similar to those of Hodgkin *et al.* were obtained.

Gutsche, Scott, and Wright (1967) reported a high incidence of the silent mutation in a population of southern Eskimos. Nineteen cases in 11 Eskimo families were ascertained as a result of apnea in 2 Eskimo children after a single low dose of succinylcholine. Prior to this survey, only 10 individuals homozygous for the silent gene had been described (Szeinberg *et al.*, 1966). The gene frequency of 0.12 in this locality of Alaska, extending from Hooper Bay to Unalakleet and centered on the lower Yukon River, led to an estimation that 1.5% of this population was sensitive to succinylcholine. The authors suggested that high frequency of the rare silent gene occurred in this, but not other, regions of Alaska because of the isolation and consequent inbreeding of the population. However, only 2 of the 11 affected Eskimo families are known to be related. Alternatively, the gene may be favored by certain characteristics of

TABLE V

MUTANTS AT CHOLINESTERASE (E) LOCUS[a]

Genotype		Phenotype						
New nomenclature[b]	Lehmann's nomenclature	New nomenclature	Previous designation	Type of enzyme present	Esterase level (rel %)	Typical dibucaine No.	Typical fluoride No.	Approximate frequency
$E_1^u E_1^u$	N-N	U	Usual	u(sual)	100	80	64	96%
$E_1^u E_1^a$	N-D	I	Intermediate	u + a(typical)	78	62	48	4%
$E_1^a E_1^a$	D-D	A	Atypical	a	25	20	23	1/3000
$E_1^s E_1^u$	S-N	U	Usual	u	65	80	64	1/150
$E_1^s E_1^s$	S-S	S	Silent; zero	None	0	—	—	1/100,000
$E_1^s E_1^a$	S-D	A	Atypical	a	20	20	23	1/8000
$E_1^f E_1^u$	F-N	UF	U_1	f(luoride-resistant) + u	80	76	52	?
$E_1^f E_1^f$	F-F	F		f	50	67	34	Very rare
$E_1^f E_1^a$	F-D	IF	I_1	f + a	60	50	30	?
$E_1^f E_1^s$	F-S	F		f	Not described yet			?
$E_2 + E_2$		C_5+		$u + C_5+$	130	80	64	5%

[a] From Motulsky (1964).

[b] New nomenclature by agreement of workers in the field (E_1 = first allele at cholinesterase (E) locus; E_1^u = usual enzyme; E_1^a = atypical, i.e., "dibucaine-resistant" allele; E_1^s = silent allele; E_1^f = "fluoride-resistant" allele; E_2+ = nonallelic cholinesterase locus (E_2) determining additional cholinesterase isoenzyme (C_5+) (Harris *et al.*, 1963).

the environment. Of 17 affected Eskimos, 8 deficient persons had detectable pseudocholinesterase activities of 2 to 8 units according to a method adapted to permit analysis of greater volumes of sera, whereas 9 individuals exhibited no activity whatever. Possibly trace pseudocholinesterase activity reflects a different mutation from that characterized by no detectable activity.

Close resemblance of most populations in their gene frequencies of atypical pseudocholinesterase implies that little selective advantage is conferred now by the various genotypes or that the pertinent environmental conditions are similar in widely different countries. Solinaceous plants such as tomatoes and potatoes possess a potent differential cholinesterase inhibitor (Orgell *et al.*, 1958) shown by Harris and Whittaker (1962b) to be the glycoalkaloid solanine. Since atypical pseudocholinesterase is less sensitive to inhibition by this naturally occurring substance than is the normal enzyme, it has been suggested that in cases of solanine poisoning the atypical genotype would be at a selective advantage. Several outbreaks of solanine poisoning have been reported (Wilson, 1959; Willimott, 1933; Harris and Cockburn, 1918).

Finally, plasma pseudocholinesterase activities are elevated in thyrotoxicosis, schizophrenia, hypertension, acute emotional disorders, after concussion and as a genetically transmitted condition without overt clinical manifestations, but associated with an electrophoretically slower moving C_4 isozyme (Harris *et al.*, 1963; Neitlich, 1966). In 1,029 male military personnel between ages 17 and 35, Neitlich (1966) discovered an individual whose plasma pseudocholinesterase activity of 1278 units was more than 3 times higher than the mean for all the volunteers. A family study revealed that the sister and daughter of the propositus had values of 1518 and 1237 plasma pseudocholinesterase units, respectively, and that his mother had 566 units. Previously Kalow and Genest (1957) and Kalow and Staron (1957) described an individual with 2.5 times the average pseudocholinesterase activity of 1556 subjects, but a family study was not performed. Harris *et al.* (1963) reported that 10% of a random sample of the British population had slightly higher than normal pseudocholinesterase activity associated with a retarded electrophoretic mobility of the main isozyme. Harris *et al.* (1963) designated this slower moving band C_5. Neitlich's pseudocholinesterase variant also exhibited slower electrophoretic mobility than the normal C_4 isozyme. However, the greatly elevated total plasma pseudocholinesterase activity of the American variants distinguished them from the variants described in England. Individuals possessing markedly elevated plasma pseudocholinesterase activity are resistant to the usual doses of suxamethonium.

D. Deficient Parahydroxylation of Diphenylhydantoin (Dilantin)

Many lipid-soluble drugs are rendered more water-soluble through metabolism by enzyme systems in liver microsomes (Gillette, 1963, 1966).

Several of these liver microsomal enzymes are oxidases requiring oxygen, NADPH, and cytochrome P-450. Characterization remains to be accomplished because these enzymes lose activity when removed from the endoplastic reticulum. Deficient parahydroxylation of Dilantin (diphenylhydantoin) reported by Kutt *et al.* (1964a) is the first example of a genetic defect of mixed function oxidases in humans.

Dilantin, one of the most commonly used anticonvulsants since its introduction by Merritt and Putnam in 1938, causes multiple toxic reactions including nystagmus, ataxia, dysarthria, and drowsiness. These have been clearly shown by Kutt *et al.* (1964b) to be dose related (Fig. 9). Yahr *et al.* (1952) stated that 77% of patients develop toxicity on a daily dose of 0.6 gm, which is not above the amount recommended by these and other authors (Yahr and Merritt, 1956).

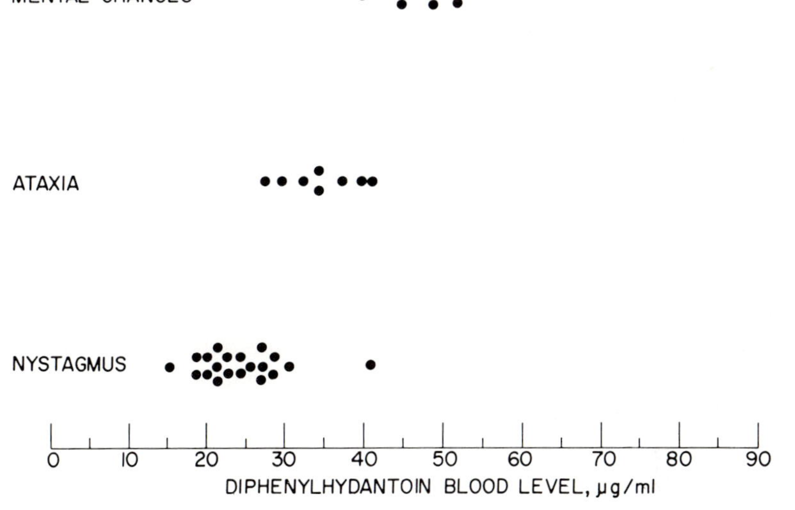

FIG. 9. The onset of nystagmus, ataxia, and mental changes in relationship to diphenylhydantoin (Dilantin) blood levels. (Reproduced from Kutt *et al.*, 1964b).

Metabolism of Dilantin proceeds by parahydroxylation of one of the phenyl groups to yield 5-phenyl-5′-parahydroxyphenylhydantoin, HPPH, which is conjugated with glucuronic acid and then eliminated in urine (Butler, 1957; Woodbury and Esplin, 1959; Maynert, 1960).

Kutt *et al.* (1964a) described a patient, W.J., in whom toxic symptoms developed on a commonly used dosage of 4.0 mg/kg, but not on a dose of 1.4 mg/kg. Their investigations established high blood levels of unchanged Dilantin and low urine levels of HPPH. A study of the family of W. J. (Fig. 10) showed 2 affected and 3 unaffected individuals. These results suggest that low activity of Dilantin hydroxylase exhibits dominant transmission.

The authors also investigated the patient's capacity to parahydroxylate other compounds such as phenobarbital and phenylalanine. These were

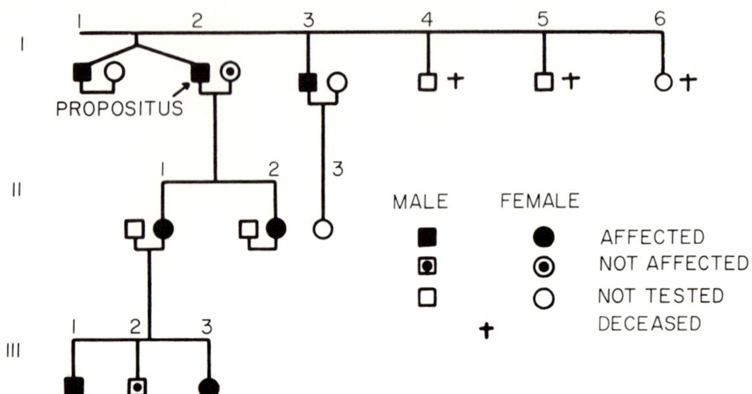

FIG. 10. Pedigree of deficient parahydroxylation of Dilantin with propositus W. J. and his affected brother C. J. and mother E. J. (Reproduced from Kutt *et al.*, 1964a.)

hydroxylated normally and apparently, therefore, by enzymes different from those that hydroxylate Dilantin. However, since urinary excretion of unaltered phenobarbital (Butler, 1956) occurs in higher amounts, reaching 30% of the daily intake, than does Dilantin, which attains only 5% of daily intake, Kutt *et al.* (1964a) suggest that phenobarbital accumulation is less likely to occur and therefore a hydroxylation defect may be masked.

The observations of Kutt *et al.* (1964a) on the family with deficient hydroxylation of Dilantin indicate that when toxic symptoms develop, particularly with low dosages, determinations of blood levels and urinary metabolites of Dilantin should be performed. If indeed the patient proves particularly sensitive to Dilantin and deficient in his hydroxylating capacity, the physician need not discontinue the drug, but should adjust its dosage to give the desired blood levels.

Another cause of Dilantin intoxication very much more prevalent than heritable deficiency of parahydroxylase activity has recently been identified by Brennan *et al.* (1968) as slow inactivation of isoniazid. All 5 patients who developed clinically evident Dilantin toxicity in a series of 29 individuals receiving Dilantin (300 mg daily for 3 weeks) were very slow isoniazid inactivators. In rat liver microsomes both isoniazid and *p*-aminosalicylic acid interfered with Dilantin parahydroxylation (Kutt *et al.*, 1968).

E. Dicoumarol Sensitivity

Solomon (1968) reported a patient hospitalized for a myocardial infarction who had a prolonged plasma dicoumarol half-life of 82 hours on a dose of 150 mg compared to normal values of 27 ± 5 hours. Although family studies were not performed because of their unwillingness to cooperate, the patient's mother suffered a spinal cord hematoma, causing permanent paraplegia on a small weekly dose of 2.5 to 5 mg of warfarin. This unfortunate accident suggests not only the possibility of hereditary transmission of dicoumarol sensitivity, but also the desirability of determining individual rates of drug metabolism prior to long-term therapy.

Warfarin and dicoumarol are extensively hydroxylated in the rat (Ikeda *et al.*, 1966; Christensen, 1966), but their metabolites in man remain to be characterized. The location of the defect in this patient with dicoumarol sensitivity may be a hepatic microsomal hydroxylase, which possibly is deficient in both him and his mother.

Genetic factors influence responsiveness to anticoagulants in rabbits (Smith, 1939; Link, 1945; Solomon and Schrogie, 1966) and in rats, where recent studies indicate that resistance to warfarin as a rodenticide is transmitted as an autosomal dominant trait (Editorial, 1966; Greaves and Ayres, 1967).

Acquired conditions can also produce increased sensitivity to coumarin anticoagulants. Most notable of these are vitamin K deficiency, increased turnover of plasma proteins, and numerous forms of liver disease impairing capacity to produce vitamin K-dependent clotting factors (O'Reilly *et al.*, 1968).

Various drugs may also increase the prothrombinopenic response to coumarin anticoagulants. Cinchopen may cause liver cell damage; phenothiazine may produce cholestasis, thereby diminishing absorption of vitamin K; phenylbutazone increases sensitivity by displacing warfarin from plasma albumin (Aggeler *et al.*, 1967); and phenyramidol inhibits the hepatic microsomal enzymes responsible for metabolism of coumarin drugs (O'Reilly and Aggeler, 1965).

F. Atypical Human Liver Alcohol Dehydrogenase

von Wartburg and Schürch (1968) have described a human variant of the enzyme that metabolizes ethanol, alcohol dehydrogenase (ADH). The atypical enzyme is exceptionally active and occurs in sufficiently high frequencies in Swiss and English populations to be designated a polymorphism. The frequency was 20% in 59 liver specimens from a Swiss population and 4% in 50 livers from an English population.

According to the difference in the pH rate profiles, the ratio of the activity at pH 10.8 to that at pH 8.8 is greater than 1 for the normal enzyme and less than 1 for the atypical enzyme. *o*-Phenanthroline, which chelates the zinc in the

ADH molecule, inhibits the normal more than the atypical ADH, whereas pyrozol inhibits the atypical more than the normal ADH. The normal ADH oxidizes *N*-butanol, benzyl alcohol, and cycloheranol faster than the atypical ADH.

Both normal and atypical ADH exhibit three distinct bands by electrophoresis on agar gel or by chromatography on ion exchange columns (von Wartburg and Schürch, 1968; Blair and Vallee, 1966). The ADH isozyme patterns of individual livers vary considerably in distribution of total activity among the three bands and some livers contain only two bands. The three normal and atypical ADH isozymes have approximately the same electrophoretic mobility on agar gel at pH 9.0 (von Wartburg and Schürch, 1968).

What significant differences exist between the atypical and normal ADH with respect to the development of alcoholism remains to be seen. Clearly these studies establish a marked difference between the two enzymes in their rates of ethanol metabolism. Family studies will also help elucidate the mode of inheritance of the trait.

The atypical ADH has 5- to 6-fold the activity of normal ADH *in vitro*, but the atypical enzyme enhances alcohol metabolism by only 40 to 50% *in vivo*, possibly because another factor such as reoxidation of coenzyme 1 becomes rate limiting (von Wartburg and Schürch, 1968). The atypical ADH also reduces acetaldol (β-hydroxybutyraldehyde) five times faster than the normal ADH.

In 23 subjects Edwards and Evans (1967) attempted to correlate, after intravenous infusion of ethanol, rates of degradation of the drug with liver ADH typed from biopsies obtained at surgery. Two of the 23 subjects had atypical ADH; in the male subject with atypical ADH, capacity to metabolize alcohol was no different from males with typical ADH, whereas in the female subject with atypical ADH, capacity to degrade ethanol was greater than in a small group of females who had atypical ADH.

VI. Genetic Conditions, Probably Transmitted as Single Factors, Altering the Way Drugs Act on the Body

A. Warfarin Resistance

O'Reilly *et al.* (1964) reported resistance to warfarin in a man who at age 71 received anticoagulants for a myocardial infarction. Other than for a reproducible reduction in his one-stage prothrombin concentration to approximately 60% of normal, the patient exhibited no abnormalities by physical or laboratory examination. Because of the patient's low prothrombin time, anticoagulants were initially withheld, but 1 month later were administered. The patient proved to be resistant, rather than sensitive, to dicoumarol. A daily dose of 20 mg of warfarin failed to achieve any prothrombinopenic response;

a daily dose of 145 mg was required to reduce the prothrombin concentration to therapeutic levels. In 105 patients on long-term anticoagulant therapy the mean daily dose of warfarin was 6.8 ± 2.8 mg (O'Reilly *et al.*, 1968). The resistant patient therefore was 49 standard deviations above the mean.

O'Reilly and associates carefully investigated the propositus and his family. Five other members of the family in three generations were also resistant to warfarin (Fig. 11). Transmission of the trait as a Mendelian dominant is suggested by the fact that all three generations and most of the members of the kindred are affected. Members of both sexes were equally affected.

Environmental conditions may also cause resistance to coumarin anticoagulant drugs. Decreased sensitivity to the prothrombinopenic effect of coumarin drugs may occur in hyperthyroid patients treated with propyl-

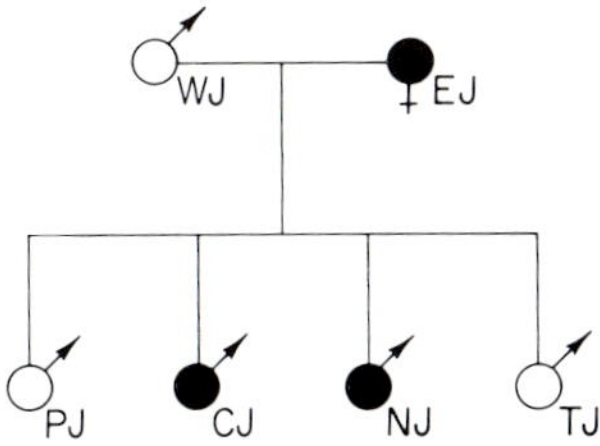

FIG. 11. Pedigree of family M, indicating the incidence of resistance to coumarin anticoagulant drugs. (Reproduced from O'Reilly and Aggeler, 1965.)

thiouracil, patients with congestive heart failure relieved by operative procedures or medications, and patients with liver disease being treated medically (Elias, 1965). Large doses of coumarin drugs are required in pregnancy to offset increased levels of vitamin K-dependent clotting factors released during pregnancy (O'Reilly *et al.*, 1968). Simultaneous administration of the natural antidote, vitamin K, and of other therapeutic agents can cause increased resistance to the coumarin anticoagulants. Barbiturates, glutethimide, chloral hydrate, and griseofulvin appear to stimulate microsomal enzymes in the liver responsible for the metabolism of coumarin anticoagulant drugs.

In order to determine the nature of the defective response to warfarin, O'Reilly *et al.* (1964) performed various pharmacodynamic studies on their patient before initiating long-term therapy. After the standard oral dose of 1.5 mg of warfarin sodium per kg of body weight, blood concentrations of the anticoagulant were determined serially. The rapid rise in plasma warfarin levels indicated that the drug was absorbed normally from the gastrointestinal tract. The concentration of warfarin attained in plasma and its rate of elimination from plasma indicated a normal volume of distribution and a normal rate of metabolism of the drug (O'Reilly *et al.*, 1968). Yet this dose of drug failed to lower prothrombin concentrations. The patient was also resistant to dicoumarol and the indanedione anticoagulant phenindione, but not to heparin. The degree of binding of warfarin to the patient's plasma proteins was identical to that of normal subjects. Electrophoretic studies showed that warfarin was bound exclusively to albumin, as in normal plasma. Warfarin was not excreted unchanged in urine or stools, even after administration of very high doses. A metabolite of warfarin was recovered from the patient's urine in amounts similar to those recovered from the urine of normal subjects given equivalent amounts of drug. While on high doses of warfarin, the patient was shown to be unusually sensitive to vitamin K, showing elevations of prothrombin time on doses of vitamin K to which normal individuals failed to respond.

The mechanism considered by O'Reilly *et al.* (1968) to be responsible for resistance to warfarin in their patient was existence of an enzyme or receptor site with altered affinity for vitamin K or for anticoagulant drugs. The former mechanism was favored because it accounted both for decreased responsiveness to anticoagulants and for increased responsiveness to vitamin K, whereas the great responsiveness of the patient to vitamin K would be difficult to explain by altered affinity for the coumarin anticoagulants.

Resistance to coumarin anticoagulants in this patient of O'Reilly *et al.* (1964) is an excellent example of a genetic defect that affects the way drugs act on the body rather than the way the body transforms or metabolizes drugs. Coumarin anticoagulants function as antimetabolites competing with the natural substrate vitamin K for receptor sites in an enzyme system responsible for synthesis of clotting factors II, VII, IX, and X (O'Reilly *et al.*, 1968). In the patient whose receptor site is so altered that its avidity for vitamin K is increased, much higher concentrations of anticoagulant are required to compete effectively with vitamin K, thereby reducing synthesis of the clotting factors and decreasing prothrombin times.

B. Primaquine Sensitivity, Favism, or Glucose-6-Phosphate Dehydrogenase (G-6-PD) Deficiency

This fascinating group of hereditary disorders transmitted as X-linked incomplete dominant traits affects nearly 100,000,000 persons and occurs in particularly high frequencies in areas of the world where malaria is endemic. In affected individuals hemolysis develops either spontaneously, after infections, or after exposure to a variety of analgesics [acetanilide, acetylsalicylic acid, acetophenetidin (phenacetin), antipyrine, aminopyrine (Pyramidon)], sulfonamides and sulfones [sulfanilamide, sulfapyridine, N_2-acetylsulfanilamide, sulfacetamide sulfisoxazole (Gantrisin), thiazolsulfone, salicylazosulfapyridine (Azulfadine), sulfoxone, sulfamethoxypyridazine (Kynex)], antimalarials [primaquine, pamaquine, pentaquine, quinacrine (Atabrine)], nonsulfonamide antibacterial agents [furazolidone, nitrofurantoin (Furadantin), chloramphenicol, *p*-aminosalicylic acid], and miscellaneous drugs [naphthalene, vitamin K, probenecid, trinitrotoluene, methylene blue, dimercaprol (BAL), phenylhydrazine, quinine, quinidine] (Beutler, 1966).

Since 1926 hemolysis was recognized in certain individuals after they received the antimalarial drug pamaquine. Cross-transfusion experiments of Dern and associates (1954a) established that primaquine-induced hemolysis was an intrinsic property of susceptible individuals, transferable with their erythrocytes to normal individuals. The next development was the discovery that the level of reduced glutathione (GSH) decreased markedly in sensitive erythrocytes several days after ingestion of various aniline derivatives and just prior to hemolysis *in vivo* (Flanagan *et al.*, 1955). A test based on reduction of GSH in erythrocytes exposed *in vitro* to acetylphenylhydrazine (Beutler, 1957) permitted identification of susceptible individuals before they ingested the drug. Genetic investigations based on this test as a probe revealed that the abnormality was inherited as an X-linked trait with intermediate dominance (Childs *et al.*, 1958). The product of the mutant gene was identified by Carson and associates (1956) as G-6-PD, which they demonstrated to be deficient in the erythrocytes of affected individuals.

Approximately 20 separate mutations at the locus on the X chromosome controlling G-6-PD synthesis have been identified; each mutation alters the properties of the G-6-PD molecule to different extents, and Table VI from Kirkman (1968) describes the physicochemical properties of some variants. An interesting variant (A^+) with more rapid electrophoretic mobility than normal G-6-PD occurs in approximately 18% of normal American Negroes. In these individuals total G-6-PD activity is normal; however, the A electrophoretic phenotype also occurs in all Negroes with G-6-PD deficiency (Kirkman and Hendrickson, 1963; Boyer *et al.*, 1962). A single amino acid substitution of aspartic acid in the common Negro variant (A^+) for asparagine in the normal (B^+) type was demonstrated by Yoshida (1967) to be responsible for the difference in electrophoretic mobility. Yoshida (1967) further showed from the number of peptide spots observed on his fingerprints that the normal G-6-PD molecule of molecular weight 230,000–240,000 was composed of six identical subunits. While Negro males possess either electrophoretic type A or B, Negro females are of type A, B, or AB, suggesting that the electrophoretic variants are also X-linked. Whether G-6-PD deficient or not, Caucasians exhibit only electrophoretic type B.

The events leading to drug-induced hemolytic anemia remain somewhat obscure. The drugs themselves are metabolized in a normal fashion by the body, but they or their hydroxylated metabolites cause damage because of

TABLE VI

VARIANTS OF HUMAN RED CELL G-6-PD[a]

Variant	Population	RBC activity (% of normal)	Electrophoretic mobility (% of normal)	K_m G-6-PD (μM)	K_m NADP (μM)	2dG-6-P utilization (%)	Thermo-stability	pH optima
Common variants, in order of diminishing activity								
Normal B	All	(100)	(100)	50–78	2.9–4.4	<4	(Normal)	Truncate
A	Negro	88	110	Normal	Normal	<4	Normal	Truncate
Athens	Greek	25	98	16–19	2.5–6.5	10–15	Slightly increased	Mildly biphasic
A⁻	Negro	8–20	110	Normal	Normal	<4	Normal	Truncate
Canton	Cantonese	4–24	104–108	20–36	2.0–2.4	4–15	Slightly reduced	Mildly biphasic
Mediterranean	Greek, Sardinians, Sephardic Jews, Asiatic Northwest Indians	0–7	100	19–26	1.2–1.6	23–37	Reduced	Biphasic
Uncommon variants, without apparent congenital nonspherocytic hemolytic disease								
"Madison"	Norwegian	100	70 (Teb) 90 (Tris)	?	?	?	?	?
Baltimore-Austin	Negro	75	90 (Tris)	68	3.1	<4	Normal	Truncate

Ibaden-Austin	Negro	72	80	62–72	3.3	<4	Normal	Truncate
Barbieri	Italian	40–50	135	Increased	Increased	?	Normal	?
Kerala	Asiatic Southeast Indians	50	75 (Teb) 90 (Tris)	23	1.5	7.4	Normal	Mildly biphasic
Tel Hashomer	Tunisian Jew	25–40	60–70	30–40	?	Normal	Normal	Mildly biphasic
Columbus	Negro	35	100	Normal	Normal	Normal	?	?
Seattle	Welsh-Scottish ? Greek	8–21	90	15–25	2.4–2.8	7–11	Normal	Mildly biphasic
West Bengal	Asiatic Indian	9	90–94	31	6.6	4	Normal	Truncate
Markham	New Guinea	1.5–10	105–108	4.4–6.3	?	162–222	?	Very biphasic
Uncommon variants, with congenital nonspherocytic hemolytic disease								
Chicago	Western Europe	9–26	100	58–76	3.1–3.7	<4	Greatly reduced	Truncate
Oklahoma	Western Europe	4–10	100	127–200	20	<4	Reduced	Narrow peak
Ohio	Italian	2–16	110	Slightly increased	Slightly increased	Normal	Greatly reduced	?
Milwaukee	Puerto Rico	0–4	90	224	?	<4	?	Narrow peak

[a] From Kirkman (1968).

increased frailty of G-6-PD-deficient erythrocytes. Normally, erythrocytes withstand oxidative compounds and maintain their glutathione in a reduced state through glutathione reductase which by means of NADPH regenerates GSH from oxidized glutathione (GSSG). NADPH is formed by both G-6-PD and 6-phosphogluconate dehydrogenase (6-PGD), the first two enzymes in the hexose monophosphate shunt or phosphogluconate oxidative pathway. This oxidative route provides only a small amount (approximately 10%) of the total metabolic energy of the erythrocyte, the major part being accounted for by the Embden-Myerhof pathway. However, the relative rates of glycolysis are appreciably altered by such factors as the pH of the suspending medium, the G-6-PD activity and the rate of TPNH oxidation. Deficiency of G-6-PD activity reduces the amount of TPNH available to the erythrocyte and thereby the concentration of GSH. GSH is apparently necessary in maintaining —SH groups on critical proteins of the erythrocytes in a reduced state (Barron and Singer, 1943); and GSH deficiency with normal G-6-PD activity causes a non-spherocytic, congenital hemolytic anemia with drug sensitivity (Oort *et al.*, 1961; Prins *et al.*, 1963). This would seem to indicate the importance of GSH in the metabolic economy of the erythrocytes; on the other hand, red cell survival is not decreased by complexing most of the GSH in erythrocytes with *N*-ethylmaleimide (Jacob and Jandl, 1962).

An investigation of the effect on mechanical fragility of exposing normal and G-6-PD deficient erythrocytes to various compounds and their metabolites suggested the following sequence of events in drug-induced hemolysis (Fraser and Vesell, 1968):

1. Metabolism of the drug to a product with greater redox properties.
2. Conversion of this metabolite to an oxidant intermediate by the erythrocyte.
3. Oxidant damage to the erythrocyte membrane, possibly by oxidation of reduced sulfhydryl groups.
4. Increased fragmentation of older erythrocytes in the circulation resulting from this membrane damage.

The metabolism of the erythrocyte is unusual in that it must function without the benefit of a nucleus. The red cell apparently is unable to synthesize protein but does synthesize certain simpler substances such as GSH, DPN, and ATP. It requires energy sources for maintaining concentration gradients of sodium and potassium and for continual reduction of methemoglobin. The glycolytic and oxidative pathways of glucose metabolism provide this energy source. But as the normal cell ages certain enzymes including G-6-PD lose activity (Marks *et al.*, 1958; Marks and Gross, 1959). In G-6-PD deficient cells, G-6-PD activity declines with age at a faster than normal rate (Marks and Gross, 1959). Clearly, therefore, older cells of individuals possessing mutations of their G-6-PD are more susceptible to lysis than younger cells.

Clinical studies of individuals bearing various G-6-PD mutations corroborate the view that older cells are more vulnerable to the hemolytic action of drugs than are younger ones. A mild form of disorder is observed in Negroes. When a Negro subject receives 30 mg primaquine daily, no hemolysis occurs for two or three days, but the urine may turn black. Further signs may not develop, but in more severe cases there may be weakness, abdominal and back pain, icterus, and black urine. Heinz (inclusion) bodies may appear in the erythrocytes (Beutler *et al.*, 1954). Anemia and reticulocytosis supervene. In approximately one week this "acute hemolytic phase" ends spontaneously, even in the face of continued drug administration, and the "recovery phase" begins (Beutler, 1966). The patient feels improved, and the abnormalities noted above regress, even though administration of drug is continued. The Coombs' test is negative; and the osmotic fragility is normal, although the mechanical fragility is increased (Fraser and Vesell, 1968). This refractory state has been attributed not to any change in the metabolism of the drug or in the reactivity of the erythrocytes, as in immunological phenomena, but rather to a change in composition of the erythrocyte population. The older, more sensitive cells with their greater relative deficiency have been eliminated. The younger remaining cells with higher G-6-PD activities resist the osmotic and oxidant effects of various drugs and their metabolites (Dern *et al.*, 1954b).

Non-Negro subjects with G-6-PD deficiency exhibit a similar, but more severe, clinical course. In some studies the anemia is not self-limited (Salvidio *et al.*, 1963); in others it is (Larizza *et al.*, 1958). In Caucasians the spectrum of drugs causing hemolysis includes fava beans and chloramphenicol and is wider than in Negro subjects (Beutler, 1966).

Attention should also be called to the greater relative deficiency of G-6-PD in Caucasian than in Negro erythrocytes (Table VI) and to the fact that Caucasians (Ramot *et al.*, 1959) but not Negroes (Marks *et al.*, 1959) lack G-6-PD in their leukocytes. In lens tissue decreases of G-6-PD activity have been reported, but in tissues where nucleated cells predominate G-6-PD activity is not decreased as much as it is in erythrocytes. Of the variants shown in Table VI those possessing more than 30% of normal G-6-PD activity in their erythrocytes exhibit no hemolytic reactions, whereas below this level there is a poor correlation between the G-6-PD activity and the severity of any accompanying hemolytic anemia (Kirkman, 1968). Caucasians with the defect are more likely than Negro subjects to hemolyze on exposure to a variety of drugs and they will do so on lower dosages.

Finally, several genetic studies should be mentioned. As Beutler (1966) illustrates with pedigrees, G-6-PD deficiency does not conform to expectations for a completely dominant sex-linked trait, in that twice as many females as males are not observed, and one parent of each affected individual does not always manifest the trait. GSH stability and enzyme deficiency frequently display intermediate values in females and the number of intermediate and affected females is not twice that of males (Gross *et al.*, 1958; Childs *et al.*, 1958; Browne, 1957; Sansone and Segni, 1957). Thus, in females there is a considerable degree of variation in the expression of the defect, a situation which pedigrees show cannot be explained by the hypothesis that severely defective females are homozygous for the trait, whereas intermediately affected females are heterozygous.

G-6-PD deficiency has been studied as an example of dosage compensation of gene activity and of the Lyon hypothesis (Davidson *et al.*, 1963a,b; Lyon, 1961; Beutler *et al.*, 1962). The Lyon hypothesis was developed to explain why females with 2 X chromosomes fail to exhibit twice the amount of information present in males since males possess only a single X chromosome. Males and females have the same levels of G-6-PD activity. Furthermore, individuals with sex chromosomal polysomy such as XXX, XXXX, XXY, and XXXY all have normal rather than increased G-6-PD activity. Lyon postulated that males and females had equal amounts of genetic information from the X chromosome because the female possessed only one active X chromosome, the other being inactivated approximately 2 weeks after fertilization. The decision as to which of the X chromosomes would remain active and which would lose activity was random at the stage of the 2-week-old embryo; however, once that decision was made all daughter cells would abide by it (Lyon, 1961). The Lyon hypothesis, now generally accepted for human X-linked traits, predicts that only half the cells of a female heterozygous for a dominant sex-linked trait would exhibit the trait. G-6-PD deficiency is in accord with this prediction, which was confirmed by studies of G-6-PD activity from skin of heterozygous females in tissue culture (Davidson *et al.*, 1963b).

Although G-6-PD deficiency is widely distributed and occurs in almost all racial groups, there are certain regions where the gene is unusually frequent. It is particularly common in areas where malaria is prevalent. Suggestions have been made that the defective gene is maintained in such high frequencies, above 60% in some locations, because in certain environments the gene confers a selective advantage. Otherwise the adverse effects of the hemolytic anemia would have tended to reduce the frequency of the gene. Motulsky (1960) and Allison and Clyde (1961) showed that malarial infections are reduced in number and severity in children possessing a gene for G-6-PD deficiency. They postulated that the defect in some way protects the erythrocyte from malarial parasites. Some conflicting data involving parasite counts have been presented (Harris and Gilles, 1961; Krautrachue *et al.*, 1961), but the hypothesis is probably correct. This remains one of the only examples in man where a specific functional benefit has been adduced for a defective gene. The picture is complicated by the observation that several other defective genes also may confer resistance to malaria; sickle cell trait and thalassemia show similar geographic distributions to those of G-6-PD deficiency and also probably protect the erythrocyte from malarial infections (Allison *et al.*, 1963; Motulsky, 1960; Allison, 1961).

Many other examples of so-called "balanced polymorphisms" have been postulated to explain the high frequency of genes such as those for diabetes mellitus and cystic fibrosis of the pancreas. A double dose of these genes proves so debilitating and disadvantageous that their elimination from the gene pool through reduced fertility of those bearing them would be expected. Their high frequency in the population suggests that their loss from the gene pool through individuals possessing both genes for the disease is balanced by increased survival advantages accruing to individuals bearing only a single defective allele. These concepts of polymorphism were discussed in 1940 by Ford, who introduced the term to refer to variants in which upward of 2% of the population would be heterozygous at a particular genetic locus; Ford recognized that such a high frequency could not be maintained by mutation alone.

Recent developments in biochemical genetics require a revision in our approach to the problem of genetic variations (Neel and Schull, 1968). General use of powerful techniques such as starch gel electrophoresis in laboratories concerned with identifying genetic differences in the proteins of large populations has revealed an unexpected wealth of inherited biochemical variations (Harris, 1968). Increasing numbers of genetically transmitted variations in proteins make it questionable whether each polymorphism confers an advantage by itself. The possibility is raised that some may be neutral or at least neutral under certain environmental conditions. The frequency of genes at a single locus may determine whether a trait is advantageous, neutral or disadvantageous. A polymorphism of an enzyme in *Drosophila* recently described by Kojima and Yarbrough (1967) illustrates frequency-dependent selection. At equilibrium there was apparent selective neutrality; below equilibrium selection favored those phenotypes containing the gene, whereas at higher frequencies selection favored phenotypes lacking the gene. Neel and Schull (1968) suggest that the relative survival value of the alleles at a given locus may be substantially modified by other aspects of the total genome and that there may be a stabilizing influence of many polymorphisms on one another.

C. Drug-Sensitive Hemoglobins

Discovery of a new hemoglobin in a 2-year-old girl and her father resulted from an investigation of life-threatening hemolytic anemia which developed after administration of sulfa drugs (Hitzig *et al.*, 1960; Frick *et al.*, 1962). The girl's severe hemolysis occurred at age 2 after she received sulfadimethoxine for a fever of unknown origin. She had a history of a milder episode at 7 months of age when sulfonamides were given for an ear infection. The father experienced repeated, but mild, occurrences of jaundice and dark urine since childhood. These episodes were not always related to drug administration. A severe hemolytic crisis ensued after he received a sulfonamide for dysuria.

Study of the hemoglobin of the father and daughter revealed the presence of an abnormal hemoglobin with electrophoretic mobility between that of hemoglobins A and S. This hemoglobin comprised 20 to 30% of the total pigment. An abnormality of the β-chain was discovered, in which arginine is substituted for the normal histidine residue (Muller and Kingma, 1961; Huisman *et al.*, 1961). This sixty-third position is particularly important because it is here that the heme group is attached to the β-chain.

Of 65 relatives, 15 exhibited the abnormal hemoglobin, which has been designated hemoglobin Zürich. It appears to be transmitted as an autosomal dominant trait (Frick *et al.*, 1962). When red cells from the father were transfused to a normal volunteer, the half-life of the transfused erythrocytes was calculated to be 11 days instead of the normal 120; administration of either sulfonamides or primaquine caused rapid disappearance of the transfused cells (Frick *et al.*, 1962). In a second family ascertained in Maryland, the severity of the hemolytic episodes was less than in the Swiss cases (Rieder *et al.*, 1965).

Other point mutations resulting in substitution of a different amino acid at the sixty-third position, or closely adjacent sites of the β-chain, result in various types of hemoglobin M, the hemoglobin composed of four β-chains instead of the normal 2 α- and 2 β-chains (Baglioni, 1963). This hemoglobin oxidizes more readily to methemoglobin and leads to hereditary methemoglobinemia (Gerald and Scott, 1966). Erythrocyte life-spans of individuals with hemoglobin M are shortened *in vivo* by administration of sulfisoxazole. Sodium nitrite precipitates hemoglobin M *in vitro* but has not been administered *in vivo* (Rigas and Koler, 1961). Hemoglobins M are transmitted as autosomal dominants and can be distinguished by atypical electrophoretic mobility under certain specified and unusual conditions (Gerald and Scott, 1966). Hemoglobin $M_{Saskatoon}$ is interesting because it represents a mutation causing a substitution at the same position in the β-chain that is altered in hemoglobin Zürich, but the residue substituted at the sixty-third position is tyrosine in hemoglobin $M_{Saskatoon}$ instead of the arginine in hemoglobin Zürich (Gerald and Efron, 1961). In patients with hemoglobin $M_{Saskatoon}$ spontaneous oxidation to methemoglobin occurs *in vivo*.

D. Taste of Phenylthiourea or Phenylthiocarbamide (PTC)

Ability to taste phenylthiourea, also called phenylthiocarbamide or PTC, is inherited as an autosomal dominant. Tasters are either heterozygous or homozygous, whereas incapacity to taste PTC is transmitted as an autosomal recessive trait (Snyder, 1932; Blakeslee, 1932; Kalmus and Hubbard, 1960). This polymorphism was discovered in 1932 when Fox, who synthesized PTC, reported that he failed to perceive a bitter taste of which a colleague working in the same room complained. The taste emanated from dust arising when the powder was poured into a container (Fox, 1932).

Harris and Kalmus (1950a) refined the test and quantitated PTC-tasting thresholds by making 14 serial dilutions of PTC with water. They alternated tumblers containing PTC in increasing concentrations with tumblers of water. Harris and Kalmus discovered that females detected PTC in greater dilutions than males, that tasting sensitivity decreased with age, and that various compounds containing the N—C═S grouping also exhibited a bimodality in taste perception. Therefore, the N—C═S group in PTC seemed responsible for differences in tasting ability (Harris and Kalmus, 1950b).

The clinical significance of ability to taste PTC lies in its relationship to thyroid disease. PTC causes goiter in the rat (Richter and Clisby, 1942). Compounds related to PTC by possessing the N—C═S group, such as the antithyroid drugs methyl and propylthiouracil, display the same bimodality in taste perception as PTC. Harris *et al.* (1949) reported that 41% of 134 patients with nodular goiter were nontasters, an observation confirmed by Kitchin *et al.* (1959) in 447 individuals submitted to thyroidectomy for various reasons. Male patients with multiple thyroid adenomas exhibited a marked increase in nontasting frequency. Kitchin *et al.* (1959) suggested that in females, cyclic changes of thyroid involution and hyperplasia occurring with the menstrual cycle were a significant cause of thyroid disease and therefore concealed the true connection of PTC-tasting and thyroid disorders. These authors also reported that toxic diffuse goiter was accompanied by markedly low frequencies of nontasters in patients of either sex. Nontasters are apparently more susceptible to athyreotic cretinism (Fraser, 1961; Shepard and Gartler, 1960) in addition to adenomatous goiter. Tasters more frequently than nontasters develop toxic diffuse goiter.

A goitrogenic substance containing the grouping S—C═N has been isolated from turnip, cabbage, brussels sprouts, kale, and rape (Greer, 1957; Clements and Wishart, 1956). The substance containing this grouping, which is closely related to the N—C═S grouping of PTC, is 1-5-vinyl-2-thio-oxazolidone, a compound generated from an inactive precursor by an enzyme in the plant. Although cooking reduces the concentration of the goitrogen, cattle during winter consume several of these plants and may transmit the goitrogen in their milk (Clements and Wishart, 1956).

Becker and Morton (1964) reported that PTC nontasters occur more frequently in open angle glaucoma than in the general population, and significantly less frequently in angle closure glaucoma.

The frequency of nontasters varies in different populations, being 31.5% in Europeans (Saldanha and Becak, 1959), 10.6% in Chinese, and 2.7% in Africans (Barnicot, 1950). The reasons for maintenance of different gene frequencies for PTC tasting in various geographical areas are obscure. Tasters and nontasters revealed no differences in their metabolism of methylthiouracil and thiopentone (Evans *et al.*, 1962). Other approaches to the enigma must be sought. Related, but as yet not submitted to genetic study, are the observations that patients with adrenal cortical insufficiency exhibit greater sensitivity than normal to taste and to olfaction, sensitivities that can be returned to normal by the administration of carbohydrate-active steroids (Henkin *et al.*, 1963; Henkin and Bartter, 1966).

E. Smell of Cyanide

Inability to smell hydrocyanic acid (HCN, prussic acid) may prove fatal. Sufficiently volatile to be used as a fumigating pesticide in closed areas, HCN is one of the most rapidly acting poisons. Inability of certain individuals to detect HCN has been recognized for many decades, and Francis (1947) claims that in 1904 he recognized his inability to smell the poison.

The studies of Kirk and Stenhouse (1953) were the first systematic investigations of this curious polymorphism. They prepared a 20% solution of HCN in water and applied this to a piece of cotton in a test tube. In 244 Australian Caucasians, Kirk and Stenhouse (1953) observed 24 nonsmellers in 132 males, an incidence of 18.2%, and only 5 nonsmellers among 112 females, an incidence of 4.46%. These data suggested transmission of failure to detect HCN as a sex-linked recessive gene. Two families reported by Kirk and Stenhouse (1953) exhibited exceptions to this mode of inheritance; but Fukumoto *et al.* (1957), in an investigation of 433 Japanese, obtained a similar incidence of 18.2% nonsmeller males and of 5.5% nonsmeller females.

Persons incapable of smelling HCN apparently can recognize the odor if they simultaneously smoke cigars or cigarettes; they then experience an extremely unpleasant taste (Francis, 1947; Sachs, 1947).

Associations of this polymorphism with various disease states remain to be investigated. The physiologic basis for differences in the receptors for olfaction in this and for taste in the PTC polymorphism is unknown.

F. Responses of Intraocular Pressure to Steroids: Relationship to Glaucoma

In a series of interesting investigations summarized in 1968, Armaly established the existence of a polymorphism in the response of ocular pressure of normal subjects to topical steroids. In 80 normal individuals he showed that elevations in intraocular pressure after local administration of 0.1% ophthalmic solution of dexamethasone 21-phosphate exhibited a trimodal distribution. The steroid was applied to the right eye daily for 4 weeks, ocular pressure was measured weekly, and elevations in pressure after 4 weeks were determined. Table VII shows the trimodal distribution of individuals according to the extent of their increases in intraocular pressure over a 4-week period. The existence of three genotypes is suggested: P^LP^L for low elevations of 5 mm Hg or less, P^LP^H for intermediate increases from 6 to 15 mm Hg, and P^HP^H for high increment in pressure of 16 or more mm Hg. This genetic hypothesis was confirmed by family studies.

Armaly (1968) also demonstrated an association between certain types of response and glaucoma. In a sample of open-angle hypertensive glaucoma and also of low-tension glaucoma the distribution of responses (Table VII) differed from that in the random sample of normal subjects shown in Table VII (Armaly, 1968). In both conditions and surprisingly in the uninvolved eye of patients with unilateral posttraumatic glaucoma there was a marked reduction in P^LP^L genotypes and a corresponding increase in P^LP^H and P^HP^H genotypes (Table VII).

Family studies of individuals with glaucoma validated the genetic hypothesis that the response of high elevations of intraocular pressure after dexamethasone administration was inherited as an autosomal recessive trait. Armaly concluded that while affliction with glaucoma can be associated with genotypes other than P^HP^H and P^HP^L, the P^H gene may be closely related to the development of the types of glaucoma listed in Table VII.

In acute angle-closure glaucoma, also called narrow-angle glaucoma, genetic factors have been described which determine chamber angles (Kellerman and Posner, 1955) as well as chamber depths (Törnquist, 1953). However, these studies revealed that environmental factors could also exert appreciable effects on chamber depths. In individuals who have inherited narrow chambers, acute attacks of glaucoma may be precipitated by dilatation of the pupils (Grant, 1955). A variety of mydriatic agents can cause these acute attacks in genetically susceptible individuals. These include various adrenergic drugs such as epinephrine, phenylephrine, ephedrine and cocaine; drugs such as atropine and scopolamine that block the effects of cholinergic nerves also may produce an attack of angle-closure glaucoma (Kalow, 1962).

VII. Conclusion

This review of hereditary factors causing clinically significant variations in human responsiveness to drugs emphasizes the great strides made in pharmacogenetics during the past decade. It is anticipated that the next decade will witness the discovery of several new hereditary conditions affecting responsive-

TABLE VII

GENOTYPE CLASSIFICATION OF DEXAMETHASONE HYPERTENSION AND FREQUENCY DISTRIBUTIONS IN DIFFERENT CLINICAL CATEGORIES[a]

Category	No. of subjects tested	Percent frequency of genotypes		
		Low $(P^LP^L)\Delta P$ < 6 mm Hg	Intermediate $(P^LP^H)\Delta P$ 6–15 mm Hg	High $(P^HP^H)\Delta P$ > 15 mm Hg
Limits of pressure rise (mm Hg)		5 or less	6–15	16 or more
Mean pressure rise (mm Hg)		1.96	10.0	19.5
Standard deviation (mm Hg)		±2.00	±2.5	[b]
Genotype		P^LP^L	P^LP^H	P^HP^H
Random sample	80	66%	29%	5%
Open-angle hypertensive glaucoma	33	6%	48%	44%
Low-tension glaucoma	15	7%	53%	40%
Normal eye in recessed-angle glaucoma	15	—	53%	47%
Normal eye in angle recession without glaucoma	4	75%	25%	—

[a] From Armaly (1968).
[b] Range in sample 18–22 mm Hg.

ness to drugs. But more important, broader clinical applications of our present knowledge are expected, thereby ensuring safer and more effective use of currently available therapeutic agents.

REFERENCES

Aebi, H. E. (1967a). *Ann. Rev. Biochem.* **36**, 271.
Aebi, H. E. (1967b). *Proc. 3rd Intern. Congr. Human Genet., Chicago*, 1966 p. 189.
Aebi, H. E., Heiniger, J. P., Butler, R., and Hassig, A. (1961). *Experientia* **17**, 466.
Aebi, H. E., Baggiolini, M., Dewald, B., Lauber, E., Suter, H., Micheli, A., and Frei, J. (1964). *Enzymol. Biol. Clin.* **4**, 121.
Aggeler, P. M., O'Reilly, R. A., Leong, L. S., and Kowitz, P. E. (1967). *New Engl. J. Med.* **276**, 496.
Allison, A. C. (1961). *Ann. N.Y. Acad. Sci.* **91**, 710.
Allison, A. C., and Clyde, D. F. (1961). *Brit. Med. J.* **i**, 1346.
Allison, A. C., Askonas, B. A., Barnicot, N. A., Blumberg, B. S., and Krimbas, C. (1963). *Ann. Human Genet.* **26**, 237.
Armaly, M. F. (1968). *Ann. N.Y. Acad. Sci.* **151**, 861.
Armstrong, A. R., and Peart, H. E. (1960). *Am. Rev. Respirat. Diseases* **81**, 588.

Axelrod, J., Cooper, J. R., and Brodie, B. B. (1949). *Proc. Soc. Exptl. Biol. Med.* **70**, 693.
Baglioni, C. (1963). *In* "Molecular Genetics" (J. H. Taylor, ed.), Pt. 1, p. 405. Academic Press, New York.
Barnicot, N. A. (1950). *Ann. Eugen.* **15**, 248.
Barron, E. S. G., and Singer, T. P. (1943). *Science* **97**, 356.
Bartlett, M. S. (1949). *Biometrics* **5**, 207.
Baur, E. W. (1963). *Science* **140**, 816.
Becker, B., and Morton, W. R. (1964). *Arch. Ophthalmol.* (*Chicago*) **72**, 323
Beutler, E. (1957). *J. Lab. Clin. Med.* **49**, 84.
Beutler, E. (1966). *In* "The Metabolic Basis of Inherited Disease" (J. B. Stanbury, J. B. Wyngaarden, and D. S. Fredrickson, eds.), pp. 1060–1089. McGraw-Hill, New York.
Beutler, E., Dern, R. J., and Alving, A. S. (1954). *J. Lab. Clin. Med.* **44**, 439.
Beutler, E., Yeh, M., and Fairbanks, V. F. (1962). *Proc. Natl. Acad. Sci. U.S.* **48**, 9.
Biehl, J. (1956). *Trans. 15th Conf. Chemotherapy Tuberc., St. Louis* p. 279.
Biehl, J. (1957). *Trans. 16th Conf. Chemotherapy Tuberc., St. Louis* p. 108.
Blair, A. H., and Vallee, B. L. (1966). *Biochemistry* **5**, 2026.
Blakeslee, A. F. (1932). *Proc. Natl. Acad. Sci. U.S.* **18**, 120.
Bönicke, R., and Lisboa, B. P. (1957). *Naturwissenschaften* **44**, 314.
Bönicke, R., and Reif, W. (1953). *Arch. Exptl. Pathol. Pharmakol. Naunyn-Schmiedebergs* **220**, 321.
Bourne, J. G., Collier, H. O. J., and Somers, G. F. (1952). *Lancet* **i**, 1225.
Bovet, D., Bovet-Nitti, F., Guarino, S., Longo, V. G., and Marotta, M. (1949). *Rend. Ist. Super. Sanita* **12**, 106.
Bovet-Nitti, F. (1949). *Rend. Ist. Super. Sanita* **12**, 138.
Boyer, S. H., Porter, I. H., and Weilbacher, R. G. (1962). *Proc. Natl. Acad. Sci. U.S.* **48**, 1868.
Brennan, R. W., Dehejia, H., Kutt, H., and McDowell, F. (1968). *Neurology* **18**, 283.
Brodie, B. B., and Axelrod, J. (1950). *J. Pharmacol. Exptl. Therap.* **98**, 97.
Brodie, B. B., and Hogben, C. A. M. (1957). *J. Pharm. Pharmacol.* **9**, 345.
Brodie, B. B., Axelrod, J., Soberman, R., and Levy, B. B. (1949). *J. Biol. Chem.* **179**, 25.
Browne, E. A. (1957). *Bull. Johns Hopkins Hosp.* **101**, 115.
Burns, J. J., Rose, R. K., Chenkin, T., Goldman, A., Schulert, A., and Brodie, B. B. (1953). *J. Pharmacol. Exptl. Therap.* **109**, 346.
Bush, G. H. (1961). *Brit. J. Anaesthesia* **33**, 454.
Butler, T. C. (1956). *J. Pharmacol. Exptl. Therap.* **116**, 326.
Butler, T. C. (1957). *J. Pharmacol. Exptl. Therap.* **119**, 1.
Carlson, H. B., Anthony, E. M., Russell, W. F., Jr., and Middlebrook, G. (1956). *New Engl. J. Med.* **255**, 118.
Carson, P. E., Flanagan, C. L., Ickes, C. E., and Alving A. S. (1956). *Science* **124**, 484.
Childs, B., Zinkham, W., Brown, E. A., Kimbro, E. L., and Torbert, J. V. (1958). *Bull. Johns Hopkins Hosp.* **102**, 21.
Christensen, F. (1966). *Acta Pharmacol. Toxicol.* **24**, 232.
Clark, S. W., Glaubiger, G. A., and La Du, B. N. (1968). *Ann. N.Y. Acad. Sci.* **151**, 710.
Clements, F. W., and Wishart, J. W. (1956). *Metab. Clin. Exptl.* **5**, 623.
Conney, A. H. (1967). *Pharmacol. Rev.* **19**, 317.
Crigler, J. F., Jr., and Gold, N. I. (1969). *J. Clin. Invest.* **48**, 42.
Davidson, R. G., Migeon, B. R., Borden, M., and Childs, B. (1963a). *Bull. Johns Hopkins Hosp.* **112**, 318.
Davidson, R. G., Nitowsky, H. M., and Childs, B. (1963b). *Proc. Natl. Acad. Sci. U.S.* **50**, 481.

Davies, R. O., Marton, A. V., and Kalow, W. (1960). *Can. J. Biochem. Physiol.* **38**, 545.
Dayton, P. G., Cucinell, S. A., Weiss, M., and Perel, J. M. (1967). *J. Pharmacol. Exptl. Therap.* **158**, 305.
Dern, R. J., Weinstein, I. M., LeRoy, G. V., Talmage, D. W., and Alving, A. S. (1954a). *J. Lab. Clin. Med.* **43**, 303.
Dern, R. J., Beutler, E., and Alving, A. S. (1954b). *J. Lab. Clin. Med.* **44**, 171.
Devadatta, S., Gangadharam, P. R. J., Andrews, R. H., Fox, W., Ramakrishnan, C. V., Selkon, J. B., and Velu, S. (1960). *Bull. World Health Organ.* **23**, 587.
Editorial (1966). *Chron. World Health Organ.* **20**, 29.
Edwards, J. A., and Evans, D. A. P. (1967). *Clin. Pharmacol. Therap.* **8**, 824.
Elias, R. A. (1965). *In* "Anticoagulant Therapy in Ischemic Heart Disease" (E. S. Nichol, ed.), pp. 443–448. Grune & Stratton, New York.
Evans, D. A. P. (1962). *Med. Hyg.* **20**, 905.
Evans, D. A. P. (1965). *Ann. N.Y. Acad. Sci.* **123**, 178.
Evans, D. A. P. (1968). *Ann. N.Y. Acad. Sci.* **151**, 723.
Evans, D. A. P., and White, T. A. (1964). *J. Lab. Clin. Med.* **63**, 387.
Evans, D. A. P., Manley, K. A., and McKusick, V. A. (1960). *Brit. Med. J.* **ii**, 485.
Evans, D. A. P., Kitchin, F. D., and Riding, J. E. (1962). *Ann. Human Genet.* **26**, 123.
Evans, D. A. P., Davison, K., and Pratt, R. T. C. (1965). *Clin. Pharmacol. Therap.* **6**, 430.
Evans, F. T., Gray, P. W. S., Lehmann, H., and Silk, E. (1952). *Lancet* **i**, 1229.
Fisher, R. A. (1954). "Statistical Methods for Research Workers," 12th Ed., Rev. Oliver & Boyd, Edinburgh and London.
Flanagan, C. L., Beutler, E., Dern, R. J., and Alving, A. S. (1955). *J. Lab. Clin. Med.* **46**, 814.
Foldes, F. F. (1968). *Ann. N.Y. Acad. Sci.* **151**, 751.
Forbat, A., Lehmann, H., and Silk, E. (1953). *Lancet* **ii**, 1067.
Ford, E. B. (1940). *In* "The New Systematics" (J. S. Huxley, ed.), pp. 493–513. Oxford Univ. Press, London and New York.
Fox, A. L. (1932). *Proc. Natl. Acad. Sci. U.S.* **18**, 115.
Francis, F. G. (1947). *Chem. Ind. (London)* **23**, 325.
Fraser, G. R. (1961). *Lancet* **i**, 964.
Fraser, I. M., and Vesell, E. S. (1968). *Ann. N.Y. Acad. Sci.* **151**, 177.
Frick, P. G., Hitzig, W. H., and Betke, K. (1962). *Blood* **20**, 261.
Fukumoto, Y., Nakajima, H., Uetake, M., Matsuyama, A., and Yoshida, T. (1957). *Japan. J. Human Genet.* **2**, 7.
Gangadharam, P. R. J., and Selkon, J. B. (1961). *Proc. 16th Intern. Tuberc. Conf., Toronto* **2**, 556.
Gerald, P. S., and Efron, M. L. (1961). *Proc. Natl. Acad. Sci. U.S.* **47**, 1758.
Gerald, P. S., and Scott, E. M. (1966). *In* "The Metabolic Basis of Inherited Disease" (J. B. Stanbury, J. B. Wyngaarden, and D. S. Fredrickson, eds.), pp. 1090–1099. McGraw-Hill, New York.
Gillette, J. R. (1963). *Progr. Drug. Res.* **6**, 11.
Gillette, J. R. (1966). *Advan. Pharmacol.* **4**, 219.
Goedde, H. W., and Altland, K. (1968). *Ann. N.Y. Acad. Sci.* **151**, 540.
Goedde, H. W., Altland, K., and Schloot, W. (1968). *Ann. N.Y. Acad. Sci.* **151**, 742.
Gow, J. G., and Evans, D. A. P. (1964). *Tubercle* **45**, 136.
Grant, W. M. (1955). *Pharmacol. Rev.* **1**, 143.
Greaves, J. H., and Ayres, P. (1967). *Nature* **215**, 877.
Greer, M. A. (1957). *Am. J. Clin. Nutr.* **5**, 440.
Gross, R. T., Hurwitz, R. E., and Marks, P. A. (1958). *J. Clin. Invest.* **37**, 1176.

Grunberg, E., Leiwant, B., D'Ascensio, L.-L., and Schnitzer, R. J. (1952). *Diseases Chest* **21**, 369.

Gutsche, B. B., Scott, E. M., and Wright, R. C. (1967). *Nature* **215**, 322.

Hamilton, H. B., and Neel, J. V. (1963). *Am. J. Human Genet.* **15**, 408.

Hammer, W., Märtens, S., and Sjöqvist, F. (1969). *Clin. Pharmacol. Therap.* **10**, 44.

Harris, F. W., and Cockburn, T. (1918). *Analyst* **43**, 133.

Harris, H. (1968). *Ann. N.Y. Acad. Sci.* **151**, 232.

Harris, H., and Kalmus, H. (1950a). *Ann. Eugen.* **15**, 24.

Harris, H., and Kalmus, H. (1950b). *Ann. Eugen.* **15**, 32.

Harris, H., and Whittaker, M. (1961). *Nature* **191**, 496.

Harris, H., and Whittaker, M. (1962a). *Ann. Human Genet.* **26**, 59.

Harris, H., and Whittaker, M. (1962b). *Ann. Human Genet.* **26**, 73.

Harris, H., Kalmus, H., and Trotter, W. R. (1949). *Lancet* **ii**, 1038.

Harris, H., Whittaker, M., Lehmann, H., and Silk, E. (1960). *Acta Genet. Statist. Med.* **10**, 1.

Harris, H., Hopkinson, D. A., Robson, E. B., and Whittaker, M. (1963). *Ann. Human Genet.* **26**, 359.

Harris, H. W. (1961a). *Proc. 16th Intern. Tuberc. Conf., Toronto* **2**, 503.

Harris, H. W. (1961b). *Trans. 20th Res. Conf. Pulmonary Diseases, Memphis* p. 39.

Harris, H. W., Knight, R. A. and Selin, M. J. (1958). *Am. Rev. Tuberc. Pulmonary Diseases* **78**, 944.

Harris, R., and Gilles, H. M. (1961). *Ann. Human Genet.* **25**, 199.

Henkin, R. I., and Bartter, F. C. (1966). *J. Clin. Invest.* **45**, 1631.

Henkin, R. I., Gill, J. R., Jr., and Bartter, F. C. (1963). *J. Clin. Invest.* **42**, 727.

Hitzig, W. H., Frick, P. G., Betke, K., and Huisman, T. H. J. (1960). *Helv. Paediat. Acta* **15**, 499.

Hodgkin, W. E., Giblett, E. R., Levine, H., Bauer, W., and Motulsky, A. G. (1965). *J. Clin. Invest.* **44**, 486.

Holmes, R. S., and Masters, C. J. (1965). *Arch. Biochem. Biophys.* **109**, 196.

Hopkinson, D. A., Spencer, N., and Harris, H. (1964). *Am. J. Human Genet.* **16**, 141.

Hughes, H. B. (1953). *J. Pharmacol. Exptl. Therap.* **109**, 444.

Hughes, H. B., Biehl, J. P., Jones, A. P., and Schmidt, L. H. (1954). *Am. Rev. Tuberc.* **70**, 266.

Hughes, H. B., Schmidt, L. H., and Biehl, J. P. (1955). *Trans. 14th Conf. Chemotherapy Tuberc., Atlanta* p. 217.

Huisman, T. H. J., Horton, B., Bridges, M. T., Betke, K., and Hitzig, W. H. (1961). *Clin. Chim. Acta* **6**, 347.

Hunt, R., and Taveau, R. de M. (1906). *Brit. Med. J.* **ii**, 1788.

Ikeda, M., Sezesny, B., and Barnes, M. (1966). *Federation Proc.* **25**, 417.

Jacob, H. S., and Jandl, J. H. (1962). *J. Clin. Invest.* **41**, 1514.

Jenne, J. W. (1965). *J. Clin. Invest.* **44**, 1992.

Jenne, J. W., MacDonald, F. M., and Mendoza, E. (1961). *Am. Rev. Respirat. Diseases* **84**, 371.

Kalmus, H., and Hubbard, S. J. (1960). "The Chemical Senses in Health and Disease." Thomas, Springfield, Illinois.

Kalow, W. (1962). "Pharmacogenetics: Heredity and the Response to Drugs." Saunders, Philadelphia, Pennsylvania.

Kalow, W., and Davies, R. O. (1959). *Biochem. Pharmacol.* **1**, 183.

Kalow, W., and Genest, K. (1957). *Can. J. Biochem. Physiol.* **35**, 339.

Kalow, W., and Gunn, D. R. (1959). *Ann. Human Genet.* **23**, 239.

Kalow, W., and Staron, N. (1957). *Can. J. Biochem. Physiol.* **35**. 1305.

Kattamis, C., Zannos-Mariolea, L., Franco, A. P., Liddell, J., Lehmann, H., and Davies, D. (1962). *Nature* **196**, 599.

Kellerman, L., and Posner, A. (1955). *Am. J. Ophthalmol.* **40**, 681.

Kirk, R. L., and Stenhouse, N. S. (1953). *Nature* **171**, 698.

Kirkman, H. N. (1968). *Ann. N.Y. Acad. Sci.* **151**, 753.

Kirkman, H. N., and Hendrickson, E. M. (1963). *Am. J. Human Genet.* **15**, 241.

Kitchin, F. D., Howel-Evans, W., Clarke, C. A., McConnell, R. B., and Sheppard, P. M. (1959). *Brit. Med. J.* **i**, 1069.

Knight, R. A., Selin, M. J., and Harris, H. W. (1959). *Trans. 18th Conf. Chemotherapy Tuberc., St. Louis*, p. 52.

Kojima, K., and Yarbrough, K. M. (1967). *Proc. Natl. Acad. Sci. U.S.* **57**, 645.

Krautrachue, M., Na-Nakorn, S., Charoenlarp, P., and Suwanakul, L. (1961). *Ann. Trop. Med. Parasitol.* **55**, 468.

Kutt, H., Verebely, K., and McDowell, F. (1968). *Neurology* **18**, 706.

Kutt, H., Wolk, M., Scherman, R., and McDowell, F. (1964a). *Neurology* **14**, 542.

Kutt, H., Winters, W., Kokenge, R., and McDowell, F. (1964b). *Arch. Neurol.* **11**, 642.

Larizza, P., Brunetti, P., Grignani, F., and Ventura, S. (1958). *Minerva Med.* **49**, 3769.

Lehmann, H., and Liddell, J. (1964). *Progr. Med. Genet.* **3**, 75.

Lehmann, H., and Ryan, E. (1956). *Lancet* **ii**, 124.

Lehmann, H., and Silk, E. (1953). *Brit. Med. J.* **i**, 767.

Lewis, R. J., Spivack, M., and Spaet, T. H. (1967). *Am. J. Med.* **42**, 620.

Link, K. P. (1945). *Harvey Lectures Ser.* **39**, 162.

Lyon, M. F. (1961). *Nature* **190**, 372.

Marks, P. A., and Gross, R. T. (1959). *J. Clin. Invest.* **38**, 2253.

Marks, P. A., Johnson, A. B., Hirschberg, E., and Banks, J. (1958). *Ann. N.Y. Acad. Sci.* **75**, 95.

Marks, P. A., Gross, R. T., and Hurwitz, R. E. (1959). *Nature* **183**, 1266.

Maynert, E. W. (1960). *J. Pharmacol. Exptl. Therap.* **130**, 275.

Meier, H. (1963). "Experimental Pharmacogenetics; Physiopathology of Heredity and Pharmacologic Responses." Academic Press, New York.

Merritt, H. H., and Putnam, T. J. (1938). *A.M.A. Arch. Neurol. Psychiat.* **39**, 1003.

Meyer, H., and Mally, J. (1912). *Monatsh. Chem.* **33**, 393.

Micheli, A., and Aebi, H. (1965). *Rev. Franc. Etudes Clin. Biol.* **10**, 431.

Mitchell, R. S., Riemensnider, D. K., Harsch, J. R., and Bell, J. C. (1958). *Trans. 17th Conf. Chemotherapy Tuberc., Memphis* p. 77.

Mitchell, R. S., Bell, J. C., and Riemensnider, D. K. (1960). *Trans. 19th Conf. Chemotherapy Tuberc.*, p. 62.

Mitoma, C., Sorich, T. J., II, and Neubauer, S. E. (1968). *Life Sci.* **7**, 145.

Motulsky, A. G. (1957). *J. Am. Med. Assoc.* **165**, 835.

Motulsky, A. G. (1960). *Human Biol.* **32**, 28.

Motulsky, A. G. (1964). *Progr. Med. Genet.* **3**, 49.

Muller, C. J., and Kingma, S. (1961). *Biochim. Biophys. Acta* **50**, 595.

Neel, J. V., and Schull, W. J. (1968). *Perspectives Biol. Med.* **11**, 565.

Neitlich, H. W. (1966). *J. Clin. Invest.* **45**, 380.

Nishimura, E. T., Hamilton, H. B., Kobara, T. Y., Takahara, S., Ogura, Y., and Doi, K. (1959). *Science* **130**, 333.

Nishimura, E. T., Carson, S. N., and Kobara, T. Y. (1964). *Arch. Biochem. Biophys.* **108**, 452.

Oort, M., Loos, J. A., and Prins, H. K. (1961). *Vox Sanguinis* **6**, 370.

O'Reilly, R. A., and Aggeler, P. M. (1965). *Federation Proc.* **24**, 1266.
O'Reilly, R. A., Aggeler, P. M., Hoag, M. S., Leong, L. S., and Kropatkin, M. L. (1964). *New Engl. J. Med.* **271**, 809.
O'Reilly, R. A., Pool, J. G., and Aggeler, P. M. (1968). *Ann. N.Y. Acad. Sci.* **151**, 913.
Orgell, W. H., Vaidya, K. A., and Dahm, P. A. (1958). *Science* **128**, 1136.
Osborne, R. H., and DeGeorge, F. V. (1959). "Genetic Basis of Morphological Variation, An Evaluation and Application of the Twin Study Method." Harvard Univ. Press, Cambridge, Massachusetts.
Perry, H. M., Jr., Sakamoto, A., and Tan, E. M. (1967). *J. Lab. Clin. Med.* **70**, 1020.
Peters, J. H. (1959). *Trans. 18th Conf. Chemotherapy Tuberc., St. Louis* p. 37.
Peters, J. H. (1960a). *Am. Rev. Respirat. Diseases* **81**, 485.
Peters, J. H. (1960b). *Am. Rev. Respirat. Diseases* **82**, 153.
Peters, J. H., Gordon, G. R., and Brown, P. (1965a). *Proc. Soc. Exptl. Biol. Med.* **120**, 575.
Peters, J. H., Miller, K. S., and Brown, P. (1965b). *Analy. Biochem.* **12**, 379.
Price, V. E., and Greenfield, R. E. (1954). *J. Biol. Chem.* **209**, 363.
Prins, H. K., Oort, M., Loos, J. A., Zürcher, C., and Beckers, T. (1963). *Proc. 9th Congr. European Soc. Haematol., Lisbon* **II/1**, 721.
Ramot, B., Fisher, S., Szeinberg, A., Adam, A., Sheba, C., and Gafni, D. (1959). *J. Clin. Invest.* **38**, 2234.
Richter, C. P., and Clisby, K. H. (1942). *A.M.A. Arch. Pathol.* **33**, 46.
Rieder, R. F., Zinkham, W. H., and Holtzman, N. A. (1965). *Am. J. Med.* **39**, 4.
Rigas, D. A., and Koler, R. D. (1961). *Blood* **18**, 1.
Robitzek, E. H., Selikoff, I. J., and Ornstein, G. G. (1952). *Quart. Bull. Sea View Hosp.* **13**, 27.
Robson, J. M., and Sullivan, F. M. (1963). *Pharmacol. Rev.* **15**, 169.
Ross, R. R. (1958). *J. Am. Med. Assoc.* **168**, 273.
Sachs, W. (1947). *Chem. Ind.* (*London*) **25**, 358.
Saldanha, P. H., and Becak, W. (1959). *Science* **129**, 150.
Salvidio, E., Pannacciulli, I., and Tizianello, A. (1963). *Proc. 9th Congr. European Soc. Haematol. Lisbon,* **II/1**, 707.
Sansone, G., and Segni, G. (1957). *Lancet* **ii**, 295.
Schmiedel, A. (1961). *Proc. 16th Intern. Tuberc. Conf., Toronto* **2**, 508.
Schroeder, W. A., Shelton, J. R., Shelton, J. B., and Olson, B. M. (1964). *Biochim. Biophys. Acta* **89**, 47.
Shepard, T. H., II, and Gartler, S. M. (1960). *Science* **131**, 929.
Shibata, Y., Higashi, T., Hirai, H., and Hamilton, H. B. (1967). *Arch. Biochem. Biophys.* **118**, 200.
Smirnov, G. A., and Kozulitzina, T. I. (1962). *Vopr. Med. Khim.* **8**, 401.
Smith, W. K. (1939). *J. Agr. Res.* **59**, 211.
Snyder, L. H. (1932). *Ohio J. Sci.* **32**, 436.
Solomon, H. M. (1968). *Ann. N.Y. Acad. Sci.* **151**, 932.
Solomon, H. M., and Schrogie, J. J. (1966). *J. Pharmacol. Exptl. Therap.* **154**, 660.
Sunahara, S. (1961). *Proc. 16th Intern. Tuberc. Conf., Toronto* **2**, 513.
Szeinberg, A., Bar-Or, R., and Sheba, C. (1963). *In* "The Genetics of Migrant and Isolate Populations" (E. Goldschmidt, ed.), p. 279. Williams & Wilkins, Baltimore, Maryland.
Szeinberg, A., Pipano, S., Ostfeld, E., and Eviator, L. (1966). *J. Med. Genet.* **3**, 190.
Takahara, S. (1952). *Lancet* **ii**, 1101.
Takahara, S., Sato, H., Doi, M., and Mihara, S. (1952). *Proc. Japan. Acad.* **28**, 585.
Takahara, S. (1954). *Laryngoscope* **64**, 685.
Takahara, S., and Doi, K. (1958). *Japan. J. Otol.* **61**, 1727.

Takahara, S., Ogura, Y., and Doi, K. (1959). *Acta Med. Okayama* **13**, 209.

Takahara, S., Hamilton, H. B., Neel, J. V., Kobara, T. Y., Ogura, Y., and Nishimura, E. T. (1960). *J. Clin. Invest.* **39**, 610.

Tanford, C., and Lovrien, R. (1962). *J. Am. Chem. Soc.* **84**, 1892.

Thorup, O. A., Jr., Carpenter, J. T., and Howard, P. (1964). *Brit. J. Haematol.* **10**, 542.

Törnquist, R. (1953). *Acta Ophthalmol. Suppl.* **39**, 1.

Vesell, E. S. (1968). *Ann. N.Y. Acad. Sci.* **151**, 900.

Vesell, E. S., and Page, J. G. (1968a). *Science* **159**, 1479.

Vesell, E. S., and Page, J. G. (1968b). *Science* **161**, 72.

Vesell, E. S., and Page, J. G. (1968c). *J. Clin. Invest.* **47**, 2657.

Vesell, E. S., and Page, J. G. (1969). *J. Clin. Invest.*, in press.

Vogel, F. (1959). *Ergeb. Inn. Med. Kinderheilk.* **12**, 52.

von Wartburg, J. P., and Schürch, P. M. (1968). *Ann. N.Y. Acad. Sci.* **151**, 936.

Weber, W. W., Cohen, S. N., and Steinberg, M. S. (1968). *Ann. N.Y. Acad. Sci.* **151**, 734.

Weiner, M., Shapiro, S., Axelrod, J., Cooper, J. R., and Brodie, B. B. (1950). *J. Pharmacol. Exptl. Therap.* **99**, 409.

Welch, R. M., Harrison, Y. E., Conney, A. H., Poppers, P. J., and Finster, M. (1968). *Science* **160**, 541.

Wenzel, D. G., and Broadie, L. L. (1966). *Toxicol. Appl. Pharmacol.* **8**, 455.

White, T. A., and Evans, D. A. P. (1967a). *Clin. Chim. Acta* **18**, 161.

White, T. A., and Evans, D. A. P. (1967b). *Experientia* **23**, 959.

White, T. A., and Evans, D. A. P. (1968). *Clin. Pharmacol. Therap.* **9**, 80.

Whittaker, V. P., and Wijesundera, S. (1952). *Biochem. J.* **52**, 475.

Willimott, S. G. (1933). *Analyst* **58**, 431.

Wilson, G. S. (1959). *Monthly Bull. Ministry Health Public Health Lab. Serv.* **18**, 207.

Wilson, I. B. (1954). *J. Biol. Chem.* **208**, 123.

Woodbury, D. M., and Esplin, D. W. (1959). *Res. Publ., Assoc. Res. Nervous Mental Disease* **37**, 24.

Wyngaarden, J. B., and Howell, R. B. (1966). *In* "The Metabolic Basis of Inherited Disease" (J. B. Stanbury, J. B. Wyngaarden, and D. S. Fredrickson, eds.), pp. 1343–1355. McGraw-Hill, New York.

Yaffee, S. J., Levy, G., Matsuzawa, T., and Baliah, T. (1966). *N. Engl. J. Med.* **275**, 1461.

Yahr, M. D., and Merritt, H. H. (1956). *J. Am. Med. Assoc.* **161**, 333.

Yahr, M. D., Sciarra, D., Carter, S., and Merritt, H. H. (1952). *J. Am. Med. Assoc.* **150**, 663.

Yata, H. (1959). *Nippon Shika Hyoron* **204**, 7.

Yoshida, A. (1967). *Proc. Natl. Acad. Sci. U.S.* **57**, 835.

The Combination of Gas Chromatography and Mass Spectrometry in the Identification of Drugs and Metabolites

Carl-Gustaf Hammar, Bo Holmstedt, Jan-Erik Lindgren, and Richard Tham

Department of Toxicology, Swedish Medical Research Council
Karolinska Institutet, Stockholm, Sweden

I. Introduction

The past quarter-century has seen a great change in the approach toward the study of drugs. Important steps include the introduction of determinations of plasma levels as a guideline for dosage, the discovery of the drug-metabolizing liver microsomal enzymes, the emerging significance of genetic variability in metabolism and pharmacologic response, and the introduction of new and more sensitive techniques such as fluorescence spectrophotometry. One would therefore be justified in calling the time from about 1945 to date the era of biochemical pharmacology. It is likely that we are now entering a period wherein physicochemical techniques will greatly influence progress in drug research. The techniques described in this review allow us to determine infinitely smaller quantities of drugs in body fluids with a much greater power of separation than ever achieved with earlier methods.

Recently an instrument combining gas chromatography with mass spectrometry has been successfully applied to the identification of many naturally occurring body constituents. This instrument with a number of accessories has been used for about two years in our laboratory for the characterization of drugs and their metabolites. The results reported in this review article are mostly based on our own experience.

The general usefulness of this instrument in research on drug metabolism is obvious. Essentially, the best known method of separation of mixtures of compounds, gas chromatography (GC), is combined with an excellent means of structural identification, mass spectrometry (MS). The mass spectrometer is capable of accurately determining the molecular weight of an unknown compound. In spite of the moderate resolution of the mass spectrometer in the combined instrument it has proved to be extremely useful. Elucidating the structure of an unknown substance is generally difficult. In the area of natural products these problems may be overcome by measuring and studying the mass spectra and fragmentation patterns of related compounds. This approach can be applied with relative ease for modern drugs, where the chemical structure is always known and synthetic analogs are usually available. Knowledge of mass spectra and fragmentation patterns forms the basis for the elucidation of the structure of the drug metabolites. Comparison of the fragmentation pattern of compounds isolated from tissues (e.g., brain, plasma) with that of appropriate reference compounds provides information for determining the structure of the drug in question and/or its metabolites.

II. Principles of Combined Gas Chromatography–Mass Spectrometry (GC-MS)

A. Gas Chromatography (GC)

The rapid development of gas chromatographic techniques during the last decade has offered a new approach to analysis of drugs and metabolites. Gas chromatographic methods for analysis of steroids, fatty acids, phenolic and nonphenolic aromatic acids, catecholamines, tryptamines, barbiturates, alkaloids, and many other substances have been described. Several handbooks and reviews have been published (Szymanski, 1964; Hammarstrand, 1966, 1967, 1968; Gudzinowics, 1967; Zlatkis, 1967; Juvet and Dal Nogare, 1968; Kern *et al.*, 1968).

In working with combined GC-MS the necessity of being familiar with ordinary GC is obvious.

1. *Detectors*

The sensitivity of the gas chromatographic technique is partly limited by the detection system that is used for recording of the separated substances emerging from the gas chromatographic column. Numerous detection systems have by now been constructed. With the commonly used hydrogen flame ionization detector it is usually easy to detect most substances in amounts in the region of 0.01 μg. Construction of detectors for analysis of smaller amounts requires not only an increase of sensitivity but also some degree of specificity of the detector. The electron capture detector has a high sensitivity but limited specificity in that it will only detect electron-capturing substances such as halogenated compounds. The mass spectrometer can also be used as a detection system, as will be described later, and the system can be adjusted to detect substances through their mass spectrometric fragmentation pattern.

2. *Liquid Phases*

The choice of a stationary phase becomes more important in the combination with MS than in conventional GC. The thermal stability of the phase at the temperature used must be very high, otherwise the "bleeding" from the phase will interfere with the interpretation of the mass spectrum of the compound. Furthermore, the bleeding may cause a contamination of the ion source of the mass spectrometer.

3. *Group Separation*

Before GC can be performed it is necessary to efficiently separate drugs and metabolites from biologic tissues, and also to attain suitable concentrations. Some important examples of such procedures are the following: Amines may be separated from urine using a Sephadex ion exchange column (Tham *et al.*, 1969). Basic metabolites of drugs in plasma may be isolated by extraction with a suitable organic solvent (Hammer and Brodie, 1967; Hammar and Holmstedt, 1968). Organic acids may be isolated from urine by extraction or by ion exchange chromatography (Tham and Holmstedt, 1965; Horning, 1968a). Alkaloids may be extracted from plants using suitable extraction procedures (Holmstedt and Lindgren, 1967).

4. *Derivative formation*

In GC analysis it is often necessary to prepare derivatives of the substances to be analyzed. The aim of derivative formation is to increase the volatility of a compound and to reduce its polarity. In addition, derivative formation may give information by causing a change in retention time.

Amines must usually be transformed to other derivatives prior to GC (Fales and Pisano, 1964). At the time of writing an important advance in the preparation of derivatives of amines suitable for GC is the formation of heptafluorobutyryl derivatives using heptafluorobutyrylimidazole (Horning *et al.*, 1968). These derivatives contain seven fluorine atoms and are thus suitable for electron capture detection. Another derivative which has been used to advantage for GC is acetylation with anhydrides containing fluorine (Hammar and Holmstedt, 1968). Many biologic amines, viz., the catecholamines, contain OH groups. In order to reduce the polarity of these compounds the OH groups may be silylated (e.g., reacted with hexamethyldisilazane with elimination of ammonia to form trimethylsilyl ethers) (Horning *et al.*, 1967; Pierce, 1968). Indoles may often be analyzed without derivative formation. Silylation may, however, be of great help in the separation of position isomers (Holmstedt *et al.*, 1964).

A technique has been described for the selective demethylation of quaternary ammonium salts, using a relatively low temperature reaction between the ammonium salt and sodium benzenethiolate (Shamma *et al.*, 1966). This method was a significant starting point from which a gas chromatographic method for the estimation of acetylcholine and other quaternary ammonium compounds was developed. The tertiary amines are volatile and amenable to estimation by GC and MS. A microestimation of acetylcholine has been developed along these lines (Jenden *et al.*, 1968; Hanin, 1968; Hanin *et al.*, 1968; Hanin and Jenden, 1969).

Acids usually have to be transformed to the corresponding methyl esters or trimethylsilyl esters (Dalgliesh *et al.*, 1966; Horning, 1968b.)

B. Combination of Gas Chromatography and Mass Spectrometry (GC-MS)

In 1964 Ryhage published a paper about the molecule separator, the principle of which was described by Becker *et al.*, 1955; (Becker, 1961). This two-step, jet-diffusing system made it possible for the mass spectrometer to directly accept the effluent from a gas chromatograph. Thus the mass spectra of compounds emerging from the gas chromatograph can be scanned without the necessity for any intermediate isolation procedure. In order to maintain the necessary vacuum in the mass spectrometer the separator removes about 99% of the helium carrier gas. More than 50% of the heavier sample molecules then pass into the ion source (Ryhage, 1967a). Separators built upon other principles have been reported (Watson and Biemann, 1964, 1965; Lipsky *et al.*, 1966a,b; Llewellyn and Littlejohn, 1966).

The mass spectrometer of the combination instrument LKB 9000,* containing a separator was specifically designed to be connected to a gas chromatograph. Accessories are a solid probe direct inlet, a heated membrane inlet, an accelerating voltage alternator (AVA), a mass marker, and a peak matcher.

* LKB-Produkter, Fack, 161 25 Bromma 1, Sweden.

Molecules entering the ion source of the mass spectrometer are ionized by electron impact. The energy of the electrons can be regulated either manually between 5 and 100 eV or automatically to a preselected value during the course of a scan. The electrons are emitted from a rhenium filament and are accelerated by a trap electrode. The sample molecules are introduced, either from the gas chromatograph through the separator or from the direct inlets. Thus the sample molecules are exposed to a bombardment of electrons of a certain energy, which will ionize and fragment the molecules. The degree of ionization and fragmentation depends upon the electron energy, the constitution of the molecules, and also upon the temperature of the ion source.

Molecules entering the mass spectrometer may or may not be fragmented. The whole molecules and their fragments may or may not be ionized. The ions may be positively or negatively charged. From these possibilities only the positively charged molecules and their positively charged fragments will be

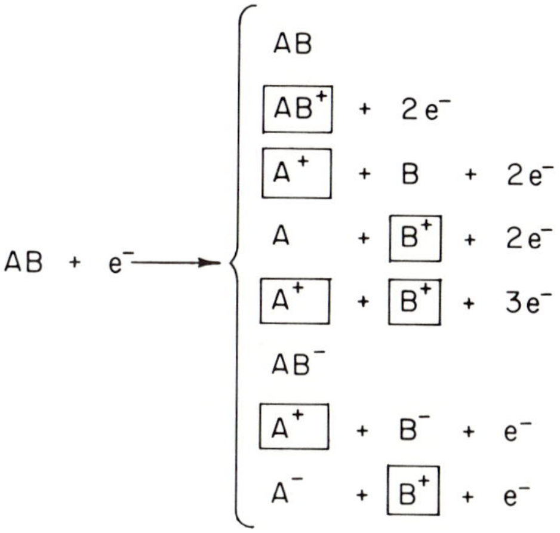

$$AB + e^- \longrightarrow \begin{cases} AB \\ \boxed{AB^+} + 2e^- \\ \boxed{A^+} + B + 2e^- \\ A + \boxed{B^+} + 2e^- \\ \boxed{A^+} + \boxed{B^+} + 3e^- \\ AB^- \\ \boxed{A^+} + B^- + e^- \\ A^- + \boxed{B^+} + e^- \end{cases}$$

FIG. 1. The main hypothetical consequences following the entry of molecule AB into the mass spectrometer; e^- = free electron; □ = ions detected.

detected (see Fig. 1). The ion-accelerating voltage is usually kept at 3.5 kV. The accelerated ions leave the ion source through the electrical focusing lenses and the exit slit and enter the analyzer tube, where, in the central section, a 60° deflection magnet is placed as is conventional in mass spectrometers of this type (see Fig. 2). Upon scanning the ions have to pass through a continuously variable magnetic field, which causes their deflection according to their individual masses (m/e values).

The relationship between the mass (m), the strength of the magnetic field (H) and the accelerating voltage (E) is expressed in the formula

$$m/e = \frac{R^2 H^2}{2E}$$

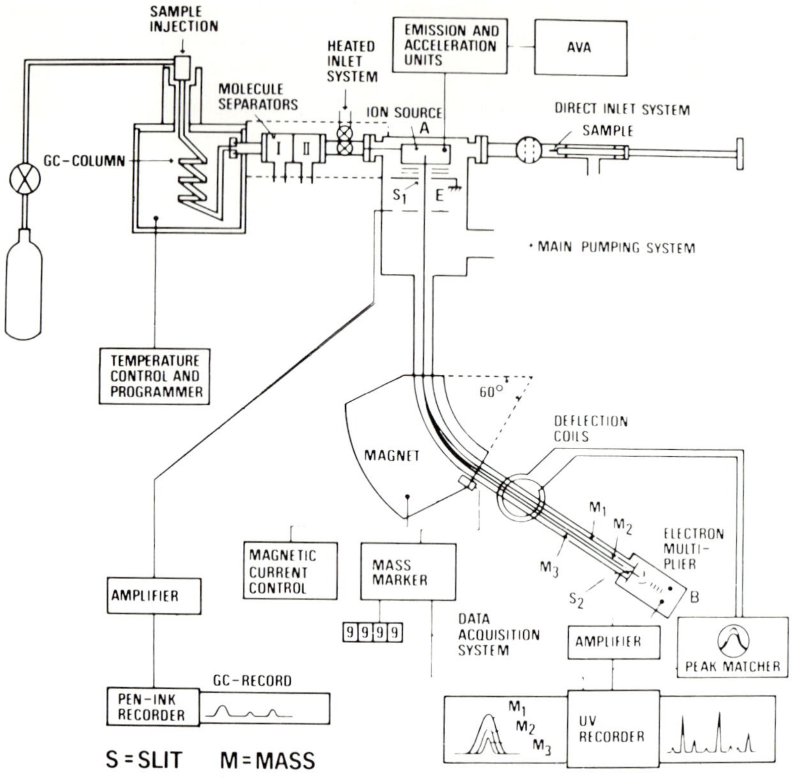

Fig. 2. Block diagram of gas chromatograph–mass spectrometer. A-B = analyzer tube; E = electrode which is hit by 20% of the ion beam; M_1, M_2, M_3: positively charged ions of high, middle, and low mass; S_1 = ion source exit slit; S_2 = collector slit.

where e = number of electrons lost (usually 1), R = radius which is constant and E which also is usually a constant. Because of this relationship only ions with a certain m/e value are able to pass through the collector slit toward the end of the tube at a certain strength of the magnetic field. By a continuous variation of the magnetic field, ions of increasing masses are successively brought into focus and hit the first dynode of the multiplier. Successive dynodes (up to 14) increase the number of secondary electrons. In this way it is possible to amplify the electrical signals resulting from the impingement of the ions by a factor of 10^3 to 10^7. These signals are further amplified by a pre-amplifier and a galvanometer amplifier before they are recorded on the direct-writing UV-oscillograph.

It is possible to scan a mass spectrum with a range of $m/e = 2$ to 1400 at an accelerating voltage of 3.5 kV; the range can be expanded to 2000 if the accelerating voltage is decreased to 2.5 kV.

The mass range $m/e = 24$–800 can be scanned in 4.2 seconds with a resolution ($M/\Delta M$) of 1000 (10% valley definition). If a resolution of 400 is acceptable the same mass range can be scanned in 1.7 seconds. Both mass range and scan speed are well suited for scanning spectra of compounds emerging from the attached gas chromatograph, since the time required for a peak of a substance to emerge from the gas chromatograph is much greater than the time required for a mass spectrometric scan to be performed. In addition the sensitivity of the mass spectrometer is usually high enough for the amounts used during ordinary GC. The required sample size is of the order 0.1 μg for columns with packings and 0.01 μg for capillary columns.

In order to utilize the combination instrument it is necessary to know the time at which the compounds emerge from the column. This is achieved by letting the effluent from the column pass continuously through the separator and into the ion source. At the beginning of the analyzer tube on the far side of the ion source exit slit an electrode is placed which is hit by about 20% of the ion beam. The signals produced by the ions are amplified by an electrometer amplifier and recorded by a pen recorder. This recording of about 20% of the total ion current is comparable to the recording of the signals from a flame ionization detector both with regard to sensitivity and selectivity. This means of detection is usually and somewhat erroneously referred to as total ion current (TIC) recording.

The great advantage of connecting a gas chromatograph to a mass spectrometer is the combination of the separation power of the gas chromatograph with the qualitative analytic ability of the mass spectrometer. Additional advantages are the relatively small amounts required and the short time in which an analysis can be performed.

From the practical point of view it is rather simple to scan and record a mass spectrum. The solution to be analyzed is injected into the gas chromatograph in the usual manner but with the valve to the mass spectrometer closed in order to prevent the solvent entering the ion source and eliminating the vacuum. When the solvent has been pumped away the valve is opened and the machine is ready for operation. When a peak that appears to be of interest is observed on the total ion current recording the scan is started by pressing a button. Appropriate sensitivity, scan speed, paper speed, and electron energy are chosen in advance. Background spectra are recorded before and after each peak. In order to obtain the true mass spectrum these background spectra are subtracted from the spectrum recorded during the elution of the compound.

C. Some Aspects of Interpretation of Mass Spectra

When the background spectrum has been subtracted the peak heights are representative of the mass numbers of a certain compound (Fig. 3). The mass

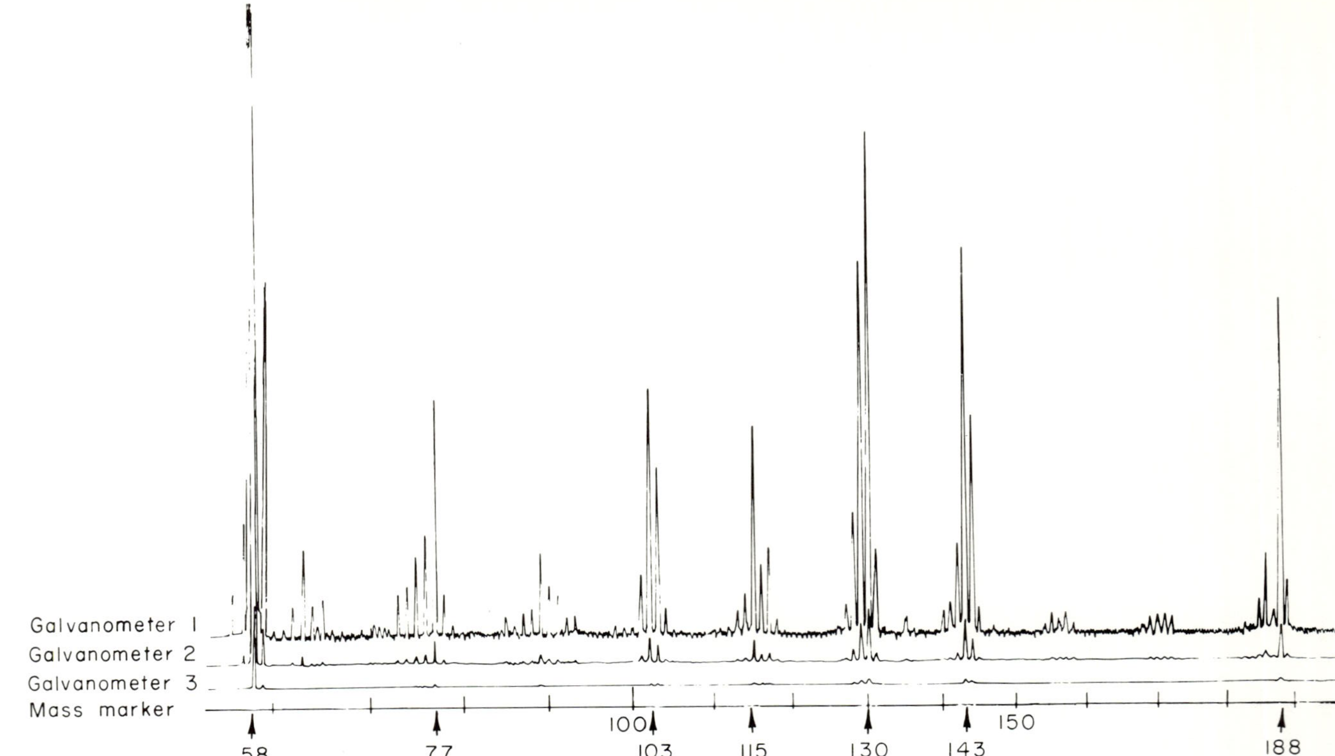

FIG. 3. Original spectrum of *N*,*N*-dimethyltryptamine (DMT), recorded on UV-sensitive paper.

number with the highest intensity is set at 100% (base peak). The intensities of the other mass numbers are calculated relative to this base peak. Plotting the intensities of the mass numbers, expressed in relative percent, against the corresponding mass numbers gives the final presentation of a mass spectrum as a bar diagram (Fig. 4). The calculations are very time-consuming but can nowadays be taken over by a computer (see Sections II,F and III,F).

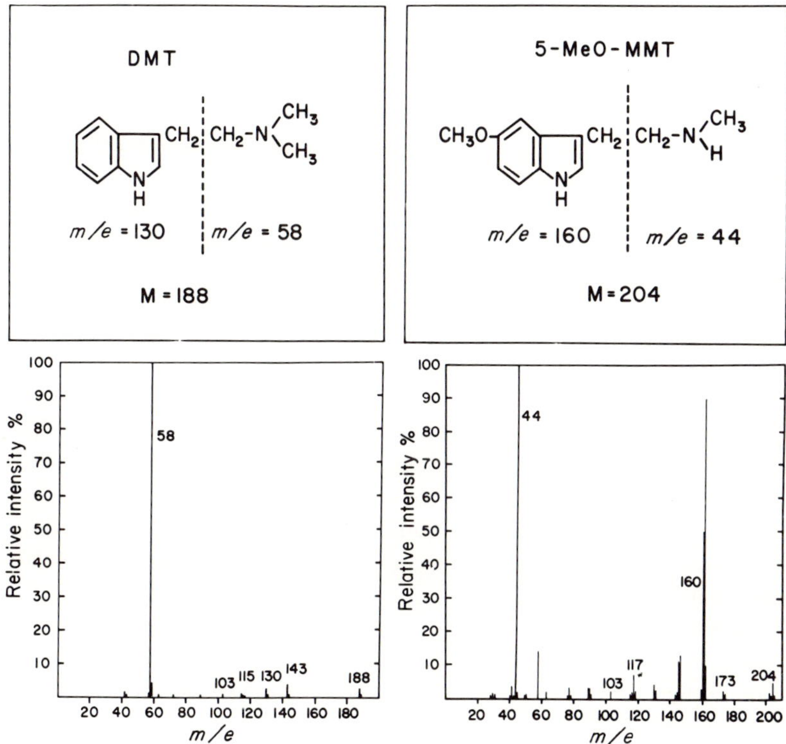

FIG. 4. Bar diagrams of mass spectra of *N*,*N*-dimethyltryptamine (DMT; compare Fig. 3) and 5-methoxy-*N*-methyltryptamine (5-MeO-MMT). Main cleavage indicated on upper part of figure.

The highest mass number in most cases represents the molecular ion and the other mass numbers represent fragments of the molecule. In this sense the mass spectrum can be used as a "fingerprint" for the molecule, the characteristics of which are the mass numbers occurring and their relative intensities. A simple example of interpretation of fragmentation pattern is given in Fig. 4, where substitution changes the fragmentation pattern of DMT and 5-MeO-MMT. For these substances the base peak is always a fragment of the side chain *m*/*e* 58 and *m*/*e* 44, respectively. The main ring structures yield (both whole and fragmented) a number of different ions, some of which are positively charged. Any single one of these positively charged ions is present in smaller amounts than the positively charged ion formed from the side chain. Hence the latter gives the mass number with the highest intensity and forms the base peak.

Prior to any work with drugs it is wise to accumulate knowledge of fragmentation pattern through mass spectrometric analysis of a series of analogs. A reference substance is necessary to obtain complete identification. Interpretation of fragmentation pattern constitutes a science of its own and has been treated by several authors (Beynon, 1960; Biemann, 1963; McLafferty, 1963; Budzikiewics *et al.*, 1964; Hill, 1966).

For practical purposes one may adhere to the procedure mentioned above. The difficulties in calculation of mass spectra obtained by means of the combination instrument may vary considerably; for example, in the extreme case the difficulty may be due to more than one molecular species being present in a single peak emerging from the GC column (i.e., poor resolution). However, a mass spectrum of a compound obtained by means of the combined GC-MS technique is generally cleaner than when the compound has been introduced directly into the mass spectrometer. This is because contaminants are separated during the GC-procedure from the compound to be scanned. Information about extraction, gas chromatographic conditions, and change of spectra due to derivative formation are helpful in the interpretation. By chemical modification of a compound its spectrum is changed and these changes may be indicative of the structure. Fragments can be made to shift toward higher mass numbers. Isotopic labeling of the compound is a much favored technique (Budzikiewics *et al.*, 1964b) and recently silylation with deuterated reagents has been introduced (McCloskey *et al.*, 1968).

It must be pointed out that some compounds have molecular ions of very low intensities or are completely lacking molecular ions. Derivative formation may be a solution to this problem and bring forth a molecular ion. Under these circumstances the fragment next to the molecular ion often constitutes the base peak.

D. Peak Matching

The LKB 9020 oscilloscope peak matching device is an accessory to the GC-MS system used to measure the ratio of the mass of an appropriate ion of an unknown compound to that of a reference agent and *vice versa*. The precise value of the unknown ion mass is then easily calculated and an empirical formula deduced (Ryhage, 1967b).

The peak matching technique is time-consuming, compared to the recording of a mass spectrum. It is necessary to isolate the compound in microgram-quantities by trapping it from the gas chromatographic effluent.

The principle of operation may be summarized as follows: In a typical operation the unknown compound is introduced by means of the direct inlet while the reference compound is simultaneously introduced through the heated inlet. Other means of introduction of both reference and unknown substances can be used. The intensity of ions of a certain mass are visualized as a Gaussian curve on the oscilloscope screen of the peak matcher. Ions of the lower mass (e.g., parent ion of the unknown compound) are brought into focus by a manual change of the magnetic field. Ions of the higher mass (e.g., reference compound) are then brought into focus by keeping the magnetic field unchanged while the accelerating voltage is decreased by manual adjustment of a high precision decade resistor, calibrated in mass ratio $1.0xxxxx$ (the x's = unknown numbers). The second to the sixth decimals are adjustable in this way. A relay is then set to switch the accelerating voltage between full and reduced representing the low and the high mass in question. This makes it possible to watch both masses simultaneously on the oscilloscope screen and to match them in order to get the sixth decimal.

The measured mass ratio between the unknown compound and the reference or *vice versa* is read and a comparatively accurate molecular weight of the unknown compound can be calculated. This mass is then compared with similar values in a reference manual (Beynon and Williams, 1963) and a possible empirical formula selected. Several possible formulas will exist due to the limited accuracy of the technique. (The accuracy is about ± 10 ppm of the mass). The knowledge of the way in which the unknown compound has been treated, i.e., extracted, aids in reducing the possibilities to a few alternatives or perhaps one. The identity may finally be established by comparing the mass spectra of the unknown to that of reference compounds selected on the basis of suitable empirical formulas.

E. Mass Fragmentography

A substance may be present in extracts in such small amounts that it is not detectable even by the total ion current. Spectra are impossible to interpret due to the relatively high background. This difficulty led us to mass fragmentography, which is essentially a technique in which the mass spectrometer is used as a chromatographic detector and advantage is taken of the physicochemical characteristics of the compounds in order to achieve separation, specificity, and sensitivity (Hammar *et al.*, 1968a). A knowledge of the fragmentation pattern of a group of compounds and the technical possibilities of focusing on three mass numbers simultaneously allowed the desired refinement of the determination.

Alternation of the accelerating voltage in the mass spectrometer was introduced by Sweeley *et al.* (1966), who used this technique in order to determine the isotope abundance in a mixture from the gas chromatographic effluent. It was possible to achieve partial separation and quantitation of the compounds by a very rapid alternation of the accelerating voltage between two adjacent mass numbers of the isotopes.

The accelerating voltage alternator unit (AVA), also called Multiple Ion Detector unit (MID), makes it possible to record the ion intensity of three mass numbers within a short time interval (Fig. 5). The intensity of the mass detected in the MS is inversely proportional to the accelerating voltage supplied to the ion source. This voltage can be selected to allow given mass numbers within a certain range to be detected. The AVA allows the voltage to be rapidly changed between three such values so that three mass numbers can be continuously recorded. Meantime the magnetic field has been kept fixed in relation to the lowest of the three selected mass numbers. Depending upon the duration of the peak emerging from the gas chromatograph, higher or lower frequencies of alternation of the accelerating voltage can be chosen. A low switching frequency allows a filter with long-time constancy to increase the signal/noise ratio, which means that with maintenance of an acceptable noise level sensitivity can be further increased. In fact, by this technique we have been able to raise the sensitivity about 10^4 times as compared to the one obtained during usual scanning of mass spectra. The information for identification obtained using mass fragmentography is, however, less than the one obtained from MS. This may be compensated for by repeated refocusing upon several different fragments of a compound at their appropriate m/e value. In this way a "partial mass spectrum" can be constructed. Compounds labeled with stable, naturally occurring and artificially introduced nonradioactive isotopes may become important in future studies of drug metabolism because of the ease with which they can be found in biologic material by use of mass fragmentography.

The intensity of the three different mass numbers may differ as well as the ordinate position of their base lines on the chart. This is due to both the high sensitivity used for registration and bleeding from the column. To accommodate all three base lines necessary for a simultaneous recording of the chosen numbers, a "buck out" or balance unit was constructed in collaboration with the LKB-Produkter. This unit was successfully used to buck out an excessive background from the column bleed.

From the practical point of view the following procedure is used: A reference substance is introduced through the direct inlet probe of the mass spectrometer and a whole spectrum is recorded. In order to get a starting point in the spectrum an easily recognized peak with a mass number as close to the desired fragment as possible is probed by manual scanning. From there on, the fragment with the lowest mass number of the two or three desired ions is brought into focus by manual changing of the magnetic field under maintenance of full accelerating voltage (3.5 kV). The mass marker of the instrument is of considerable help in this initial procedure. By keeping the magnetic field constant

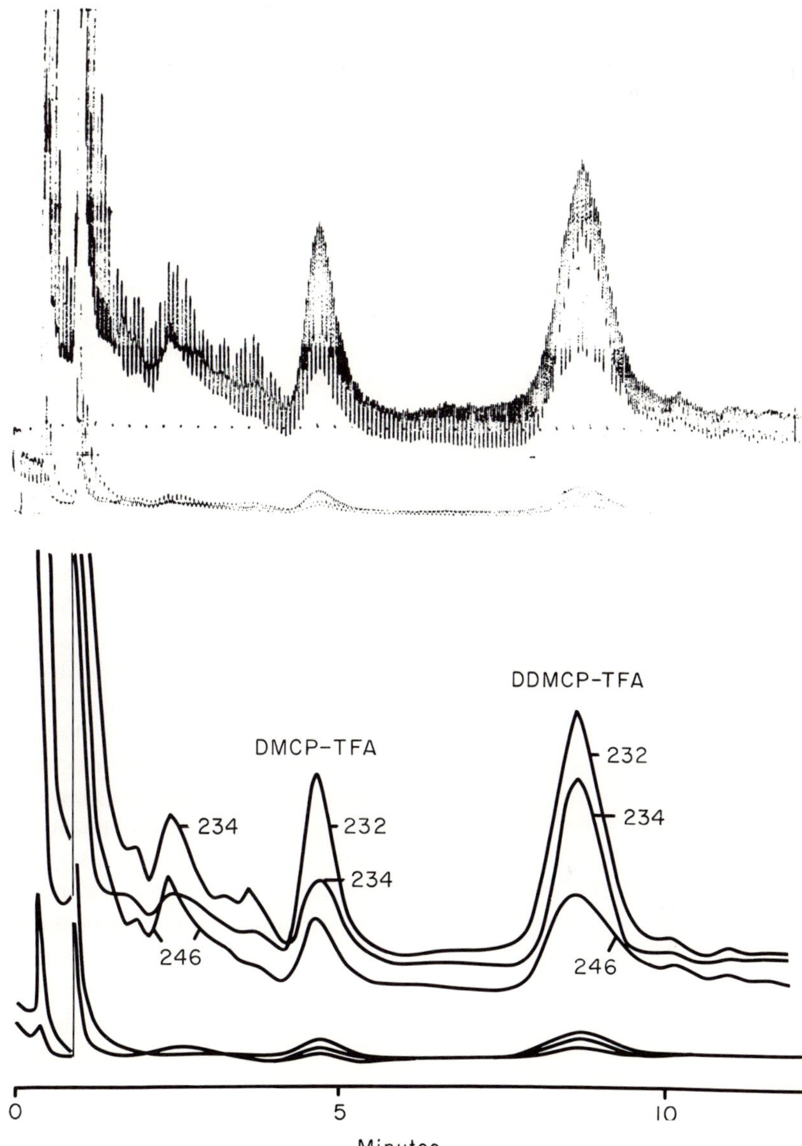

FIG. 5. Mass fragmentogram of extract of red blood cells which have been treated with β-glucuronidase. Patient receiving 75 mg chlorpromazine daily. Conditions: 0.75% Versamid 900 on silanized Chromosorb G (100–120 M); column temperature 236°C. Ionization energy 50 eV, trap current 240 μA, multiplier voltage 2.5 kV; focusing upon fragments corresponding to $m/e = 232$, 234, and 246 (see Fig. 13). Upper panel: original mass fragmentogram. Lower panel: The three curves, each representing a mass number, are drawn from the original fragmentogram (DMCP-TFA and DDMCP-TFA = trifluoroacetate of des- and didesmethylchlorpromazine). (Courtesy of Analytical Biochemistry.)

and decreasing the accelerating voltage first with one, then another potentiometer the desired ions representing higher mass numbers are then selected. The two higher masses are selected by watching the deflection of the galvanometers. In this case the mass marker can no longer be used due to the fact that it is connected with the strength of the magnetic field which is kept constant.

The mass spectrometer is thus set to monitor continuously the three mass numbers of the compounds emerging from the gas chromatograph. The recording is made on UV-sensitive paper run at slow speed (2.5 cm/min) and the resulting curve has certain similarities to an ordinary gas chromatogram (Fig. 5, upper panel). However, three deflection lines become visible as a result of the alternating accelerating voltage. To make the original recording more readable a transparent paper may be superimposed and the curves drawn (Fig. 5, lower panel).

F. Data Processing

A logical extension of the integrated gas chromatography–mass spectrometry systems is the inclusion of computer analysis. To evaluate a mass spectrum from the recording on the UV-sensitive paper and construct a bar diagram takes a long time, sometimes several hours. It therefore comes as no surprise that various solutions to the computerization and digitalization of mass spectra have been attempted. Several reasons exist for following this line of research, as pointed out by Biemann and Hites (1968).

The efficient use of a gas chromatograph–mass spectrometer combination results in the recording of a large number of mass spectra which then have to be processed, evaluated, and interpreted. If conventional recording systems (i.e., oscillographs) are employed, one is thus practically limited to taking individual spectra when a fraction of interest emerges from the gas chromatograph. This procedure requires continuous decision-making during the course of the experiment and leads to the loss of valuable, often unexpected, information represented by small GC peaks, shoulders, or data revealed only when comparing the mass spectra of consecutive segments of a chromatographic fraction.

The generation of the data directly in digital form may not only permit a wide variety of presentations but also open the way for efficient, automatic evaluation of the spectra. They can be presented in tabular form (using the line printer of the computer) or as "bar graphs," produced by an incremental plotter driven by the computer.

Because of the large number of spectra that can be recorded it is practically impossible to interpret all of them individually and the use of the computer for this task is therefore a logical consequence. In the future the automatic identification may be achieved by searching a collection of authentic mass spectra, stored in the secondary memory of a computer, for identical or similar spectra. A system of this kind is obviously most useful for problems that involve a number of gas chromatograms of very complex mixtures rather than an occasional one involving only one or very few components of interest. The former situation may often arise when investigating samples of natural origin as encountered in pharmacologic and toxicologic problems. A data acquisition system which continuously samples the output of a mass spectrometer, manufactured by Radiation Inc. in the United States, has been used by Hites and Biemann at the Massachusetts Institute of Technology. A cyclic magnetic scan of the mass spectrometer and reference compounds for calibration of the mass number were used (Hites and Biemann, 1967, 1968).

A different approach has been used by Ryhage *et al.* at the Karolinska Institute, to whom we are indebted for the following brief description of the system (Jansson *et al.*, 1968).

A mass spectrum digitizer has been developed and used together with the LKB 9000 gas chromatograph–mass spectrometer. The digital data are recorded by an incremental tape recorder. The electronic mass marker senses a change in the magnetic field at constant accelerating voltage and generates a trigger pulse for each mass number. The recording speed of the system is limited by the incremental tape recorder (max. 300 peaks/sec). The trigger pulse starts the analog to digital signal conversion as well as the recording onto the magnetic tape. The mass marker of the LKB 9000 is used for calibration of the mass numbers, which means that spectra can be taken at random rates without reference compounds. The digitally recorded mass spectra are given to a computer (IBM 1800) where background spectra are subtracted from the actual mass spectra and the results are conveniently readable in table form or can be plotted as bar graphs.

Other solutions to the computerization of mass spectra have been presented (Frazer, 1968). Low-cost, general purpose computers like PDP-8 (Digital Equipment) can be coupled via suitable interfaces to mass spectrometers (Reynolds *et al.*, 1967).

It seems very likely that the combination instruments of gas chromatograph–mass spectrometer in the future will also include a computer.

III. Applications of Combined Gas Chromatography–Mass Spectrometry (GC-MS)

A. Structural Determination of Alkaloids in Plants

Prior to the 1960's, the conventional methods used for isolation and structure determination of alkaloids (extraction, column chromatography, countercurrent distribution, and chemical degradations) were limited to the major plant constituents, which could be isolated in large quantities. Minor components and trace materials either remained undetected or were not available in quantities sufficient for degradative work. Such minor components may be decisive in the understanding of biosynthetic pathways. Because of the great sensitivity and specificity of GC-MS it was apparent that this method of analysis could be most useful in the complete analysis of a plant extract.

As an example of the use of GC-MS with regard to plant material may be mentioned studies of the active components of psychotomimetic South American plants containing indole alkaloids (Holmstedt and Lindgren, 1967).

Recently we had occasion to reexamine the alkaloid content of the leaves of the malphigiaceous vine *Banisteriopsis rusbyana*, used for preparation of the Amazonian hallucinatory drink *ayahuasca* (*caapi*, *yajé*). In an earlier investigation this plant proved to contain a large amount of the hallucinogen *N*,*N*-dimethyltryptamine (Poisson, 1965). By GC-MS we also found this substance to be the principal alkaloid but in addition we could identify as minor components *N*-methyl-tryptamine, 5-methoxy-*N*,*N*-dimethyltryptamine, and 5-hydroxy-*N*,*N*-dimethyltryptamine (Agurell *et al.*, 1968). Furthermore we found an unknown compound emerging from the GC column with a retention time between that of *N*,*N*-dimethyltryptamine and 5-methoxy-*N*,*N*-dimethyltryptamine. When analyzed in the LKB 9000 gas chromatograph–mass spectrometer, this peak proved to have a molecular weight of 186, viz. two mass units less than *N*,*N*-dimethyltryptamine. The prominent peaks of the mass spectrum were *m*/*e* 143 (base peak) and *m*/*e* 128. The losses from the parent ion are 43 and 58 mass units, respectively. If a structure such as in Fig. 6 is assumed it can be

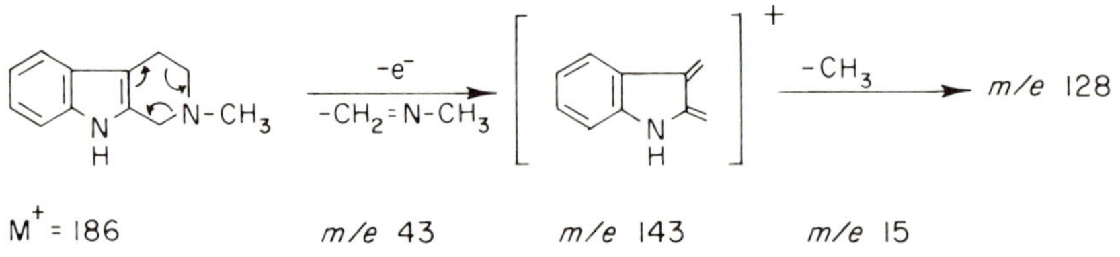

FIG. 6. Fragmentation pattern of 2-methyl-tetrahydro-β-carboline.

readily reconciled with the mass spectrometric data. Accordingly this compound, *N*-β-methyltetrahydrocarboline, was synthesized from *N*-methyltryptamine and found to be identical in all respects with the naturally occurring compound.

An investigation was also made of another plant, *Anadenanthera peregrina*, used for the preparation of snuffs inhaled by some South American Indians to produce hallucinations. The bark of this plant contains a high amount of 5-methoxy-*N*,*N*-dimethyltryptamine. In addition to this substance the existence of five other compounds was proved (Agurell *et al.*, 1969). Some of them were easily identified as simple indoles but one of the remaining substances had a molecular weight of 230. The mass spectrum of this alkaloid (Fig. 7, left, upper panel) showed certain similarities to that of tetrahydroharmine

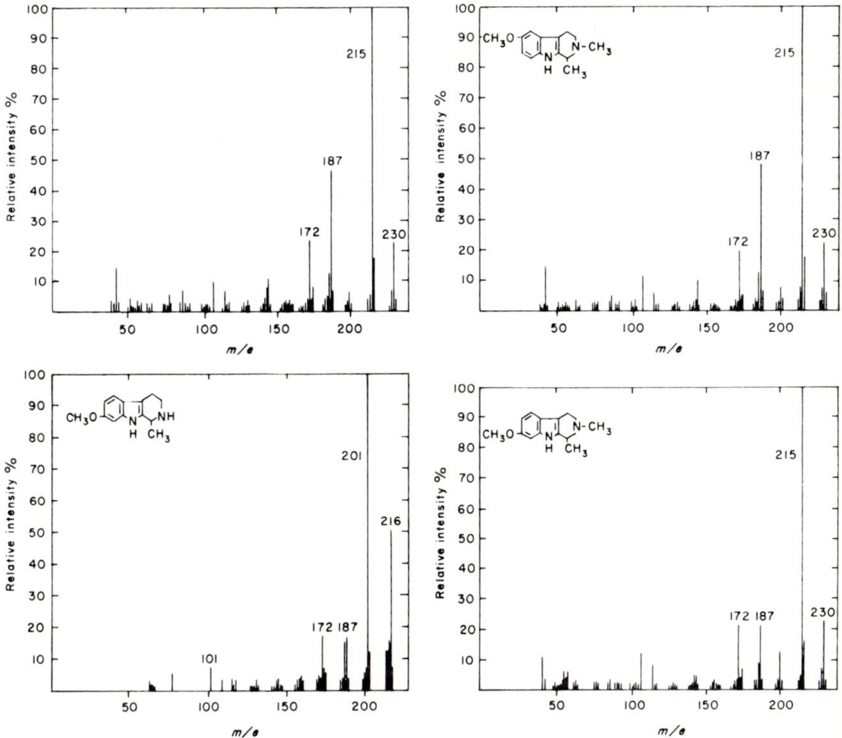

Fig. 7. Left, upper panel: mass spectrum of compound present in *Anadenanthera peregrina*; lower panel: mass spectrum of tetrahydroharmine. Right, upper panel: mass spectrum of 1,2-dimethyl-6-methoxy-1,2,3,4-tetrahydro-β-carboline; lower panel: mass spectrum of 2-methyl-tetrahydroharmine.

(Holmstedt and Lindgren, 1967), but the molecular weight was 14 mass units higher. The mass spectrum of tetrahydroharmine, which does not possess an *N*-methyl group, shows a base peak at M^+-15 due to the loss of the C-methyl group (Fig. 7, left, lower panel). Prominent peaks in the spectrum are at m/e 187 and m/e 172, which is in agreement with the fragmentation mechanism suggested above for 2-methyltetrahydro-β-carboline. The fragmentation pattern of the unknown alkaloid in *Anadenanthera peregrina* is analogous to that of tetrahydroharmine except for the loss of 43 mass units, presumably due to the presence of an *N*-methyl group. This would indicate a structure as in Fig. 7 (right, upper panel). Accordingly 1,2-dimethyl-6-methoxy-1,2,3,4-tetrahydro-β-carboline was synthesized in addition to 2-methyltetrahydroharmine (Fig. 7, right, lower panel). When the mass spectra of these two compounds are examined closely it is seen that they are very much alike with the exception of the intensity of the fragment at m/e 187. In this respect the alternative given in

Fig. 7 (right, upper panel) shows identity with the unknown plant alkaloid, giving the structure 1,2-dimethyl-6-methoxy-1,2,3,4-tetrahydro-β-carboline. Further proof for the position of the methoxy group was given in this case by ultraviolet and fluorescence spectra. Insufficient quantities of the compound were available for infrared examination.

It is important to know that the two position isomers were found almost impossible to separate on several different gas chromatographic columns and that the only major difference in the mass spectrum was the intensity of the fragment at *m/e* 187. This demonstrates that caution ought to be exercised in identification of unknowns even when as sophisticated techniques as GC-MS are used.

B. Identification of Histamine Metabolites in Urine

One of our aims has been to develop a method for identification and estimation of 1-methylimidazole-4-acetic acid in human urine. This compound in all likelihood is the main metabolite of histamine and estimation of the excretion in urine ought to give a good idea about the release of histamine *in vivo*.

Studies on urinary metabolites of subcutaneously injected ^{14}C-labeled histamine have shown that this amine is metabolized along two different pathways in man (Schayer and Cooper, 1956). One involves *N*-methylation of the imidazole ring to 4-(2-aminoethyl)-1-methylimidazole (1,4-methylhistamine), the major part of which then undergoes oxidative deamination to 1-methylimidazole-4-acetic acid (1,4-MeImAA). According to these experiments, no detectable amounts of the isomeric 1-methylimidazole-5-acetic acid (1,5-MeImAA) are excreted by humans. The other pathway of degradation involves direct oxidative deamination of histamine to imidazoleacetic acid (ImAA).

In order to develop a method for analysis of 1,4-MeImAA the gas chromatographic properties of the substance and similar compounds viz. 1,5-MeImAA and ImAA were studied (Tham and Holmstedt, 1965; Tham, 1966a,b). The free acids were converted into methyl esters before GC.

Gas chromatographic analysis of the purified urine extracts treated to form methyl esters revealed several peaks. One peak with a relative retention time coinciding with that of the methyl ester of 1,4-MeImAA was found. The identity of the peak was established by mass spectrometry of the effluent from the gas chromatographic column (Tham and Holmstedt, 1965). The mass spectrum of the compound in the urine extract having the retention time of 1,4-MeImAA (methyl ester) was identical with the mass spectrum of authentic 1,4-MeImAA (methyl ester) (Fig. 8, left panel). The mass spectrum showed a molecular ion peak at *m/e* 154 and other ion peaks at *m/e* 95, 68, 54, and 42. The main metabolite of exogenously administered histamine, 1,4-MeImAA, was thus identified as a normal urinary constituent of healthy man.

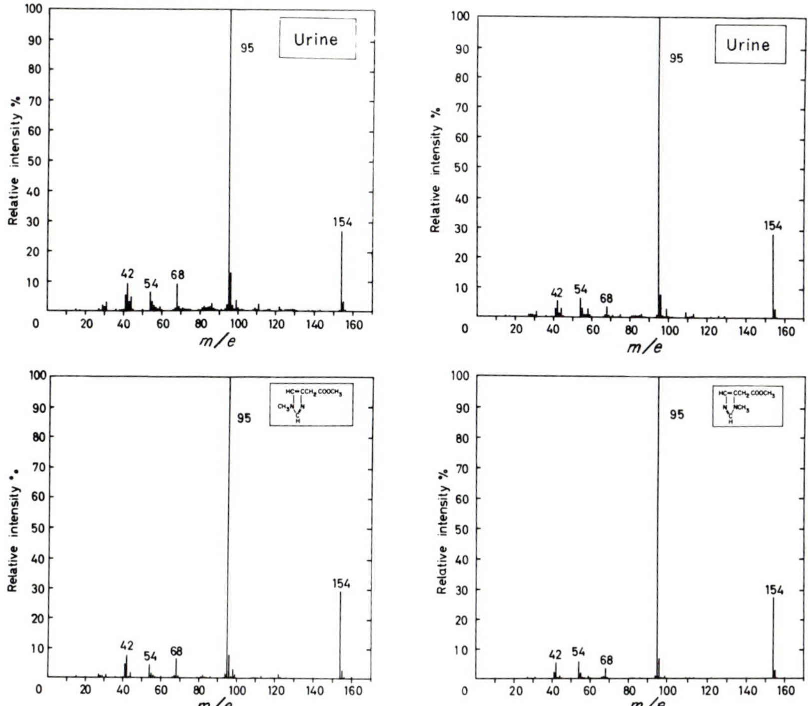

FIG. 8. Left, upper panel: mass spectrum of the gas chromatographic peak in urine extract coinciding with that of authentic 1,4-MeImAA (methyl ester) (for abbreviations see text); lower panel: mass spectrum of the methyl ester of authentic 1,4-MeImAA. Right, upper panel: mass spectrum of the gas chromatographic peak in urine extract coinciding with that of authentic 1,5-MeImAA (methyl ester); lower panel: mass spectrum of the methyl ester of authentic 1,5-MeImAA. Conditions: 10% EGA on silanized Gas Chrom P (100–120 *M*); column temperature 175°C. (Courtesy of *Journal of Chromatography*.)

In gas chromatograms of urine extracts, a peak with the retention time of authentic methyl ester of 1,5-MeImAA could also be seen (Fig. 9). The mass spectrum of the chromatogram component in the urine corresponding to this isomer, recorded as described above, was identical with that of authentic 1,5-MeImAA (methyl ester) (Fig. 8, right panel) (Tham and Holmstedt, 1965). The finding was rather surprising since previous investigators had shown that ring methylation of histamine occurs only at the nitrogen remote from the side chain (Schayer and Cooper, 1956).

The methyl esters of both 1,4-MeImAA and 1,5-MeImAA thus gave similar mass spectra. In fact, it would be difficult to differentiate between them by mass spectra alone. The combination with GC in this case overcomes the problem because of the gas chromatographic separation.

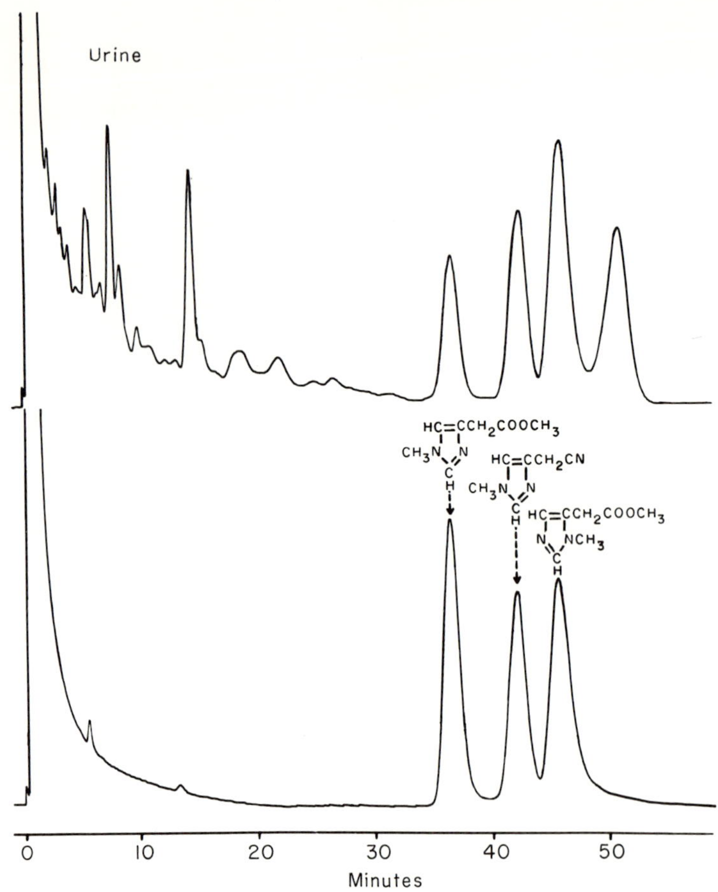

FIG. 9. Upper panel: gas chromatogram of urine extract; internal standard (1-methylimidazole-4-acetonitrile) had been added. Lower panel: gas chromatogram of a mixture of the methyl esters of 1,4-MeImAA and 1,5-MeImAA and of the internal standard. Conditions: 10% EGA on silanized Gas Chrom P (100–120 *M*); column temperature 182°C. (Courtesy of *Journal of Chromatography*.)

C. IDENTIFICATION OF AN UNKNOWN ACID IN HUMAN URINE USING THE COMBINATION INSTRUMENT AND THE PEAK MATCHING DEVICE

In studying the urinary excretion of histamine metabolites by patients with various diseases some observations were made concerning the gas chromatographic peaks, representing nonimidazolic acids. It was especially evident that one of the peaks, always appearing in the chromatograms of healthy man, was unusually high in the chromatograms of urine from patients with burns and with some allergic diseases (Tham, 1966b) (Fig. 10).

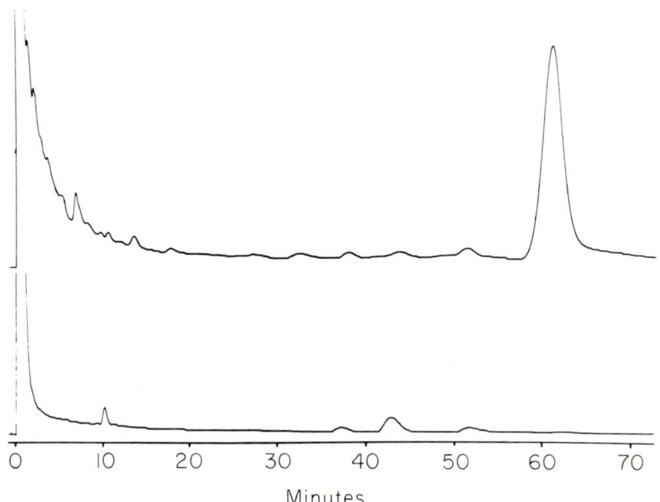

FIG. 10. Gas chromatography of urine extracts. Upper panel: urine from a patient with a severe burn; the high peak represents the unknown compound referred to in text; the small peaks represent different imidazolic acids; the size of these peaks correspond to a 24-hr excretion of 2–4 mg. Lower panel: urine from a healthy man. Conditions: 10% EGA; column temperature 185°C. (Courtesy of *Biochemical Pharmacology*.)

A mass spectrum recorded from the gas chromatographic effluent corresponding to the unknown peak revealed a molecular ion peak at m/e 143, a base peak at m/e 84, and other peaks at m/e 56, 41, and 28 (Fig. 11, upper panel). In order to get further information small amounts were isolated by means of a stream-splitter system.

The effluent from the column was collected in a coiled teflon tube. The compound condensed as a white powder in the teflon tube and could be dissolved in a small amount of methanol. About 1 mg of the substance so obtained was introduced into an Atlas SM 1 high-resolution mass spectrometer (i.e., not the LKB combined GC-MS) and a peak matching of the molecular ion ($m/e = 143$) was carried out. This gave the empirical formula $C_6H_9O_3N$ (Tham *et al.*, 1968).

With the accumulated information it could be suggested that the identity of the unknown substance could be pyroglutamic acid methyl ester. Relative retention times compared with authentic substance on two different columns were identical. A mass spectrum recorded from the effluent corresponding to the unknown peak in urine showed close resemblance to the mass spectrum of the methyl ester of authentic pyroglutamic acid (Fig. 11, lower panel). However, it has been demonstrated that glutamic acid is very easily converted to pyroglutamic acid (Tham *et al.*, 1968). Authentic glutamic acid was added to urine, subjected to ion exchange extraction, and esterification. Thereafter GC yielded a very high peak corresponding to pyroglutamic acid. It is evident that

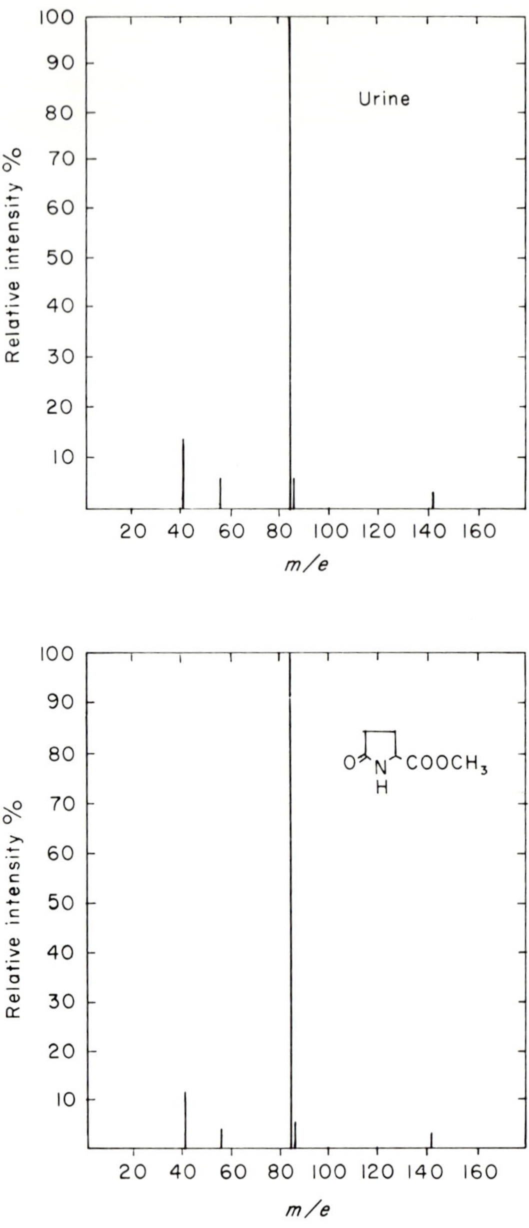

Fig. 11. Upper panel: mass spectrum of the unknown gas chromatographic peak in urine extracts from a patient with a severe burn. Lower panel: mass spectrum of the methyl ester of synthetic pyroglutamic acid. (Courtesy of *Biochemical Pharmacology*.)

glutamic acid may be converted to pyroglutamic acid in urine during the procedure of analysis.

This set of experiments demonstrates how an unknown peak in a urine extract can be identified by a combination of GC, GC-MS, and peak matching.

D. Mass Fragmentography of Chlorpromazine Metabolites in Plasma

Mass fragmentography has been used to advantage in studies of the basic metabolites of chlorpromazine in plasma (Hammar *et al.*, 1968a).

A typical example of a mass fragmentogram obtained from the plasma of a patient treated with this drug is presented in Fig. 12. Mass numbers charac-

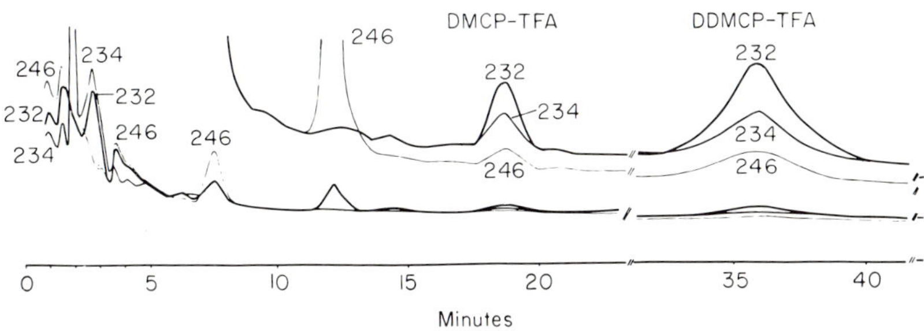

Fig. 12. Mass fragmentograms of plasma extracts. Patient receiving 200 mg chlorpromazine daily. Conditions: same as in Fig. 5 except for column temperature 220°C, ionization energy 70 eV, trap current 120 μA, multiplier voltage 2.9 kV; focusing upon fragments corresponding to m/e = 232, 234, and 246 (see Fig. 13) (DMCP-TFA and DDMCP-TFA = trifluoroacetate of des- and didesmethylchlorpromazine). (Courtesy of *Analytical Biochemistry*.)

teristic of the ring system were used: 232, 234, and 246 (Fig. 13). Two metabolites of chlorpromazine, monodesmethyl- and didesmethylchlorpromazine, were easily recognized by their retention times and by the relative intensities of the three mass numbers. Earlier in the fragmentogram an increased intensity of mass number 246 can be observed. Since the other two mass numbers do not increase correspondingly, this response can scarcely be due to a derivative of a 2-chlorophenothiazinyl compound. The beginning of the mass fragmentogram shows compounds that are incompletely resolved. Temperature programing resolved this accumulation of compounds but did not reveal any with the characteristic relative intensities of the three selected mass numbers. None of the peaks showed a simultaneous rise of all three mass numbers.

The side chains differ in one methylene group, e.g., 14 mass units, and can also be used for detection. Refocusing on the trifluoroacetylated side chains of desmethylchlorpromazine and didesmethylchlorpromazine increases the

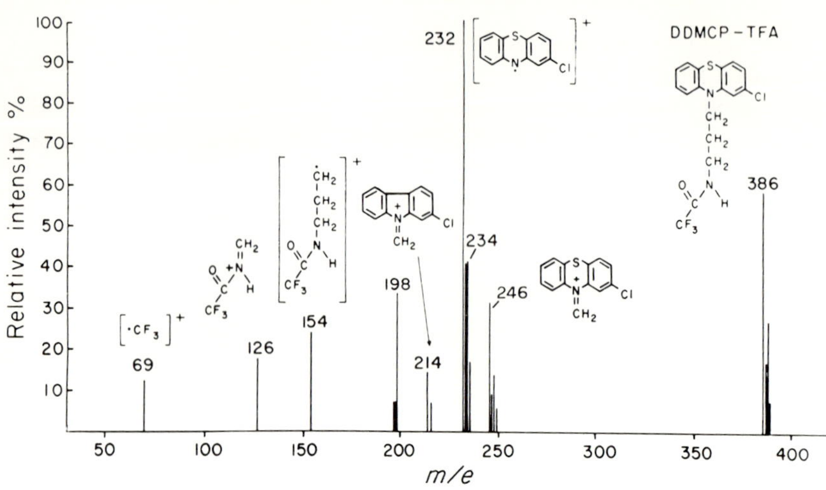

FIG. 13. Mass spectrum and fragmentation pattern of trifluoroacetate of didesmethylchlorpromazine (DDMCP-TFA). (Courtesy of *Analytical Biochemistry*.)

specificity of the determination (Fig. 14). Furthermore, in Fig. 15 the molecular ion and its isotope have been brought into focus (desmethylchlorpromazine, left fragmentogram, and didesmethylchlorpromazine, right fragmentogram). By adding the information provided by the different mass fragmentograms

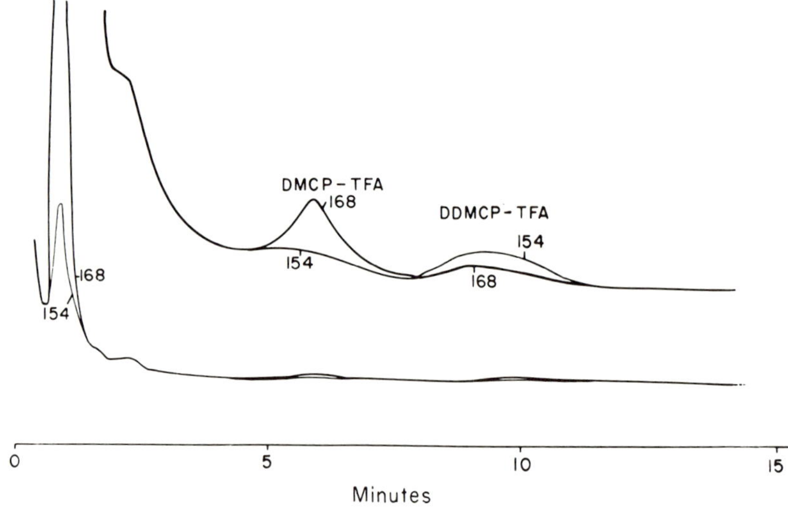

FIG. 14. Mass fragmentogram of plasma extract. Patient receiving 400 mg chlorpromazine daily. Conditions: same as in Fig. 5 except for column temperature 232°C, ionization energy 50 eV, trap current 240 μA, multiplier voltage 3.3 kV; focusing upon the m/e values corresponding to side chains of the two trifluoroacetylated desmethylated chlorpromazine metabolites. (Courtesy of *Analytical Biochemistry*.)

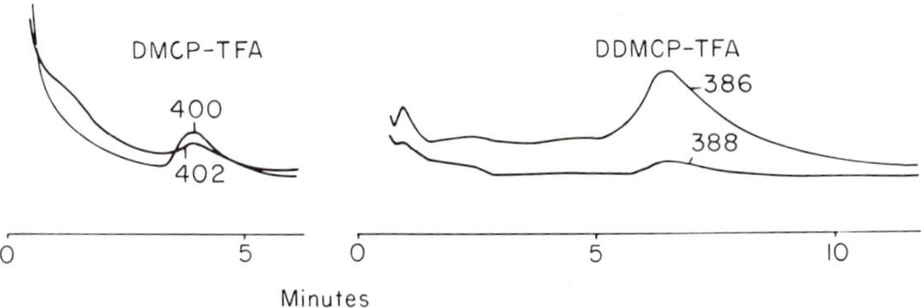

FIG. 15. Mass fragmentogram of the same basic extract as in Fig. 14. GC and MF conditions: same as in Fig. 14 except for column temperature at 238°C; Focusing upon m/e values corresponding to molecular ions and isotopic mass numbers of trifluoroacetylated desmethylchlorpromazine (left) and didesmethylchlorpromazine (right). (Courtesy of *Analytical Biochemistry*.)

one obtains for the compound with the retention time of didesmethylchlorpromazine the following mass numbers: 154, 232, 234, 246, 386, and 388 (compare Fig. 13). The relative intensities are the same as those of the reference compound. This means that in addition to the retention time, a complete agreement exists between the reference compound and the metabolite with regard to the fragments representing the side chain, the ring skeleton, and its naturally occurring chlorine isotope 37, the ring skeleton plus one methylene group, and the molecular ion with its isotope.

When these requirements are fulfilled it can be firmly stated that there is a complete identity between a reference and a metabolite, especially since none of the mass numbers used gives rise to peaks when plasma from people not given chlorpromazine is treated in the same way. The other metabolite, desmethylchlorpromazine, also gave complete agreement with the reference with regard to retention time and the fragments present including the molecular ion. In the same way chlorpromazine itself and 2-chlorophenothiazinylpropionic acid have been identified in plasma extracts (Hammar *et al.*, 1968a).

In addition to the possibility of identifying metabolites by mass fragmentography it may be used for quantitation. Amounts of chlorpromazine of 10^{-12} gm (3×10^{-15} moles) have been measured.

It may be concluded that the possibility of utilizing certain fragments or ions for detection allows a unique means of selectivity, which can easily be changed in such a way that either a single compound or a family of related compounds can be recorded. By refocusing, "partial mass spectra" characteristic of the compounds may be obtained in spite of the fact that the amounts available are too small to give a complete mass spectrum. The technique allows a tremendous gain in sensitivity.

The following criteria are used to characterize a compound: the retention time of the compound (GC part of the combined instrument), the presence of all the investigated mass numbers, and the characteristic ratio between their intensities (MS part of the combined instrument).

E. Chemical Identification of Acetylcholine in Rat Brain

The definitive identification of acetylcholine in fresh rat brain by means of combined gas chromatography–mass spectrometry has recently been reported (Hammar *et al.*, 1968b). After demethylation of the quaternary amine the

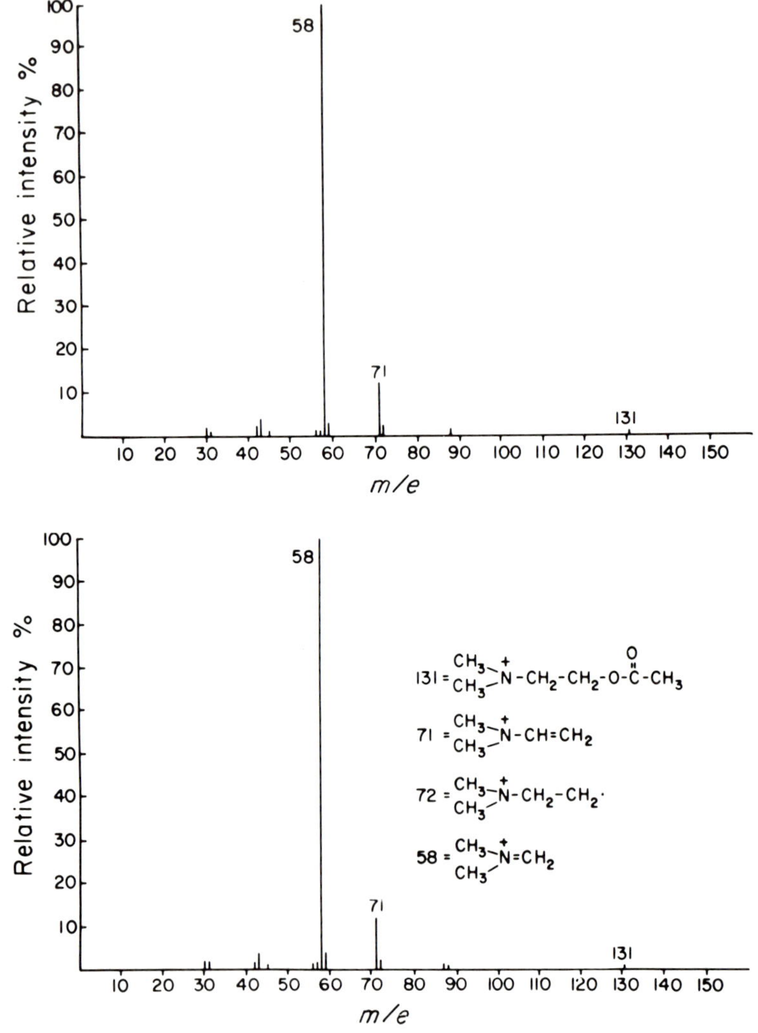

Fig. 16. Mass spectra obtained for dimethylaminoethyl acetate (DMAEA). Upper panel: demethylated rat brain extract. Lower panel: synthetic DMAEA. (Courtesy of *Nature*.)

procedure for microanalysis described earlier was employed (Jenden *et al.*, 1968; Hanin and Jenden, 1969).

Figure 16 (upper panel) shows the mass spectrum obtained from a rat brain extract recorded at the summit of the gas chromatographic peak with the same retention time as that of synthetic dimethylaminoethyl acetate (DMAEA). The spectrum recorded from the reference compound is presented below for comparison. The similarities of the two spectra are such that one could conclude that the compounds are identical. The molecular ion (m/e 131) is discernible. The base peak (m/e 58) is attributable to the dimethylmethylenimmonium ion. This peak and the peaks at m/e 71 and 72 are common to the acetate, propionate, and butyrate of dimethylaminoethanol. The corresponding three choline esters are all converted quantitatively to their tertiary amines

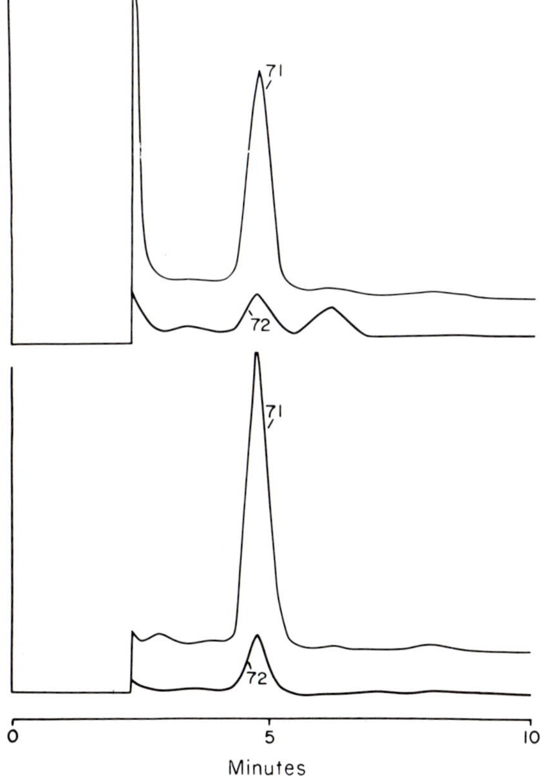

FIG. 17. Mass fragmentograms. Upper panel: demethylated rat brain extract. Lower panel: synthetic DMAEA. GC conditions: 75% Polypak 1 and 25% silanized Gas Chrom P, coated with 1% *N*,*N*-bis(2-succinimidoethyl)-*N*-dodecylamine; column temperature 128°C. MF conditions: focusing upon $m/e = 71$ and 72; ionization energy 50 eV, multiplier voltage 1.9 kV. (Courtesy of *Nature*.)

under the reaction conditions employed, and the propionate and butyrate appear as chromatographic peaks following the acetate when the choline esters are added to brain homogenates (Hanin, 1968; Hanin *et al.*, 1968). Rat brain extracts, to which choline esters have not been added, upon demethylation and gas chromatographic determination show only a peak corresponding to the product of demethylation of acetylcholine. These findings therefore indicate that propionylcholine and butyrylcholine are absent in rat brain extracts.

Advantage can also be taken of the fragments in the mass spectrum common to esters of choline ($m/e = 58$, 71, 72) by applying mass fragmentography (Hammar *et al.*, 1968a). Figure 17 shows the mass fragmentograms of ions m/e 71 and 72. The major peak observed following injection of the treated brain extract is attributable to dimethylaminoethyl acetate, which shows, in comparison with a standard, similar relative intensities for the two ions at the same retention time. In the rat brain extract a minor peak was observed at m/e 72 (Fig. 17, upper panel) following that corresponding to synthetic DMAEA. This peak was not associated with an m/e 71 peak and its retention time was different from that of any of the three esters studied. It was therefore not attributable to any of them. Propionylcholine and butyrylcholine are apparently absent in the brain extract.

Further evidence for the presence of acetylcholine and the absence of propionyl- and butyrylcholine under the conditions used is presented in Fig. 18. The mass spectrometer was focused only on m/e 58, the base peak for all three esters. The very high sensitivity used and the high signal/noise ratio obtained under these conditions should allow detection of the compounds in minute quantities. Even when the sensitivity was increased 250 times after the DMAEA peak had been eluted, no peaks appeared at the retention times expected for the homologs.

From these experiments it may be concluded that acetylcholine is definitely present in rat brain extracts. On the other hand, propionylcholine and butyrylcholine are not present in rat brain in significant amounts (<1 ng/gm).

F. Identity of "Hog": Solving the Structure of an Unknown Hallucinogen by Use of the Combination Instrument

During the summer of 1968 we obtained information concerning what appeared to be a different type of hallucinogenic drug, the slang name of which was "hog." The account that follows is a detective story showing how GC-MS techniques led to the identification of the active principle in the preparation.

The substance was given to a judge in New York by a person who received it from a young man studying for a doctorate in California. The effect of this drug was described by this young man as rather weird and he indicated that because

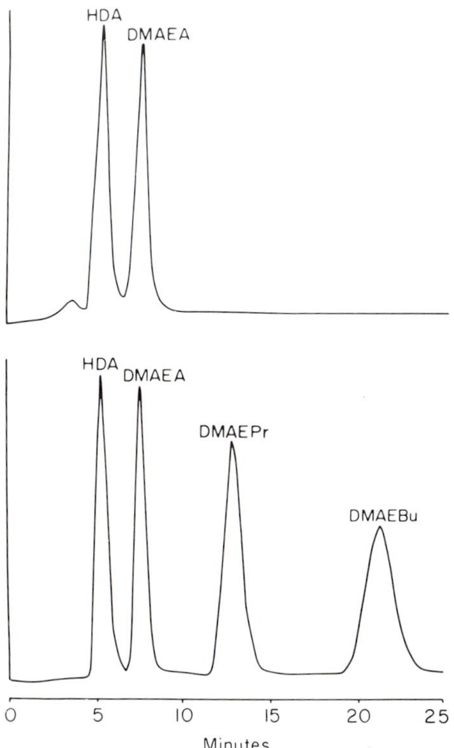

FIG. 18. Mass fragmentograms. Upper panel: demethylated rat brain extract. Lower panel: synthetic hexyldimethylamine, dimethylaminoethyl acetate, propionate, and butyrate, respectively. GC conditions: same as in Fig. 17, except for column temperature 110°C. MF conditions: same as in Fig. 17 except focusing upon $m/e = 58$. (Courtesy of *Nature*.)

its effects were so bizarre and more satisfying than "acid," it had become "the rage of the Hippie community." According to an analysis report from a police laboratory "there was no narcotic, barbiturate, amphetamine, or hallucinogenic drug present." A 20-mg sample of the white powdered drug was forwarded to us and we proceeded to analyze it by means of the combination instrument.

The powder was subjected to an amine extraction (Lindgren *et al.*, 1969). Gas chromatography of the resulting methanol solution revealed only a single peak. Additional components were excluded by programing the temperature from 100°C up to 280°C.

The next step was to record a mass spectrum of the compound corresponding to the gas chromatographic peak. In this case the absolute intensity of each mass number as well as the mass number was printed on data cards for operation on an IBM 1800 digital computer, programed to calculate the relative intensity and plot the mass spectrum on a plotter. The spectrum obtained showed a molecular ion of 243 (M^+) and prominent peaks at *m/e* 84, 91, 115, 129, 130, 143, 158 (base peak), and 200 (Fig. 19, upper panel).

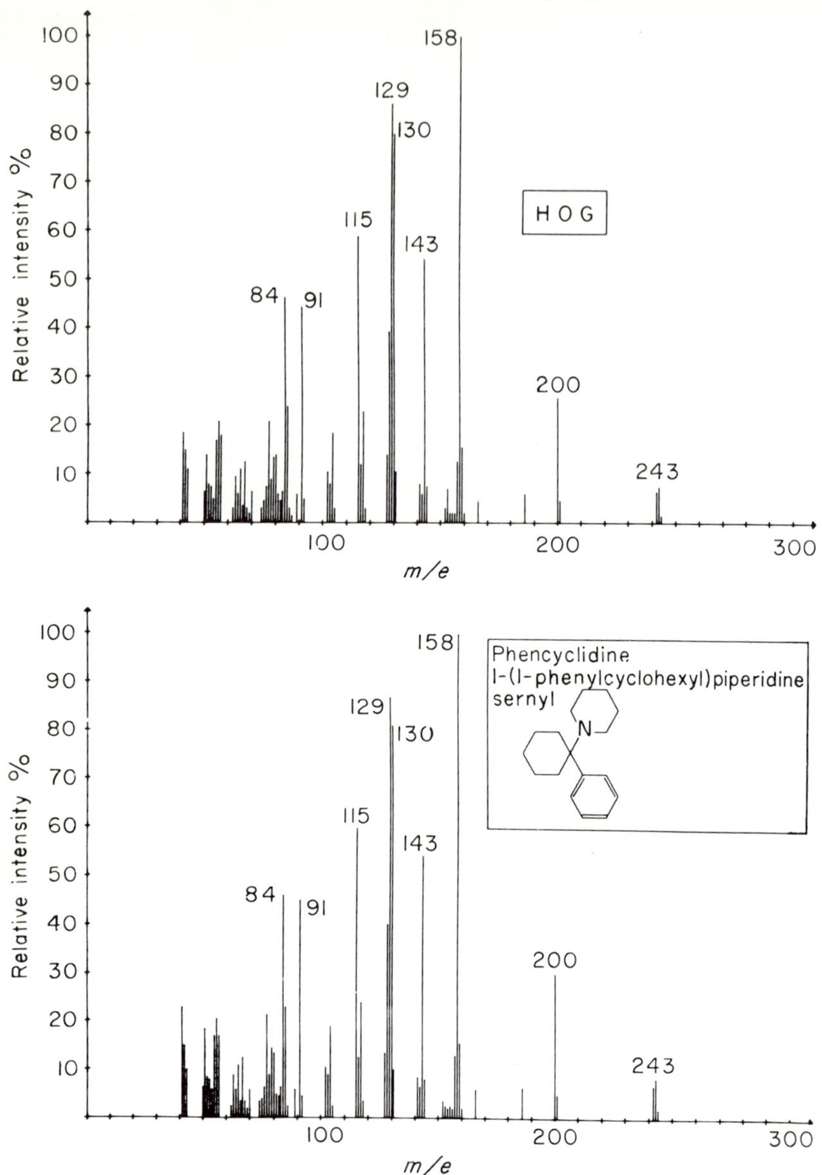

FIG. 19. Mass spectra of gas chromatographic peak from "hog" (upper panel) and phencyclidine (lower panel).

The ratio of the mass of the unknown ion to that of the reference ion can be accurately measured with the peak matcher.

In the case of hog the molecular ion of the normal mass 243 was matched against the molecular ion of *n*-heptadecane (M = 240.281687). The results were as follows:

$$\text{Hog} \qquad M = 243.......$$

$$N\text{-Heptadecane} \quad M = 240.281687$$

$$\frac{M_{Hog}}{240.281687} = 1.012133$$

$$M_{Hog} = 243.197025$$

The measured ratio of 1.012133 thus gave the unknown a molecular weight of 243.197. The reference tables of Beynon and Williams (1963) were then consulted. Under mass 243 are listed 108 possibilities. The values closest to 243.197 were as follows:

Alternative	Empirical formula		Molecular weight
A	$C_{10}H_{23}N_6O$	=	243.1933
B	$C_{11}H_{23}N_4O_2$	=	243.1829
C	$C_{11}H_{25}N_5O$	=	243.2059
D	$C_{12}H_{25}N_3O_2$	=	243.1947
E	$C_{13}H_{25}NO_3$	=	243.1834
F	$C_{13}H_{27}N_2O_2$	=	243.2072
G	$C_{14}H_{27}O_3$	=	243.1960
H	$C_{16}H_{23}N_2$	=	243.1861
I	$C_{17}H_{25}N$	=	243.1987

A very simple rule states that all organic molecules having an even molecular weight must contain an even number (0, 2, 4, etc.) of nitrogen atoms, and all those having an odd molecular weight, an odd number (1, 3, 5, etc.) of nitrogen atoms. The rule holds for all compounds containing carbon, hydrogen, nitrogen, oxygen, sulfur, and the halogens, and can also be applied when many of the less frequently encountered atoms are present. The rule does not hold if bonds other than covalent ones are included (Beynon, 1960).

Thus the empirical formulas A, B, F, and H are eliminated owing to this rule. The two values in the reference tables closest to the measured value are 243.1960 with the empirical formula of $C_{14}H_{27}O_3$ and 243.1987 corresponding to the empirical formula $C_{17}H_{25}N$. The former one is impossible to construct and cannot exist except as a fragment and the latter one is probable after an amine extraction. The difference in mass between the unknown and the most probable compound $C_{17}H_{25}N$ is 7 ppm.

Peak matching can be carried out not only on the molecular ion but also on the fragments.

If the assumption is made that the unknown compound is $C_{17}H_{25}N$ then the mass of the molecular ion minus one hydrogen should be 243.1987 − 1.0078 = 242.1909. The mass observed using the peak matcher was 242.1893. The predicted and observed values lie within 7 ppm of each other. The presumed measurement error is therefore almost constant for this technique. Measurement of the weight of the fragment $m/e = 158$ with the peak matcher gave 158.1094 and the closest Beynon and Williams (1963) table value was 158.1095 with the empirical formula of $C_{12}H_{14}$. The difference in measured mass from the closest value in the Beynon and Williams table now amounted to only 1 ppm.

Measured masses		Nearest values derived from tables of Beynon and Williams	
Whole mass number from MS scan	Decimals obtained using peak matcher	Empirical formula	Mass
243	0.1970	$C_{17}H_{25}N$	243.1987
242	0.1893	$C_{17}H_{24}N$	242.1909
200	0.1465	$C_{14}H_{18}N$	200.1439
166	0.1519	$C_{11}H_{20}N$	166.1596
158	0.1094	$C_{12}H_{14}$	158.1095

The MS scan has (1) a fragment $m/e = 84$ which may be characteristic of a piperidine moiety, (2) a fragment $m/e = 158$ indicating a phenylcyclohexyl moiety, and (3) another fragment $m/e = 166$ indicating a cyclohexylpiperidine moiety.

A table of compounds reported to have psychotropic activity revealed that one drug indeed contained all these three ring systems and also had a nominal molecular weight of 243 (Usdin and Efron, 1967). This compound is phencyclidine or 1-(1-phenylcyclohexyl)-piperidine. An appropriate quantity of phencyclidine was then processed in the manner used for hog. Gas chromatographic measurement yielded similar retention times for this reference and hog and the mass spectrum obtained showed identity with the unknown substance (Fig. 19, lower panel).

The identity of hog was thus established as phencyclidine, marketed under the name Sernyl. It has been used in the treatment of neurotic patients, anxiety states with depressive mood swings, and also as an intravenous anesthetic (Lindgren *et al.*, 1969). It is no longer in general use because of unpleasant side effects such as loss of balance, dissociation with respect to time and place, visual hallucinations, and delusions. The latter properties apparently make this obsolete drug attractive to certain people.

Our experience with hog shows that the structure of a completely unknown compound supplied in a quantity of a few milligrams can be solved. The elements that made this possible are the following: (1) Establishing through extraction and gas chromatography that only one component of amine character was present; (2) recording of the mass spectrum of this compound; (3) measurement of the masses of the molecular ion and certain fragments; (4) selection of the most likely empirical formulas for these fragments; and finally (5) a high index of suspicion coupled with a knowledge of the relevant literature.

IV. Conclusions

The correct choice of a sensitive and appropriate gas chromatographic technique nowadays can achieve rapid separation of components in complex mixtures such as biologic extracts. However, in qualitative analysis the identification of an unknown compound cannot be based entirely upon its relative retention time on different stationary phases. Other methods of chemical identification, such as infrared spectrometry (IR), ultraviolet spectrometry (UV), and nuclear magnetic resonance spectrometry (NMR) can be utilized for additional information. In order to obtain an IR or an NMR spectrum the compound has to be isolated in rather large quantities (0.1–10 mg). This is a disadvantage and in most cases makes drug analyses impossible in body fluids where only small amounts of compounds are available for chemical identification. In such cases advantage cannot be taken of the techniques mentioned above, but it is possible to further improve the sensitivity of GC by the additional dimension of a direct combination with MS. Our main effort during the past years has been the application of the combined GC-MS method to the study of drugs and their metabolites.

In order to utilize the combined GC-MS technique a previous familiarity with ordinary GC technique is imperative. It is of great importance to optimize the resolution of the GC peaks by an appropriate choice of stationary phase, column length, and temperature, as well as other parameters such as derivative formation. In the combination with MS the choice of stationary phase and column temperature becomes of special importance, due to the bleeding of the phase, which always takes place, giving rise to a background spectrum and under unfavorable circumstances to contamination of the ion source.

The great advantage of the combination of the techniques of GC and MS is the exploitation of the separation power of a GC system coupled to the extremely high selectivity of an MS system. The smallest amounts needed for the scanning of a mass spectrum are in the range of 10–100 ng and the time required for the practical procedure is relatively short. It must be pointed out that this combined technique gives so much information that it is possible to achieve a positive identification of a compound by comparing it to a reference substance. This is not the case when ordinary GC alone is used.

Although the sensitivity of the combined technique may seem to be high there are situations when it is insufficient. In some drug metabolic studies the amounts available are too small for the scanning of complete mass spectra. It may still be possible, however, to identify a compound by means of a technique which we have called mass fragmentography. In this technique advantage is taken of some of the physicochemical characteristics of a compound or a group of compounds by simultaneous recording of up to three mass numbers representing either the molecular ion or fragments of the molecule. By recording additional characteristic fragments it is possible to obtain information allowing the construction of a "partial mass spectrum," in spite of the fact that the amounts present are insufficient for the scanning of a complete spectrum. This method gives a gain in sensitivity of about 1000–10,000 times as compared to ordinary GC-MS. The selectivity can be altered by changing the mass numbers monitored; this distinguishes mass fragmentography from detectors used in ordinary GC-system.

The problem of identifying a completely unknown substance may be overcome by the use of the peak matching technique. This requires the isolation of the compound by trapping it from the GC effluent. The amount needed is in the range of a few micrograms or less. The nominal molecular weight will be known from a previously scanned spectrum. A reference substance with an accurate molecular weight as close as possible to the unknown is chosen. By matching these two weights against each other the mass ratio between them is measured and a more accurate molecular weight with decimals is calculated. By comparing this calculated mass to masses listed in tables it is possible to select a few probable empirical formulas of which ordinarily most can be eliminated based upon knowledge of the extraction procedure. The final establishment of the identity is achieved by comparison of the spectrum of the unknown compound to that of the supposed one. In an analogous way peak matching can be performed on fragments, thus giving information about their empirical formulas. Peak matching is extremely useful in the interpretation of fragmentation patterns. Peak matching may also be of importance as a basis for mass fragmentography, where parts of a molecule are used to characterize either a single compound or a family of metabolites.

The combined gas chromatography–mass spectrometry method and mass fragmentography allow the analysis of drugs in body liquids in very small concentrations. These techniques will no doubt open new fields in clinical pharmacology and toxicology by permitting the measurement of therapeutic plasma levels of many compounds. Further developments may lead to human pharmacologic studies of drugs such as morphine and digitalis, which have been used for centuries with only a limited knowledge of the relationship between their pharmacokinetics and their clinical effects. In the future the sensitivity of the techniques mentioned in this review, coupled with the possibility of determining stable isotopes, will permit early experiments in man. Tracer doses of drugs labeled with stable isotopes could safely be given even in cases where unstable (i.e., radioactive) isotopes are generally avoided, e.g., in pregnant women and newborns. The appropriate species for further animal experimentations could then be selected on the basis of the knowledge of metabolic patterns in man, eliminating needless and costly experimentation with several species of animals. Correlating the pattern of metabolism with the pharmacologic effects of drugs may also lead to the discovery in man of new active drug metabolites, which again do not need extensive testing in animals before clinical trials. It is not unlikely that in the future the pattern of circulating metabolites of any given drug may prove to be as important as the plasma levels of a single compound when correlated with therapeutic effects and side effects. The techniques described in this review, together with computer analysis, will be the best means to elucidate these problems.

ACKNOWLEDGMENTS

The research work in this review has largely been supported by the Swedish Medical Research Council, project No. B69-40X-199; the National Institute of General Medical Sciences, Bethesda, Maryland, (GM 13978); the National Institute of Mental Health, Bethesda, Maryland (MH 12007); and by the Knut and Alice Wallenberg Foundation, Stockholm, Sweden.

We thank Dr. Ragnar Ryhage, Dept. of Mass Spectrometry, Karolinska Institutet, Stockholm, and the LKB-Produkter, Fack, 161 25, Bromma 1, Sweden, for valuable support and collaboration.

Most of the blood samples have been obtained by courtesy of Assistant Professor Folke Sjöqvist, Division of Clinical Pharmacology, Dept. of Pharmacology, Karolinska Institutet, Stockholm, whom we thank for a fruitful collaboration. We want to express our thanks to Professor David A. Price Evans for helpful suggestions during the preparation of the manuscript. Finally, we thank all collaborators and assistants in the department for their unfailing work during the past years.

REFERENCES

Agurell, S., Holmstedt, B., and Lindgren, J. E. (1968). *Am. J. Pharm.* **140**, 148.

Agurell, S., Holmstedt, B., Lindgren, J. E., and Schultes, R. E. (1969). *Acta Chem. Scand.* **23**, 903.

Becker, E. W. (1961). *In* "Separation of Isotopes" (H. London, ed.), pp. 360–367. Newnes, London.

Becker, E. W., Bier, K., and Burghoff, H. Z. (1955). *Z. Naturforsch.* **10**a, 545.

Beynon, J. H. (1960). "Mass Spectrometry and Its Applications To Organic Chemistry." Elsevier, Amsterdam.

Beynon, J. H., and Williams, A. E. (1963). "Mass and Abundance Tables for Use in Mass Spectrometry." Elsevier, Amsterdam.

Biemann, K. (1963). "Mass Spectrometry—Organic Chemical Applications." McGraw-Hill, New York.

Biemann, K., and Hites, R. A. (1968). *Intern. Symp. Chromato-mass Spectrometry, May, Moscow.*

Budzikiewics, H., Djerassi, C., and Williams, D. H. (1964a). "Interpretation of Mass Spectra of Organic Compounds." Holden-Day, San Francisco, California.

Budzikiewics, H., Djerassi, C., and Williams, D. H. (1964b). "Structural Elucidation of Natural Products by Mass Spectrometry. Vol. I: Alkaloids." Holden-Day, San Francisco, California.

Budzikiewics, H., Djerassi, C., and Williams, D. H. (1964c). "Structural Elucidation of Natural Products by Mass Spectrometry. Vol. II: Steroids, Triterpenes and Related Classes." Holden-Day, San Francisco, California.

Dalgliesh, C. E., Horning, E. C., Horning, M. G., Knox, K. L., and Yarger, K. (1966). *Biochem. J.* **101**, 792.

Fales, H. M., and Pisano, J. J. (1964). *In* "Biomedical Applications of Gas Chromatography" (H. A. Szymanski, ed.), pp. 39–87. Plenum Press, New York.

Frazer, J. W. (1968). *Anal. Chem.* **40**, 27.

Gudzinowics, B. J. (1967). "Gas Chromatographic Analysis of Drugs and Pesticides." Dekker, New York.

Hammar, C. G., and Holmstedt, B. (1968). *Experientia* **24**, 98.

Hammar, C. G., Holmstedt, B., and Ryhage, R. (1968a). *Anal. Biochem.* **25**, 532.

Hammar, C. G., Hanin, I., Holmstedt, B., Kitz, R. J., Jenden, D. J., and Karlén, B., (1968b). *Nature* **220**, 915.

Hammarstrand, K. (1966). "Gas Chromatographic Analysis of Fatty Acids." Varian Aerograph, Walnut Creek, California.

Hammarstrand, K. (1967). "Gas Chromatographic Analysis of Steroids." Varian Aerograph, Walnut Creek, California.

Hammarstrand, K. (1968). "Gas Chromatographic Analysis of Carbohydrates." Varian Aerograph, Walnut Creek, California.

Hammer, W. M., and Brodie, B. B. (1967). *J. Pharmacol. Exptl. Therap.* **157**, 503.

Hanin, I. (1968), Ph.D. Thesis, Univ. of California, Los Angeles, California.

Hanin, I., and Jenden, D. J. (1969). *Biochem. Pharmacol.* **18**, 837.

Hanin, I., Jenden, D. J., and Lamb, S. I. (1968). *Proc. Western Pharmacol. Soc.* **11**, 144.

Hill, H. C. (1966). "Introduction to Mass Spectrometry." Heyden, London.

Hites, R. A., and Biemann, K. (1967). *Anal. Chem.* **39**, 965.

Hites, R. A., and Biemann, K. (1968). *Anal. Chem.* **40**, 1217.

Holmstedt, B., and Lindgren, J. E. (1967). *In* "Ethnopharmacologic Search for Psychoactive Drugs" (D. H. Efron, ed.), *U.S. Public Health Serv. Publ.* **1645**, 339–373.

Holmstedt, B., Vanden Heuvel, W. J. A., Gardiner, W. L., and Horning, E. C. (1964). *Anal. Biochem.* **8**, 151.

Horning, M. G. (1968a). *In* "Theory and Application of Gas Chromatography in Industry and Medicine" (H. S. Kroman and S. S. Bender, eds.), pp. 135–146. Grune & Stratton, New York.

Horning, M. G., (1968b). *In* "Biomedical Applications of Gas Chromatography" (H. A. Szymanski, ed.), Vol. 2, pp. 53–86. Plenum Press, New York.

Horning, M. G., Moss, A. M., and Horning, E. C. (1967). *Biochim. Biophys. Acta* **148**, 597.

Horning, M. G., Moss, A. M., Boucher, E. A., and Horning, E. C. (1968). *Anal. Letters* **1**, 311.

Jansson, P. Å., Melkersson, S., Ryhage, R., and Wikström, S. (1968). *16th Ann. Conf. Mass Spectrometry Allied Topics, ASTM Committee E–14, May, Pittsburgh, Penna.*

Jenden, D. J., Hanin, I., and Lamb, S. I. (1968). *Anal. Chem.* **40**, 125.

Juvet, R. S., Jr., and Dal Nogare, S. (1968). *Anal. Chem.* **40**, 33R.

Kern, H., Schilling, P., and Müller, S. H. (1968). "Gas Chromatographic Analysis of Pharmaceuticals and Drugs." Varian Aerograph, Walnut Creek, California.

Lindgren, J. E., Hammar, C. G., Hessling, R., and Holmstedt, B. (1969). *Am. J. Pharm.* In press.

Lipsky, S. R., Horvath, C. G., and McMurray, W. J. (1966a). *Anal. Chem.* **38**, 1194.

Lipsky, S. R., Horvath, C. G., and McMurray, W. J. (1966b). *Anal. Chem.* **38**, 1585.

Llewellyn, P. M., and Littlejohn, D. P. (1966). *Pittsburgh Conf. Anal. Chem. Appl. Spectry.*

McCloskey, J. A., Stillwell, R. N., and Lawson, A. M. (1968). *Anal. Chem.* **40**, 233.

McLafferty, F. W. (1963). "Mass Spectrometry of Organic Ions." Academic Press, New York.

Pierce, A. E. (1968). "Silylation of Organic Compounds." Pierce Chem. Co., Rockford, Illinois.

Poisson, J. (1965). *Ann. Pharm. Franc.* **23**, 241.

Reynolds, W., Bridges, J., Coburn, T., and Tucker, R. (1967). *Biomed. Symp. Proc.* p. 77.

Ryhage, R. (1964). *Anal. Chem.* **36**, 759.

Ryhage, R. (1967a). *Arkiv Kemi* **26**, 305.

Ryhage, R. (1967b). *15th Ann. Conf. Mass Spectrometry Allied Topics, ASTM Committee E–14, May, Denver, Colo.*

Schayer, R. W., and Cooper, J. A. D. (1956). *J. Appl. Physiol.* **9**, 481.

Shamma, M., Deno, N. C., and Remar, J. F. (1966). *Tetrahedron Letters* **13**, 1375.

Sweeley, C. C., Elliott, W. H., Fries, I., and Ryhage, R. (1966). *Anal. Chem.* **38**, 1549.

Szymanski, H. A. (1964). "Biomedical Applications of Gas Chromatography." Plenum Press, New York.

Tham, R. (1966a). *J. Chromatog.* **23**, 207.

Tham, R. (1966b). *Scand. J. Clin. Lab. Invest.* **18**, 603.

Tham, R., and Holmstedt, B. (1965). *J. Chromatog.* **19**, 286.

Tham, R., Nyström, L., and Holmstedt, B. (1968). *Biochem. Pharmacol.* **17**, 1735.

Tham, R., Moss, A. M., Horning, M. G., and Horning, E. C. (1969). To be published.

Usdin, E., and Efron, D. H. (1967). "Psychotropic Drugs and Related Compounds." *U.S. Public Health Serv. Publ.* **1589**.

Watson, J. T., and Biemann, K. (1964). *Anal. Chem.* **36**, 1135.

Watson, J. T., and Biemann, K. (1965). *Anal. Chem.* **37**, 844.

Zlatkis, A. (1967). "Advances in Gas Chromatography." Preston Tech. Abstr. Co., Evanston, Illinois.

Drugs and the Mechanism of Insulin Secretion

JOHN STEPHEN KIZER AND RUBIN BRESSLER

Departments of Medicine and Physiology and Pharmacology,
Duke University Medical Center,
Durham, North Carolina

I. Introduction

In 1889, it was first demonstrated that pancreatectomized dogs developed a disease, the features of which closely resembled those of diabetes mellitus (1). These demonstrations and the subsequent elucidations of the dominant regulatory role of insulin in intermediary metabolism (2) have caused an overwhelming amount of investigative attention to be directed to the diabetic pancreas and its insulin. When insulin assays became available and it was discovered that many diabetics maintained respectable plasma levels of the hormone, speculation developed that diabetes mellitus was in actuality a relative insulin deficiency with either the synthesis of a defective hormone or the presence of an antagonist being the heritable defect. Abnormal insulins have in fact been reported sporadically in juvenile (3) and adult diabetics (4); however, Kimmel and Pollock examined the insulin isolated from a large number of diabetic pancreases at autopsy and found that the amino acid composition was in agreement in all cases with the known structure of human insulin, with one exception—that being a one-residue alteration at a locus known to be associated in other species with no loss of activity (5). The question of insulin antagonists, however, is still unresolved.

Although it is commonly observed that there is an absolute insulin deficiency in the late diabetic, much confusion concerning the status of the insulin secretory mechanism of the early diabetic resulted from reports of an augmented insulin response to a standard glucose tolerance test in early maturity onset diabetes. Recently Karam *et al.* (6), Pfeiffer (7), and others (8) have clearly shown that there are two patient populations among the early diabetics, one normal in weight and one overweight. Abnormally high fasting plasma insulin levels and supranormal responses to a glucose tolerance test are characteristic of the obese patient irrespective of whether he is nondiabetic or an early diabetic (9, 10). Malaisse *et al.* have demonstrated this phenomenon experimentally in mice and have shown that the pancreatic insulin store and secretory capacity vary in direct proportion to body weight (11). Further studies (7, 9, 12–15) have compared the insulin response of the nondiabetic patient and the early diabetic patient of similar weight and concluded that at no time is the insulin response of the diabetic superior to that of the nondiabetic control. Furthermore, the insulin reserve of the early diabetic is decreased (16), suggesting that the diabetic pancreas is already working to capacity. In attempting to relate the rate of glucose removal (K) of normal volunteers to the changes in insulin secretion during repeated 60-minute intravenous glucose tolerance tests, Garcia *et al.* (17) found a highly significant correlation between K and the fraction of insulin released in the 0–10 minute interval, but no significant correlation between K and the total insulin release (0–60 minutes). The implications of this relationship between K and the initial insulin release can be seen in the studies of Seltzer *et al.* (9, 10), Luft (18), Cerasi and Luft (19), Shochat and Willansky (20), and Karam *et al.* (21), all of whom have observed that the early diabetic insulin response is delayed and lacks the immediate initial release which characterizes the normal response. This insulin response is so characteristic of all stages of diabetes mellitus that Seltzer has advocated that the primary lesion of diabetes is a "biochemical inertia of the pancreatic β-cell" (10).

Since it is well established, therefore, that whatever else if anything the diabetic disease state encompasses, a primary defect in the continued storage and secretion of insulin by the diabetic pancreas must be included, it is the intent of this monograph to extensively review those agents which have been found to stimulate the secretion of insulin and to discuss the possible mechanism of its normal release in the nondiabetic and abnormal release in the diabetic.

II. Glucose, Hexoses, and Pentitols

Whether used to stimulate the pancreas *in vivo* or the isolated perfused pancreas, glucose provokes an immediate release of insulin (22–26). Using the isolated perfused rat pancreas, Grodsky has shown that a finite time is required for the appearance of insulin in the eluate following glucose pulses and that the insulin response parallels the glucose levels, but with a 30-second lag at all phases. At the termination of the glucose pulse, the insulin level returns to baseline, also within 30 seconds (27, 28). When the isolated pancreas is perfused continuously for 10 minutes with a constant level of glucose, the rate of insulin release increases immediately (within 30 seconds) with a rapid fall to a lower, relatively more stable rate for the duration of the infusion and then returns promptly to baseline levels at the termination of the infusion (29). Throughout the period of infusion, the pancreas is still capable of increasing its output, as evidenced by the additional insulin release in response to a cross-stimulation by tolbutamide (29). In the normal human, the *in vivo* insulin response to a given level of glucose may be further enhanced by the combined administration of tolbutamide, glucose, and glucagon (16). *In vitro* studies of isolated rat islets have supported these latter observations and suggest that the total pancreatic insulin store is depleted by approximately 5% by an immediate stimulus (30). After stimulation of the isolated perfused pancreas with a maximal glucose infusion, there is a slight loss of responsiveness to immediate reinfusion with lower glucose concentrations, suggesting that intracellular feedback may be of some importance (29).

Following the possibility suggested by this work of Grodsky that insulin secretion by the β-cell may occur in two distinct phases, the first involving the rapid release of preformed insulin and the second requiring insulin synthesis, Howell and Taylor (31) incubated slices of rabbit pancreas in media containing leucine-^{3}H and then measured the specific activity of the insulin released in response to glucose stimulation. At low glucose concentrations, there was a small but measurable release of labeled insulin. When the glucose concentration was increased, there was little additional labeled insulin released in the first hour in contrast to the second and third hours during which there was a marked release of labeled insulin. More recently Curry *et al.* (32) have pursued this question further by studying the insulin response of the isolated rat pancreas to prolonged infusions of glucose (40–70 min). They demonstrated an immediate increase in the insulin release followed by a rapid fall to nearly baseline levels within approximately 5 minutes. This initial decline was then followed by a gradual increase in assayable insulin such that by 40 minutes the rate of insulin release was of the same magnitude as the initial spike. Administration of puromycin had no effect on the initial phase but decreased the insulin response during the second phase by 33% and appeared to be increasingly effective with time. It would seem, therefore, that the synthesis of new insulin is an essential aspect of insulin secretion.

Recently, evidence has accumulated indicating that glucose must be metabolized to stimulate the secretion of insulin. Mannoheptulose and 2-deoxyglucose, two sugars which competitively inhibit the phosphorylation (33) of glucose and the phosphohexose isomerase and glucose-6-phosphate dehydrogenase reactions (35, 36), respectively, will inhibit the secretion of insulin in response to a glycemic stimulus (22, 34, 37–40) as will glucosamine (41). In isolated mouse pancreatic acinar tissue the rate of glucose oxidation does not increase when incubated in media containing glucose in concentrations increasing from 27.5 to 450 mg/100 ml, whereas under similar conditions in isolated islets, the rate of glucose oxidation increases proportionately (40). Furthermore, this increase in glucose oxidation is blocked by mannoheptulose and acetyl glucosamine (38, 40, 41), and a block in oxidation is accompanied by a decrease in insulin release (38). As a corollary, it is apparent that glucose must freely enter the β-cell for it to control the rate of insulin secretion. Accordingly, studies utilizing 3-*O*-methyl glucose and phloridzin, which compete with glucose for active transport into the cell (42, 43), have failed to demonstrate any decrease in the rate of insulin secretion or rate of glucose oxidation of the β-cell in response to glucose stimulation (38, 40). These results suggest that perhaps some product of the glycolytic or hexose monophosphate (HMP) pathway is responsible for the initiation of the secretory event, although Malaisse (34) concludes that the kinetics of phosphorylation alone cannot account for the kinetics of insulin release since the rate of phosphorylation is nearly maximal at a glucose concentration of 1 mM, whereas little insulin is released at similar concentrations. The case for the metabolism of glucose being the trigger for insulin release has been strengthened by the demonstration of the HMP pathway in the β-cell (44) and by the observation that sugars such as mannose (23, 39, 41, 45, 46), fructose (23, 41, 45, 46), and ribose (36, 41, 47) are effective stimuli of insulin release, whereas xylose (36, 45), arabinose (23, 36, 45) and galactose (23, 39, 45, 46) are not. Further studies have also shown xylitol (36, 48), ribitol (36), glutamate (40), fumarate (40), and pyruvate (40) to be capable of causing insulin release from the β-cell in contrast to sorbitol, arabitol, and mannitol, which are not (36). Recently, Hellerström (41) has found significant increases in the respiratory rate of isolated mice islets incubated with glucose, mannose, fructose, or ribose, but no such increase when incubated with galactose, allose, altrose, tagatose, L-glucose, 2-deoxyglucose, talose, xylose, and lyxose.

Furthermore, 2-deoxyglucose has proven to be an ineffective inhibitor of the insulinogenic response to xylitol, indicating that xylitol is not being metabolized to glucose-6-phosphate in effecting insulin release (36).

This latter finding coupled with the previously outlined observations that many diverse substrates are able to trigger the release of insulin strongly suggests the hypothesis that an increased respiratory rate irrespective of the stimulus somehow is able to alter the intracellular milieu such that the β-cell is caused to release its insulin stores.

III. Fatty Acids and Ketone Bodies

The prominence of hyperketonemia in the uncontrolled diabetic and the theoretic regulatory role of plasma free fatty acid (FFA) concentrations (45, 49, 50) in metabolism have stimulated attempts to qualify and quantify the metabolic effects of increased plasma levels of FFA and ketones. Early studies had shown that intravenous infusions of β-hydroxybutyric acid, acetoacetic acid, or their sodium salts into the dog were followed by rapid decreases in the blood glucose concentration, a 50% decrease in hepatic glucose output, and a 50% fall in the plasma nonesterified fatty acids (51). Mebane *et al.* pursued these studies further and failed to reproduce their observations in depancreatized dogs, indicating the necessity of the presence of pancreatic tissue for the elicitation of these results (52). Subsequent analyses of pancreatic and peripheral venous blood in dogs infused with either long- and short-chain fatty acids or ketones have shown significant elevations in the immunoreactive insulin (52–55). Also of interest is the demonstration in sheep that propionate and butyrate are more potent stimulators of insulin secretion than is glucose (56). It has been postulated that in starvation the elevated FFA and ketones would either maintain or slightly increase pancreatic insulin output, thereby indirectly conserving protein and glucose and preventing the uncontrolled overproduction of ketone bodies by the liver as seen in the insulin-dependent diabetic in ketosis (57).

Recently, Balasse and Ooms sought to duplicate these effects of hyperketonemia in the normal human subject. Intravenous infusion of β-hydroxybutyrate reproduced the falls in blood glucose and FFA concentrations as observed in the dog, but there was no concomitant modification of the peripheral insulin level. It was these authors' conclusion that the pancreas did not participate in the observed phenomenon (58). Sanbar *et al.* (59) were unable to detect any alteration of the peripheral insulin levels in dogs treated with intravenous infusions of octanoate in concentrations less than 3.0 mM, although the insulin content of pancreatic venous blood was increased several fold. Octanoate infusions in concentrations greater than 3.0 mM, however, produced significant and detectable elevations of peripheral insulin levels. They concluded that short-chain fatty acids did indeed provoke the secretion of insulin, but the small magnitude of this increased release was undetectable peripherally due to the entrapment of insulin by the liver (59).

Guided by this hypothesis, Greenberger *et al.* administered medium-chain triglycerides orally to cirrhotic patients some of whom had had portocaval shunts. This procedure produced elevated plasma levels of octanoate and additionally elevated peripheral insulin levels, apparently because of the decreased liver mass and the shunting of pancreatic venous blood into the systemic circulation (60).

In vitro incubation of isolated rat islets with low concentrations of glucose and octanoate, butyrate, or citrate increases the secretion of insulin by the β-cell, and intracellular concentrations of glucose-6-phosphate parallel these increases (61). These observations prompted their observers, Montague and Taylor, to conclude that some pathway other than glycolysis (perhaps the HMP shunt) might mediate the insulin release under these particular conditions since citrate depresses glycolysis (62, 63). Such findings would exclude the mediation of insulin secretion by some specific glycolytic intermediate only if the β-cell were to possess none of the enzymes of gluconeogenesis, or if these organic acids were not metabolized.

Whether fatty acids or ketones must first be metabolized in order to induce insulin release has yet to be studied, but such a finding would be logically expected and would strengthen the notion that an overall increase in the metabolism of the β-cell or an increase in the individual activity of any one of several different pathways is the initial event in insulin secretion—with some pathways perhaps more potent than others.

IV. Enteroinsular Axis

In 1964, it was postulated that a fundamental difference exists between orally and intravenously administered glucose tolerance tests. The basis for this proposal stemmed from observations by McIntyre *et al.* that a given oral glucose load resulted in lower plasma glucose levels and higher peripheral insulin levels than an equivalent amount of glucose infused intravenously (64). That such a difference was indeed real was further emphasized by the finding that an oral glucose load was capable of reversing the block of insulin release by epinephrine, whereas intravenous glucose was not (65). Such observations prompted many investigators to conclude that in response to an oral meal an intestinal hormone must be released capable of stimulating the release of insulin in anticipation of the actual hyperglycemia or amino acidemia.

In 1965, it was reported by Samols *et al.* that plasma immunoreactive glucagon-like activity rose in response to oral glucose stimulation (66). Following the obvious implication of this observation he was also able to show that pancreatic glucagon was a potent stimulus to insulin secretion (67, 68). Subsequently, this observation has been amply documented (69–71). Samols' finding of increased glucagon immunoreactivity after an oral glucose stimulus was in obvious conflict with the established concept of glucagon as being gluconeogenic. Accordingly, Unger *et al.* carefully examined these results in the dog (72). They, too, found an increase in the glucagon immunoreactivity after oral glucose, but actual measurements of pancreatic venous plasma revealed a decrease in the glucagon activity. In addition the peripheral elevation of the glucagon-like activity persisted after pancreatectomy. A jejunal extract was prepared which stimulated insulin release and shared the immunologic reactivity of glucagon but was devoid of glycogenolytic activity and could not increase the levels of hepatic cyclic 3′,5′-AMP. It was concluded that there was indeed a glucagon-like intestinal hormone released after an oral meal, but that this hormone differed significantly from pancreatic glucagon.

Secretin has been repeatedly demonstrated to be a rapid and effective stimulus of insulin release (69–78) and does so with little or no increase in arterial blood glucose concentration (69, 73, 76) or glucagon-like activity (75). Furthermore, the effectiveness of this hormone is unaltered by the prior administration of epinephrine (79).

Pancreozymin, serotonin, and gastrin have all been found to stimulate insulin secretion (77), although the efficacy of gastrin is disputed (69). Pancreozymin is approximately three times as potent as secretin, but unlike secretin, it also releases pancreatic glucagon, which may account for this difference in potency (74).

From these observations it appears amply documented that intestinal hormones do in fact mediate an anticipatory response of the pancreas to an oral meal. The evaluation of the relative importance of each, however, awaits further *in vitro* studies.

V. Amino Acids

Investigations into the mechanism of leucine-induced hypoglycemia demonstrated this amino acid to be capable of increasing plasma levels of insulin in man (80). Subsequently, Floyd and his co-workers reported that either a protein meal or an infusion of the 10 essential amino acids resulted in a marked increase in insulin secretion and was not dependent on the presence of leucine. Their studies also showed that not all the amino acids were of equal potency in mediating this response—arginine being as effective as a mixture of the 10 essential amino acids, with lysine, leucine, phenylalanine, and histidine being respectively less effective (81). Since leucine is not gluconeogenic, it has been concluded that gluconeogenesis is not essential for this increase in insulin release, and that amino acids are undoubtedly a physiologic stimulus (82). That some similarity between the mechanism of insulin release mediated by amino acids and glucose may exist is suggested by the fact that administration of the two in concert provides a greater increase in insulin activity than either ingested alone (83). Further implicative evidence is the blunting of the insulin response to amino acids as well as glucose in normal-weight, adult-onset diabetics (84–86). Although Berger and Vongaraya have reported increased insulin responses in the maturity-onset diabetic in comparison to normal after the ingestion of a protein meal (87), they did not eliminate the obese diabetic from their study—individuals known to have increased insulin responses to glucose as well as arginine ingestion (88).

The awareness of the physiologic importance of the enteroinsular axis and the potent insulinogenic capacity of glucagon encouraged Ohneda and Unger to characterize the response of circulatory glucagon to amino acids infused either intravenously or intraduodenally (89). They found that hyperamino acidemia did indeed release pancreatic glucagon, an effect which could be augmented by pancreozymin. Intraduodenal amino acid infusion, however, provoked no increase in glucagon-like activity measured in the mesenteric vein. Furthermore, hyperglycemia prevented the hyperglucagonemia in response to amino acids and pancreozymin administered either individually or in concert. It was suggested by these authors that the prevention of hypoglycemia during hyperamino acidemia was an important physiologic function of glucagon (89). An additional implication of these results is that glucagon is not mediating the amino acid-induced hyperinsulinemia since the insulinogenic effect of glucose and amino acids infused together intravenously would not be expected to be additive if glucose inhibits pancreatic glucagon secretion. Accordingly, Floyd *et al.* were able to demonstrate the synergistic effect of intravenously administered amino acids and glucose (90) and concluded that the magnitude of insulin secretion induced by a particular amino acid or group of amino acids depended on this synergism between that particular amino acid and glucose as well as on the total amount ingested.

Recently evidence has come to the fore indicating that there is a difference in mechanisms by which leucine and the other amino acids stimulate insulin release. In healthy subjects either with an islet tumor or pretreated with chlorpropamide leucine will stimulate insulin release and the others will not. Subjects pretreated with diazoxide, however, are still responsive to the other amino acids, but not to leucine (91).

VI. Glucagon

Glucagon can stimulate the secretion of insulin by the pancreas both *in vitro* and *in vivo* (23, 28, 40, 67, 69, 70, 92–96). With respect to time, Samols *et al.* found that the insulin response to glucagon infusion in man was more rapid than to glucose (94) and also more quickly dissipated (67). Although the initially high rate of insulin secretion gradually declines during a continuous 3-hour glucagon infusion in man, an added pulse of glucagon will still provoke an increase in measurable immunoreactive insulin (95). A 5 μg/minute infusion of glucagon has been reported to be a more potent stimulus of insulin secretion in man than 650 mg of glucose (95). In the isolated perfused pancreas, Grodsky and Bennett demonstrated that in the absence of glucose in the perfusate, a glucagon pulse was followed by an increase in insulin output within 30 seconds.

This rate of insulin secretion paralleled the changes in glucagon and returned to baseline within 30 seconds after cessation of the infusion (27, 28). The similarity of these results to those obtained for glucose are remarkable. Although Grodsky was able to demonstrate these results in the absence of glucose, other authors have found that glucagon in a concentration of 2.0 μg/ml will stimulate insulin release from slices of rabbit pancreas only at high glucose concentrations (93, 96), whereas glucagon in a concentration of 5.0 μg/ml will provoke insulin release even at low glucose concentrations. Furthermore, the insulinogenic effect of glucagon can be blocked by mannoheptulose (37).

The secretions of insulin in response to glucagon, therefore, is not only dependent on the presence of either glucose (or perhaps glycogen in its absence), but the magnitude of the rate of secretion also depends on the magnitude of their availabilities.

VII. Tolbutamide

The sulfonylureas—tolbutamide, acetohexamide, hydroxyhexamide, and chlorpropamide—have been shown to stimulate the prompt release of pancreatic insulin *in vivo* in both normals and mild diabetic patients (7, 24, 29, 40, 97, 99) and from the isolated pancreas *in vitro* (98). In the isolated perfused rat pancreas, a 2-minute tolbutamide pulse provokes a prompt release of insulin within 30 seconds which terminates 30 seconds after the disappearance of the stimulus, and the magnitude of this release appears to be concentration-related (99). During a continuous 60-minute tolbutamide infusion after the initial increase in insulin release, the rate of secretion declines rapidly to baseline levels within 4–5 minutes and remains at that level for the duration of the infusion (32, 99). The action of tolbutamide is weak in comparison to glucose in high concentrations (100), the enhancement of insulin release by glucose being approximately 5–10 times that of tolbutamide (24). Tolbutamide is also capable of causing pancreatic tissue already maximally stimulated by glucose to further increase its insulin output (16). Unlike glucose, which is capable of inducing not only the release of insulin but also its synthesis, tolbutamide is incapable of stimulating insulin synthesis and appears to release only preformed stores (24, 32), which may amount to 40% of the total granular insulin store (101). After stimulation by tolbutamide the pancreas is refractory to stimulation by glucose or tolbutamide (7, 100).

In the normal, pancreatic insulin stores are replenished within approximately 90 minutes. In contrast, the diabetic pancreas is refractory to glucose and tolbutamide for 8–29 hours, further evidence indicating the inability of the diabetic β-cell to rapidly replenish its insulin stores (7)—a capacity necessary for both phases of insulin release.

It has been observed that long-term sulfonylurea therapy in early diabetics leads to an improved glucose tolerance test without elevations of the plasma insulin levels (102). This has led several authors to hypothesize that chronic sulfonylurea therapy resulted in islet hypertrophy (103), but this has not been found experimentally (104). Furthermore, the rate of insulin release during fasting and in response to progressive hyperglycemia is not significantly enhanced or modified by tolbutamide (105–108). The fasting blood glucose concentration is significantly reduced by the sulfonylureas, however (108). It may be, therefore, that the long-term efficacy of the sulfonylureas stems not from their ability to release insulin but rather from their ability to reduce hepatic glucose output, inhibit lipolysis, and increase insulin-mediated peripheral utilization of glucose (102, 103, 109). Glucose is not required for the stimulation of insulin release by tolbutamide (96), nor will the presence of mannoheptulose inhibit its action (100). Diazoxide will inhibit the insulinogenic response to glucose (110, 111) but has no effect on the action of tolbutamide (111–113).

Tolbutamide, therefore, is not a true insulinogenic agent, being capable only of depleting most of the granular insulin reserve without affecting its replacement.

VIII. Other Hormones

Corticotropin (ACTH) provokes a rapid release of insulin from the isolated perfused rat pancreas (23). The insulinogenic response to ACTH is apparently delayed somewhat in comparison to the response to glucose (114). In the dog, an infusion of ACTH into the pancreatic artery leads to an increase in the plasma insulin levels measured in both the pancreatic vein and femoral artery (115).

Investigation into the mechanism of corticotropin-induced hypoglycemia in the mouse has disclosed that the hormone produces hyperketonemia, hyperfatty acidemia and hyperinsulinemia, all concomitantly. This increase in insulin activity is approximately 5–10 times baseline values and is inhibited by the simultaneous administration of D-mannoheptulose (116). Also, omission of glucose from slices of rabbit pancreas *in vitro* eliminates the insulinogenic response to corticotropin (92). The dose of ACTH producing maximum hypoglycemia in the mouse (5 μg) is nearly 1000 times that necessary to stimulate the adrenals and a 1.6 ng dose is able to stimulate adrenal cortical activity without elevations of insulin activity (117). Such observations would appear to deny ACTH any physiologic role in the regulation of insulin release *in vivo*. The hyperinsulinemia provoked by corticotropin is lost in the adrenalectomized mouse, but administration of corticosteroids will restore it (117). *In vitro* studies of the rat pancreas have shown that the release of insulin in response to glucose is not altered by the acute addition of methylprednisone to the incubation medium (118). Insulin secretion by the rat pancreas *in vivo* in response to hyperglycemia is diminished (up to 60%) by prior adrenalectomy and is increased by pretreatment with cortisone for 2–5 days (118). These hormonal manipulations are not accompanied by significant changes in pancreatic insulin content—an observation that prompted Malaisse to conclude that glucocorticoids act chronically in a permissive manner to enhance the sensitivity of the β-cell to stimulation by glucose (118).

In vitro, thyroid-stimulating hormone (THS) will also provoke the release of insulin by isolated pieces of rat pancreas, an effect dependent on the concentration of glucose in the medium (92). In contrast, the acute addition of thyroxine to such a preparation in no way modifies the insulinogenic response to glucose (119). In normal rats, the insulin response to hyperglycemia is diminished (up to 34%) by prior thyroidectomy, but thyroxine administration can restore the normal response (119). These modifications of insulin release in the thyroidectomized rat occur in the face of normal pancreatic insulin stores. Induction of hyperthyroidism, on the other hand, will not only deplete pancreatic insulin content but also impair pancreatic responsiveness to hyperglycemia (119).

Studies of the insulin response to growth hormone have been infrequent; however, Campbell and Rastogi (120) have studied this action of growth hormone fairly completely in the dog. Administered in a daily dosage of 2 mg/kg over a period of 1–2 weeks, growth hormone increases both the fasting plasma insulin level (up to 10 times) and the rate of insulin release in response to progressive increases in glycemia (up to 8 times) with prolonged maximal rates of release. This effect is manifest after only 1 day of treatment and disappears within 4 days after its cessation. In this instance, as is the case with the glucocorticoids, growth hormone apparently acts permissively, enhancing the sensitivity of the β-cell to stimulation by glucose.

Of further interest, is the finding that some of the prostaglandins (notably the E's) are capable of insulin release (121, 122) as is the placental lactogenic hormone (123). Two other peptide hormones, oxytocin and vasopressin, however, are ineffective (92).

IX. Pharmacologic Agents

Infusion of norepinephrine into man will blunt the insulinogenic effect of hyperglycemia and of tolbutamide, an effect which is subsequently reversed by withdrawal of the catecholamine (124). Conversely, infusion of isoproterenol in low doses stimulates the secretion of insulin without measurable changes in blood glucose concentrations and in the presence of nicotinic acid, a potent inhibitor of lipolysis (125, 126). Higher doses of isoproterenol (6 μg/min) further enhance insulinogenesis and lipolysis (in the absence of nicotinic acid) but elevate plasma glucose levels as well (126). Addition of propranolol to the infusion in small amounts (0.08 mg/min) blocks all these actions of isoproterenol but does not block the insulinogenic effect of glucagon (126). Addition of adrenergic amines to pieces of rat pancreas *in vitro* inhibits the insulin secretory response to glucose, and β-adrenergic blockers do not modify these results. On the other hand, α-adrenergic blockers are capable of reversing this inhibition and in fact augment the insulinogenic action of glucose when administered in concert with epinephrine (127). Mixed with an α-adrenergic-blocking agent, isoproterenol is an extraordinarily potent insulin secretagogue when added to the incubation medium with pieces of rat pancreas. This insulinogenic action is not detectable, however, in the absence of glucose in the medium and is dependent on the concentration of glucose (127).

The physiologic significance of these observations is interesting. In the fasting intact animal, the hypercatecholaminemia induced by hypoglycemia would stimulate hepatic glycogenolysis and lipolysis, and inhibit the secretion of insulin (128, 129), thereby switching the metabolic machinery to the use of fatty acids as the primary substrate while conserving glucose for use by the brain. Were the animal then to be refed, the oral ingestion of glucose would overcome the epinephrine-induced hypoinsulinemia (39, 65) and indirectly inhibit lipolysis and hepatic glucose output and stimulate the utilization of glucose.

Recently, the glucose tolerance tests of depressed patients have been observed to show significant improvement during antidepressive therapy with monoamine oxidasive (MAO) inhibitors (130). In the mouse, the intraperitoneal injection of 0.4 mg of tranylcypromine, a nonhydrazine MAO inhibitor, provokes a marked increase in the rate of insulin secretion, an effect which is potentiated by pretreatment with phentolamine, unaffected by reserpine, and inhibited by MJ1999, a potent β-adrenergic blocker (122). While declining to explain the MAOI-induced hypoglycemia on the basis of these results, Bressler *et al.* were able to conclude, nevertheless, that an inadequacy of the adrenergic homeostatic mechanism was not the proper explanation.

In the acutely adrenalectomized rat fasted for 48 hours, a 15 mg intravenous injection of theophylline elicits a rapid and significant elevation of plasma insulin, an effect which is greatly enhanced by the concomitant administration of epinephrine and an α-adrenergic blocker. In the presence of epinephrine and a β-blocker, however, theophylline is ineffectual (131). Further studies have shown the potent insulinogenic effect of theophylline and caffeine *in vitro* (40, 92, 132) and demonstrated the enhancement of their effect by further addition of glucagon or tolbutamide to the incubation mixture (132). This stimulatory potential of theophylline is abolished by the omission of glucose from or the addition of mannoheptulose or 2-deoxyglucose to the incubation medium (92). Furthermore, theophylline was found to stimulate insulin secretion in the absence of glucose only if glycogen could be demonstrated in the β-cell, and this effect was abolished by 2-deoxyglucose but not mannoheptulose (92).

The importance of adrenergic receptors in the mediation of insulin secretion is further highlighted by the observation that the inhibitory effect of diazoxide is partially reversed by α-adrenergic blockade (110), and the insulinogenic effect of prostaglandin E_1 is blocked by MJ1999 (122).

In the dog cervical vagotomy decreases the insulin content of portal vein plasma without significantly modifying plasma glucose concentrations and vagal stimulation increases immunoreactive insulin levels as much as 10 times. This response gradually declines, however, although glucagon is still able to cause a prompt increase in the rate of insulin secretion (133). Bethanecol or metacholine administered parenterally to the anesthetized dog elicits a rapid and significant elevation of immunoreactive insulin in pancreatic venous and femoral arterial plasma. Pretreatment with local pancreatic infusions of atropine abolished this response. Although infusions of metacholine or benthanecol induce an elevation of plasma glucose, this elevation follows the hyperinsulinemia (134). *In vitro*, cholinergic drugs will stimulate insulin release from slices of rat pancreas, an effect which is suppressed by the simultaneous administration of atropine (127). Of additional importance is the independence of this stimulatory effect on the concentration of glucose in the medium (127).

X. Insulin Synthesis and Storage

Like all proteins, the synthesis of insulin is commonly considered to take place in the rough endoplasmic reticulum (135). It has only recently been learned that insulin is apparently initially synthesized as a single chain protein or "proinsulin," which is then subsequently transformed to active insulin by enzymatic removal of a 32-residue polypeptide chain connecting the A and B chains of the future insulin molecule (136). When and exactly how this cleavage occurs is as yet unknown. After synthesis, the insulin is thought to be stored in membrane-bound sacs or granules, which form in the region of the Golgi apparatus and subsequently migrate to the periphery of the cell (135, 137, 138). In the granule, the insulin is precipitated by the presence of zinc in high concentrations (139). When the β-cell is stimulated the granules marginate about the internal lamina of the plasma membrane, and the membranes of a small number of the granules fuse with the plasma membrane. Rupture then occurs and the granule is expelled into Disse's space where it rapidly dissolves. As more of the granules are released, increasing numbers of microvilli are formed from the cytoplasm on either side of the now empty sacs (135, 137).

This hypothesis of emiocytosis has had its opponents as well as proponents. Findlay *et al.* were unable to detect any fusion of granular and plasma membranes after stimulation of rabbit β-cell with tolbutamide or glucose (138); others have declared the β-granule to be nonessential for the release of insulin (101).

Electron microscopy of β-cells stimulated with tolbutamide show depletion of granules but little activity in the Golgi region, an observation considered to support the idea that tolbutamide releases only preformed insulin stores and is incapable of stimulation of insulin synthesis (137).

Insulin does not regulate its own release. Chronic administration of exogenous insulin to the mouse will decrease total extractable pancreatic insulin, but its withdrawal does not blunt the islet's response to hyperglycemia (140). It may very well be that the decreased storage of insulin is not due to a feedback inhibition by insulin itself, but rather to the chronic reduction of the blood glucose by the exogenous insulin (140).

XI. Cations

In recent years, exhaustive attempts have been made to clarify the role of various extracellular cations in the insulin secretory process *in vitro*.

The addition of potassium to slices of rabbit pancreas in a concentration greater than 8 meq/liter will augment the insulinogenic action of glucose (23, 27, 141, 142) or tolbutamide (143) and will also stimulate insulin release in the absence of glucose and independently of any change in the osmolarity or sodium concentration of the medium (96). Associated with the stimulation of insulin release by glucose is an increased uptake of potassium (^{42}K) from the medium, a finding not obtained when tolbutamide is used (143). Howell has also found that under conditions of increased β-cell secretory activity, fluxes of K^+ do occur but are apparently nonessential for the hormonal release to occur (143).

Omission of K^+ from or addition of ouabain (10^{-5} M) to the incubation medium with slices of rabbit pancreas, manipulations which lead to the inhibition of the sodium-potassium membrane pump, will also stimulate insulin secretion in the absence of glucose (96). In addition, the insulinogenic actions of glucose, glucagon, L-leucine, tolbutamide, K^+, or ouabain are inhibited by the omission of Na^+ from the incubation medium (96).

In vitro stimulation of insulin secretion from adult or fetal rat pancreas by glucose, tolbutamide, ouabain, or K^+ is abolished by the omission of calcium from the incubation medium (27, 98, 141, 142) and inhibited by elevation of the calcium concentration to 10.2 meq/liter (141). Stimulation of insulin by glucose occurs at calcium concentrations as low as 0.2 meq/liter, increases proportionately as the calcium concentration is increased, and becomes maximal at concentrations of approximately 2–5 meq/liter (98, 142, 144). The action of tolbutamide is also dependent on the presence of extracellular calcium, but unlike glucose, its effect is enhanced by progressive increases of the calcium concentration up to 10 meq/liter (144). Calcium is necessary for both of the two phases of insulin secretion described by Curry *et al.*, but the absence of calcium does not adversely effect protein synthesis in the pancreas (32).

Recently, in studying the role of extracellular calcium in catecholamine release from the adrenal medulla, Jaanus found that propranolol, considered to be a classic β-adrenergic-blocking agent, was capable of inhibiting the stimulatory action of acetylcholine. It was his conclusion that in pharmacologic doses propranolol was acting as a local anesthetic to inhibit intracellular calcium fluxes and thereby inhibiting catecholamine release (145). In the mouse 0.25 mg of propranolol [doses approximately 10^4 times greater than those used by Porte (126)] will inhibit the insulinogenic effect of tolbutamide, glucose, ACTH, and glucagon (146). Replacement of calcium by an equivalent amount of barium (5 meq/liter) will transiently stimulate the secretion of insulin, an effect which is inhibited by calcium or large concentrations of magnesium (24 meq/liter) (141). Such observation led to the conclusion that irrespective of the stimulus to the release of insulin, there is an absolute requirement for the presence of extracellular calcium for the response to occur, but that this requirement for calcium may be fulfilled at least partially by other divalent cations.

The presence of extracellular magnesium is not a prerequisite for insulin secretion to occur and in fact high concentrations (24 meq/liter) are inhibitory (141).

XII. Cyclic 3′,5′-AMP

The metabolism of glucose as a necessary prerequisite for its insulinogenic effect has been emphasized, as has the recognition that an increase in the activity of any one of several different metabolic pathways may also serve as a necessary and sufficient stimulus. The diverse metabolic substances which can serve as stimuli to the insulin-secretory process suggest that some fundamental product of intermediary metabolism is responsible, irrespective of whether substrate utilization occurs via the HMP pathway, glycolysis, or fatty acid oxidation. Such basic metabolic products might be NADH, NADPH, or ATP; in fact all three of these substrates are capable of stimulating insulin secretion *in vitro* (147, 148). An alternative hypothesis, however, is that intermediates of the glycolytic or of other pathways mediate the insulinogenic action of the various substrates. It has been shown that the activity of the HMP shunt does not increase rapidly enough in response to glucose to account for the kinetics of insulin secretion (149), but this observation does not rule out its participation under other circumstances. An intermediate in the glycolytic pathway, fructose-1,6-diphosphate, has been found capable of stimulating lipolysis in isolated fat cells (150) and there is the possibility that it may mediate the secretory response of the β-cell as well. Against such a possibility is the fact that citrate infusions are known to inhibit phosphofructokinase (62), and xylitol has been shown to stimulate the release of insulin in the presence of 2-deoxyglucose (36). Such evidence would indicate that at least under these conditions fructose-1,6-diphosphate is not the effective stimulus to insulin release. 2,3-Diphosphoglyceric acid controls the level of adenosine monophosphate deaminase in the red cell (151) and may be capable of serving to control the enzymes involved in insulinogenesis. Such an hypothesis is engaging since there is rapid interconversion among intermediates of fructose metabolism (152), the HMP shunt, and the glycolytic pathway via the triose phosphates (153). In addition, these glycolytic intermediates might be expected to be elevated during utilization of fatty acids or ketone bodies as substrates if the β-cell were capable of gluconeogenesis. A choice between these hypotheses does not have to be made, and, in fact, both may be correct, emphasizing that the initial first step in insulin secretion may be a nonspecific increase in some aspect of the cell's metabolic activity.

In recent years intensive investigation has developed the concept that cyclic 3′,5′-adenosine monophosphate is an important intracellular messenger. Serotonin (154), glucagon, TSH, and vasopressin have been found to increase intracellular levels of cyclic 3′,5′-AMP and are considered to bring about some of their various actions via this mechanism (92, 154–158). In the adrenal cortex, the initial response to ACTH is the elevation of cyclic 3′,5′-AMP followed by activation of phosphorylase and a subsequent increase in secretory activity (159, 190). The prostaglandins are also considered to mediate their cellular effects through elevations of intracellular cyclic 3′,5′-AMP (121). Addition of epinephrine to epididymal fat pads *in vitro* increases intracellular cyclic 3′,5′-AMP while stimulating lipolysis (161). Theophylline and caffeine, inhibitors of phosphodiesterase, the enzyme responsible for the breakdown of cyclic 3′,5′-AMP (162), also increase intracellular cyclic 3′,5′-AMP and will enhance the lipolytic action of epinephrine (161). Epinephrine and theophylline are able to facilitate neuromuscular transmission, an action also considered to be mediated by intracellular cyclic 3′,5′-AMP (163). In general, it is considered that α-adrenergic agents decrease whereas β-adrenergic agents increase the levels of intracellular cyclic 3′,5′-AMP (164).

The cellular levels of cyclic 3′,5′-AMP are controlled by the membrane-bound enzyme, adenylcyclase (27, 158), which mediates its synthesis, and phosphodiesterase which effects its degradation (as noted above) (162).

The cellular effects of cyclic 3′,5′-AMP are legion. It was first recognized as the mediator of the glycogenolytic effects of epinephrine by activation of muscle phosphorylase (165, 166). Among other things, the activity of the key glycolytic enzyme, phosphofructokinase, the rate of glucose oxidation, and cellular permeability are all increased by elevation of intracellular cyclic 3′,5′-AMP (157, 167). (For reviews see 154–158.)

It has been recently proposed by Rasmussen and Tennenhouse that hormones which stimulate adenylcyclase do not mediate their effects by the intracellular influence of cyclic 3′,5′-AMP per se, but rather do so by formation of cyclic 3′,5′-AMP from membrane-bound ATP, thereby enhancing cellular permeability to calcium by virtue of the hydrolysis of membrane calcium-ATP complexes (168).

Such speculations prompted investigation into the biologic properties of cyclic 3′,5′-AMP itself. Cyclic AMP will mimic the lipolytic effects of epinephrine on isolated fat cells *in vitro* (161) and will stimulate the release of insulin from the isolated rabbit pancreas, also *in vitro* (23, 92, 114). This insulinogenic effect of cyclic 3′,5′-AMP can be abolished by the omission of glucose or calcium from the incubation mixture (92). Furthermore, the stimulatory effect of theophylline is inhibited by 2-deoxyglucose in the presence of demonstrable β-cell glycogen or by mannoheptulose in its absence (92). From such evidence it seems that the mechanism proposed by Rasmussen for the action of adenylcyclase is untenable for the β-cell, since not only can cyclic 3′,5′-AMP itself stimulate insulin secretion, but also those agents which activate adenyl cyclase cannot release insulin in the absence of glucose or glycogen as a substrate.

The question of how an increase in the metabolism of the β-cell is coupled to the insulin secretory mechanism remains as yet unanswered.

XIII. β-Cell Secretion Hypothesis

The dependence of the insulin secretory process on the presence of certain extracellular cations and the similarity of the β-cell cytoplasmic granules to the synaptic vesicles of neurons suggest that the β-cell and perhaps other secretory cells are functioning as quasi-nerve cells.

Stimulation of the adrenal medulla results in an extracellular increase of specific vesicle proteins paralleling the increases in catecholamine release, evidence that Kirshner has considered to support the concept that catecholamines are released from granules or storage sacs directly to the exterior of the cell (169). This process is calcium-dependent and requires ATP (169, 170). Similarly, the transmission across the myoneural junction is also calcium-dependent (171, 172).

It has been demonstrated that acetylcholine will stimulate catecholamine release from the adrenal medulla even in the absence of extracellular sodium or potassium, indicating that an intracellular flux of calcium is of primary importance in the extrusion of the granular contents (173). This result was obtained under extremely severe *in vitro* conditions, and its physiologic significance may be open to question. Under more physiologic conditions, Baker and Blaustein have found that the Ca^{++} uptake by crab nerve is very dependent on the intracellular concentration of sodium (174). They concluded that small cellular influxes of Na^+ could lead to marked changes in cellular calcium which would be of metabolic significance.

The importance of a cellular influx of calcium for the release of the synaptic vesicle or β-cell granule is reminiscent of the stimulation of muscle contraction by the release of calcium from the sarcoplasmic reticulum (175, 176), and suggests the possibility of a Ca^{++} dependent ATPase. Such an ATPase has been found in synaptic vesicles (177), and apparently in the leukocyte (178). Woodin and Wieneke have theorized that a cellular influx of calcium resulted from the administration of a staphylococcal leukocidin which induced depolarization of the cell. They further hypothesized that this increase in intracellular calcium activated the granular ATPase which subsequently effected the hydrolysis of membrane Ca-ATP complexes and led to the extrusion of the contents of the granule, as if the granule were digesting its way out of the leukocyte (178). Such a concept now appears somewhat simplistic. In the frog synapse, the rate of transmitter release is dependent on the presence of divalent cations and on the ability of these cations to enter the axonal membrane (179). The divalent cations (Mg^{++} and Be^{++}) which penetrate the cell poorly will inhibit an increase in the rate of transmitter release in response to an action potential (179). In the absence of Ca^{++}, however, Mg^{++} may partially substitute for Ca^{++} and lanthanum^{+++} and thorium^{++} are even more effective in facilitating transmitter release than calcium (179). It has also been found that artificial membranes will adhere in the presence of these cations—those cations with the higher valence being the most effective (179). From these observations Blioch *et al.* have theorized that one function of the cellular influx of calcium would be to reduce the electrical repulsion forces between synaptic vesicle and plasma membrane leading to their fusion (179).

The demonstration of a calcium-dependent ATPase in synaptic vesicles confers no information about the process to which it is coupled, but merely suggests that the utilization of ATP is stimulated by increases of calcium within the cell. One result of a cellular influx of calcium might be the activation of a membrane transport to pump calcium back outside the cell. Such a pump does exist in the human red cell (180) and in isolated sarcoplasmic reticulum (181). It may also be that calcium stimulates the energy-dependent incorporation of labeled phosphate into phospholipids (182), suggesting that another function of increased intracellular calcium may be the stimulation of membrane turnover.

Recently Dean and Matthews undertook to study the membrane potential fluctuations of the β-cell in response to glucose, tolbutamide, and leucine. In unstimulated cells they found that the membrane potential averaged about –20 millivolts (mV) and was subject to small, rapid, random fluctuations. Within 2 minutes after exposure to tolbutamide rhythmic action potentials of 1–4 mV occurred with a periodicity of 0.950 second. After 40 minutes the membrane potential decreased to approximately −10 mV, action potential production ceased, and no repolarization was apparent 90 minutes after the drug had been washed out. Similarly, islets treated with glucose or L-leucine provoked action potentials within 2 minutes. These action potentials, however, were irregular in comparison to those induced by tolbutamide and often occurred in bursts. In contrast to tolbutamide, removal of glucose or leucine was followed by a return of the membrane potential to its resting state. Moreover, continued stimulation by glucose or leucine was not accompanied by the cessation of action potential production seen at 30–40 minutes with tolbutamide (183).

These data suggest that insulin secretion may occur as follows: As previously discussed, the rate of glucose oxidation by the β-cell is linearly related to the extracellular glucose concentration even at very high concentrations. Hyperglycemia, therefore, would augment the metabolic rate of the β-cell and elevate intracellular levels of NADH, NADPH, ATP, or some other intermediate whose immediate or secondary effect would be to either inhibit the sodium-potassium pump or so affect the sodium and potassium membrane conductances that the cell would depolarize. Accompanying the sodium influx would be an influx of calcium which could have two effects. The first of these would be to neutralize the repulsion between granules and plasma membranes, perhaps by neutralizing the negative charges on one of them, and thereby cause adhesion between the granule and plasma membrane as proposed for the synaptic vesicle by Blioch *et al.* (179). Fusion of the two membranes would be followed by the stimulation by calcium of local membrane synthesis and turnover leading to degeneration of the area of fusion and extrusion of the granular contents to the exterior of the cell. Increased phospholipid synthesis and incorporation of the granule membrane into the plasma membrane would explain the increased number of microvilli seen on the secretory surface of active β-cells. Subsequently, the calcium influx would also stimulate a membrane pump leading to the expulsion of calcium from the cell. Decrease of the sodium conductance would follow and cause repolarization of the cell. Finally, the removal of intracellular calcium and repolarization of the cell would then lead to restoration of the membrane to a resting state capable of immediately releasing a second granule if the insulinogenic stimulus remained.

Tolbutamide is known to cause only a transient release of insulin, after which the β-cell remains refractory. This suggests several things. First, continued depolarization of the cell is effective in releasing insulin only if the intracellular insulin pool is being replenished by synthesis, which tolbutamide does not stimulate. Second, the refractoriness to tolbutamide may be due not only to depleted insulin stores but also to the prolonged depolarization. Third, tolbutamide must have an irreversible effect on membrane conductance. The failure of the ability of the β-cell to produce action potentials in response to prolonged exposure to tolbutamide indicates that in addition to a direct effect on sodium conductance, tolbutamide must be capable of adversely affecting the sodium pump, leading to the eventual intracellular buildup of sodium with a concomitant fall in membrane potential.

On the other hand, the reversibility of the depolarization induced by glucose suggests that not only is the mediator of insulin secretion in these conditions intracellular but also is capable of being removed (through further metabolism).

The release of insulin by acetylcholine would occur by primary depolarization of the β-cell without stimulating insulin synthesis, just as is the case for tolbutamide. It would not be expected, however, to produce a prolonged depolarization after removal since the β-cell most likely should be able to effect its degradation fairly rapidly. Furthermore, acetylcholine would not be expected to inhibit the Na-K membrane pump.

Finally leucine may exert a direct membrane effect similar to that found in HeLa cells (184), resulting in an inhibition of the Na-K membrane pump and an initiation of the cellular events mediating the release of insulin.

REFERENCES

1. Mering and Minkowski, *Arch. Exptl. Pathol. Pharmakol. Navnyn-Schmiedebergs* **26**, 371 (1889).
2. Banting, F. G., and Best, C. H., *J. Lab. Clin. Med.* **7**, 251 (1922).
3. Elliott, R. B., O'Brien, D., and Roy, C. C., *Diabetes* **14**, 780 (1965).
4. Roy, C., Shapcott, D. J., and O'Brien, D., *Diabetologia* **4**, 133 (1968).
5. Kimmel, J. R., and Pollock, H. G., *Diabetes* **16**, 687 (1967).
6. Karam, J. H., Grodsky, G., Pavalatos, F., and Forsham, P., *Lancet* **i**, 286 (1965).
7. Pfeiffer, E., *in* "Tolbutamide After Ten Years" (W. J. H. Butterfield and W. van Westering, eds.) p. 127. Excerpta Med. Found., Amsterdam, 1967.
8. Bagdade, J. D., Bierman, E. L., and Porte, D., Jr., *J. Clin. Invest.* **46**, 1549 (1967).
9. Seltzer, H. S., Allen, E. W., Herron, A. L., and Brennan, N. T., *J. Clin. Invest.* **46**, 323 (1967).
10. Seltzer, H. S., and Allen, E. W., *J. Lab. Clin. Med.* **62**, 1014 (1963).
11. Malaisse, W., Malaisse-Lagae, F., and Coleman, D., *Metab. Clin. Exptl.* **17**, 802 (1968).
12. Simpson, R. G., Benedetti, A., Grodsky, G. N., Karam, J. H., and Forsham, P. H., *Diabetes* **17**, 684 (1968).
13. Forbath, N., and Hetenyi, G., Jr., *Diabetes* **15**, 778 (1966).
14. Ricketts, H. T., Cherry, R. A., and Kirstein, L., *Diabetes* **15**, 880 (1966).
15. Howell, S. L., and Taylor, K. W., *Lancet* **i**, 128 (1966).
16. Ryan, W. G., and Schwartz, T. B., *Diabetes* **16**, 514 (1967). Abstr.
17. Garcia, M. J., Soeldner, J. S., Gleason, R. E., and Williams, R. F., *J. Clin. Invest.* **45**, 1010 (1966). Abstr.
18. Luft, R., *New Engl. J. Med.* **279**, 1086 (1968).
19. Cerasi, E., and Luft, R., *Diabetes* **16**, 651 (1967).
20. Schochat, G., and Willansky, D., *Metab. Clin. Exptl.* **17**, 928 (1968).
21. Karam, J. H., Pavalatos, F., and Forsham, P., *Lancet* **i**, 290 (1965).
22. Vance, J. E., Buchanan, K. D., Challoner, D. R., and Williams, R. H., *Diabetes* **17**, 187 (1968).
23. Sussman, K. E., Vaughn, P. D., and Timmer, R. F., *Diabetes* **15**, 521 (1966). Abstr.

24. Seltzer, H. S., *J. Clin. Invest.* **41**, 289 (1962).
25. Williams, R. H., and Ensinck, J. W., *Diabetes* **15**, 623 (1966).
26. Grodsky, G. N., Bennett, L. L., Smith, D. F., and Nemechek, K., *Diabetes* **16**, 509 (1967). Abstr.
27. Grodsky, G. N., and Bennett, L. L., *J. Clin. Invest.* **45**, 1018 (1966). Abstr.
28. Grodsky, G. N., and Bennett, L. L., *Diabetes* **15**, 521 (1966). Abstr.
29. Grodsky, G. N., Bennett, L. L., Smith, D. F., and Nemechek, K., *in* "Tolbutamide After Ten Years" (W. J. H. Butterfield and W. van Westering, eds.), p. 11. Excerpta Med. Found., Amsterdam, 1967.
30. Malaisse, W. J., Malaisse-Lagae, F., and King, S., *J. Lab. Clin. Med.* **71**, 56 (1968).
31. Howell, S. L., and Taylor, K. W., *Biochem. J.* **102**, 922 (1967).
32. Curry, D. L., Bennett, L. L., and Grodsky, G. N., *Endocrinology* **83**, 572 (1968).
33. Coore, H. G., and Randle, P. J., *Biochem. J.* **91**, 56 (1964).
34. Malaisse, W. J., Lea, N. A., and Malaisse-Lagae, F., *Metab. Clin. Exptl.* **17**, 126 (1968).
35. Wick, A. N., Drury, D. R., Nakada, H. I., and Wolfe, J. D., *J. Biol. Chem.* **224**, 963 (1957).
36. Montague, W., Howell, S. L., and Taylor, K. W., *Nature* **215**, 1088 (1967).
37. Simon, E., Kraicer, P. F., and Shelessnyack, N. C., *Nature* **197**, 1264 (1963).
38. Ashcroft, S. J. H., and Randle, P. J., *Lancet* **i**, 278 (1968).
39. Karam, J. H., Grasso, S. G., Wegienka, L. C., Grodsky, G. N., and Forsham, B. H., *Diabetes* **15**, 571 (1966).
40. Ashcroft, S. J. H., Coll-Garcia, E., Gill, J. R., and Randle, P. J., *Diabetologia* **4**, 178 (1968). Abstr.
41. Hellerström, C., *Diabetologia* **4**, 178 (1968). Abstr.
42. Crofford, O. B., and Renold, A. E., *J. Biol. Chem.* **240**, 3237 (1965).
43. Alvardo, F., and Crane, R. K., *Biochim. Biophys. Acta* **56**, 170 (1962).
44. Field, A. B., Johnson, P., Herring, B., and Weinberg, A. N., *Nature* **185**, 468 (1960).
45. Grodsky, G. N., *Diabetes* **15**, 281 (1966).
46. Jarrett, R. J., and Keen, H., *Metab. Clin. Exptl.* **17**, 155 (1968).
47. Goetz, F. C., Manuy, J. W., and Zoske, A. R., *Diabetes* **16**, 511 (1967). Abstr.
48. Hiratta, Y., Fujisawa, M., Sata, H., Asano, T., and Katsaki, S., *Biochem. Biophys. Res. Commun.* **24**, 471 (1966).
49. Randle, P. J., Garland, P. B., Hales, C. N., and Newsholme, E. A., *Lancet* **i**, 785 (1963).
50. Randle, P. J., *Postgrad. Med. J.* **40**, 457 (1964).
51. Mebane, D., and Madison, L. L., *J. Clin. Invest.* **41**, 1383 (1962). Abstr.
52. Madison, L. L., Mebane, D., Unger, R. H., and Lochner, A., *J. Clin. Invest.* **43**, 408 (1964).
53. Greenough, W. B., Crespin, S. R., and Steinberg, D., *Lancet* **ii**, 1237 (1967).
54. Madison, L. L., Seyffert, W. A., Unger, R. H., and Barker, B., *Metab. Clin. Exptl.* **17**, 301 (1968).
55. Seyffert, W. A., and Madison, L. L., *Diabetes* **16**, 765 (1967).
56. Editorial, *Nutr. Rev.* **25**, 342 (1962).
57. Madison, L. L., Unpublished observations, 1967.
58. Balasse, E., and Ooms, H. A., *Diabetologia* **4**, 133 (1968).
59. Sanbar, S. S., Hetenyi, G., Forbath, N., and Evans, J. R., *Metab. Clin. Exptl.* **14**, 1311 (1965).
60. Greenberger, N. J., Tzagournis, N., and Graves, T. N., *Metab. Clin. Exptl.* **17**, 796 (1968).

61. Montague, W., and Taylor, K. W., *Nature* **217**, 853 (1968).
62. Garland, P. B., Randle, P. J., and Newsholme, E. A., *Nature* **200**, 169 (1963).
63. Mansour, T. E., *Pharmacol. Rev.* **18**, 173 (1966).
64. McIntyre, N., Holdsworth, C. A., and Turner, D. S., *Lancet* **ii**, 20 (1964).
65. Langs, H. N., and Friedberg, D., *Clin. Res.* **14**, 283 (1966). Abstr.
66. Samols, E., Marri, G., Tyler, J., and Marks, B., *Lancet* **ii**, 1257 (1965).
67. Samols, E., Marri, G., and Marks, B., *Lancet* **ii**, 415 (1965).
68. Brech, W. J., Kaess, H., Schlierf, G., and Rohs, M., *Klin. Wochschr.* **46**, 449 (1968).
69. Jarrett, R. J., and Cohen, N. M., *Lancet* **ii**, 861 (1967).
70. Deckert, T., *Acta Endocrinol.* **57**, 578 (1968).
71. Jarrett, R. J., and Cohen, N. M., *Diabetologia* **4**, 175 (1968).
72. Unger, R. H., Ohneda, A., Valverde, I., Eisentraut, A. N., and Exton, J., *J. Clin. Invest.* **47**, 48 (1968).
73. Dupre, J., *Lancet* **ii**, 672 (1964).
74. Ketterer, H., Ohneda, A., Dupre, J., Eisentraut, A. N., and Unger, R. H., *J. Lab. Clin. Med.* **68**, 888 (1966). Abstr.
75. Dupre, J., Rojas, L., White, J. J., Unger, R. H., and Boch, J. C., *Lancet* **ii**, 26 (1966).
76. Unger, R. H., Ketterer, H., Eisentraut, A. N., and Dupre, J., *Lancet* **ii**, 24 (1966).
77. Pfeiffer, E. F., and Raplis, S., *Klin. Wochschr.* **46**, 337 (1968).
78. Unger, R. H., and Eisentraut, A. N., Unpublished observations, 1967.
79. Nelson, J. K., Rabinowitz, D., and Merimee, T. J., *Diabetologia* **4**, 174 (1968).
80. Floyd, J. C., Jr., Fajans, S. S., Knopf, R. F., and Conn, J. W., *J. Clin. Invest.* **42**, 1714 (1963).
81. Floyd, J. C., Jr., Fajans, S. S., Knopf, R. F., Rull, J., and Conn, J. W., *Clin. Res.* **13**, 323 (1965). Abstr.
82. Floyd, J. C., Jr., Fajans, S. S., Conn, J. W., Knopf, R. F., and Rull, J., *J. Clin. Invest.* **45**, 1487 (1966).
83. Rabinowitz, D., Merimee, T. J., Maffezzoli, R., and Burgess, J. A., *Lancet* **ii**, 454 (1966).
84. Floyd, J. C., Jr., Fajans, S. S., Conn, J. W., Thiffault, C., Knopf, R. F., and Guntsche, E., *Endocrinology* **28**, 266 (1968).
85. Merimee, T. J., Burgess, J. A., and Rabinowitz, D., *Lancet* **i**, 1300 (1966).
86. Floyd, J. C., Jr., Fajans, S. S., Thiffault, C., Knopf, R. F., Guntsche, E., and Conn, J. W., *Clin. Res.* **14**, 280 (1966). Abstr.
87. Berger, S., and Vongaraya, N., *Diabetes* **15**, 303 (1966).
88. Copinschi, G., Wegienka, L. C., Hane, S., and Forsham, P. H., *Metab. Clin. Exptl.* **16**, 485 (1967).
89. Ohneda, A., Parada, E., Eisentraut, A. N., and Unger, R. H., *J. Clin. Invest.* **47**, 2305 (1968).
90. Floyd, J. C., Fajans, S. S., Pek, S., Thiffault, T. C. A., Knopf, R. F., and Conn, J. W., *Diabetes* **16**, 510 (1967). Abstr.
91. Fajans, S. S., Floyd, J. C., Knopf, R. F., Guntsche, E. M., Rull, J. A., Thiffault, C. A., and Conn, J. W., *Endocrinology* **27**, 1600 (1967).
92. Malaisse, W. J., Malaisse-Lagae, F., and Mayhew, D., *J. Clin. Invest.* **46**, 1724 (1967).
93. Turner, D. S., and McIntyre, N., *Lancet* **i**, 351 (1966).
94. Samols, E., Marri, G., and Marks, V., *Diabetes* **15**, 855 (1966).
95. Crockford, P. N., Porte, D., Jr., Wood, F. C., Jr., and Williams, R. H., *Metab. Clin. Exptl.* **15**, 114 (1966).
96. Hales, C. N., and Milner, R. D. G., *J. Physiol.* (*London*) **194**, 725 (1968).
97. Yu, T., Berger, L., and Gutman, A. B., *Metab. Clin. Exptl.* **17**, 309 (1968).

98. Hales, C. N., and Milner, R. D. G., *Diabetologia* **3**, 47 (1967).
99. Grodsky, G. N., Bennett, L. L., Smith, D. S., and Nemechek, K., *Diabetes* **16**, 509 (1967). Abstr.
100. Malaisse, W. J., Malaisse-Lagae, F., Mayhew, D. A., and Wright, P. H., *in* "Tolbutamide After Ten Years" (W. J. H. Butterfield and W. van Westering, eds.) p. 49. Excerpta Med. Found., Amsterdam, 1967.
101. Creutzfeldt, W., Fririchs, H., and Creutzfeldt, C., *in* "Tolbutamide After Ten Years" (W. J. H. Butterfield and W. van Westering, eds.) p. 34. Excerpta Med. Found., Amsterdam, 1967.
102. Chu, P. C., Conway, N. J., Krouse, H. A., and Goodner, C. J., *Ann. Internal. Med.* **68**, 757 (1968).
103. Davidoff, F., *New Engl. J. Med.* **278**, 148 (1968).
104. Sussman, K. E., Stjernholm, M., and Vaughn, P. D., *Diabetes* **16**, 511 (1967). Abstr.
105. Crofford, O. B., and Renold, A. E., *J. Biol. Chem.* **240**, 3237 (1967).
106. Chiumello, G., Del Guercio, M. J., and Bidone, G., *Diabetes* **17**, 133 (1968).
107. Nielson, R. L., Reeves, R. L., and Crampton, J. H., *Diabetes* **16**, 542 (1966). Abstr.
108. Wales, J. K., Grant, A. M., and Wolff, F. W., *Lancet* **i**, 1137 (1967).
109. Stone, D. V., and Brown, J. D., *in* "Tolbutamide After Ten Years" (W. J. H. Butterfield and W. van Westering, eds.), p. 202. Excerpta Med Found., Amsterdam, 1967.
110. Wong, K. K., Synchovicz, S., Stauv, N. S., and Tabachmick, I. I. A., *Life Sci.* **6**, 2285 (1967).
111. Howell, S. L., and Taylor, K. W., *Lancet* **i**, 128 (1966).
112. Blackard, W. G., and Aprill, C. N., *J. Lab. Clin. Med.* **69**, 960 (1967).
113. Seltzer, H. S., and Crout, J. R., *Diabetes* **15**, 523 (1966). Abstr.
114. Sussman, K. E., and Vaughn, P. D., *Diabetes* **16**, 449 (1967).
115. Ohsawa, M., Kuzuya, T., Tanioka, T., Kanazawa, Y., Ibayoshi, H., and Nakao, K., *Endocrinology* **81**, 975 (1967).
116. Genuth, S., and Lebovitz, H. E., *Endocrinology* **76**, 1093 (1965).
117. Lundquist, I., and Rerup, C., *Acta Endocrinol.* **56**, 713 (1967).
118. Malaisse, W. J., Malaisse-Lagae, F., McCraw, E. F., and Wright, P. H., *Proc. Soc. Exptl. Biol. Med.* **124**, 924 (1967).
119. Malaisse, W. J., Malaisse-Lagae, F., and McCraw, E. F., *Diabetes* **16**, 643 (1967).
120. Campbell, J., and Rastogi, K. S., *Diabetes* **15**, 749 (1966).
121. Bergeström, S., Carlson, F. A., and Weeks, J. R., *Pharmacol. Rev.* **20**, 1 (1968).
122. Bressler, R., Vargas-Cordon, M., and Lebovitz, H. E., *Diabetes* **17**, 617 (1968).
123. Kalkhoff, R., Schalch, D. S., Walker, J. L., Beck, P., Kipnis, D. N., and Daughaday, W. H., *Trans. Assoc. Am. Physicians* **77**, 270 (1964).
124. Porte, D., and Williams, R. F., *Science* **152**, 1248 (1966).
125. Porte, D., Jr., *Diabetes* **15**, 543 (1966). Abstr.
126. Porte, D., Jr., *Diabetes* **16**, 150 (1967).
127. Malaisse, W. J., Malaisse-Lagae, F., Wright, D. H., and Ashemore, J., *Endocrinology* **80**, 975 (1967).
128. Abramson, E. A., and Arky, R. A., *Diabetes* **17**, 141 (1968).
129. Abramson, E. A., Arky, R. A., and Woaber, K. A., *Lancet* **ii**, 1386 (1966).
130. Adnitt, P. I., *Diabetes* **17**, 628 (1968).
131. Turtle, J. R., Littleton, G. K., and Kipnis, D. M., *Nature* **213**, 723 (1967).
132. Lambert, A. E., Jeanrenaud, B., and Renold, A. E., *Lancet* **i**, 819 (1967).
133. Frohman, L. A., Ezdinli, E. Z., and Javid, R., *Diabetes* **15**, 522 (1966). Abstr.
134. Kaneto, A., Kajinuma, H., Kosaka, K., and Nakao, K., *Endocrinology* **83**, 651 (1968).
135. Lacy, P. E., *New Engl. J. Med.* **276**, 187 (1967).

136. Chance, R. E., Ellis, R. N., and Bromer, W., *Science* **161**, 165 (1968).
137. Williamson, J. R., Lacy, P. E., and Gisham, J. W., *Diabetes* **10**, 460 (1961).
138. Findlay, J. A., Gill, J. R., Irvin, G., Lever, J. D., and Randle, P. J., *Diabetologia* **4**, 150 (1968).
139. Falkmer, S., and Pihl, E., *Diabetologia* **4**, 239 (1968).
140. Chu, P. C., and Goodner, C. J., *Endocrinology* **82**, 296 (1968).
141. Hales, C. N., and Milner, R. D. G., *J. Physiol.* (*London*) **199**, 177 (1968).
142. Grodsky, G. N., and Bennett, L. L., *Diabetes* **15**, 910 (1966).
143. Howell, S. L., *Diabetologia* **4**, 177 (1968). Abstr.
144. Curry, D. L., Bennett, L. L., and Grodsky, G. N., *Am. J. Physiol.* **214**, 174 (1968).
145. Jaanus, S. D., Miele, E., and Rubin, R. P., *Brit. J. Pharmacol.* **31**, 319 (1967).
146. Bressler, R., Vargas-Cordon, M., and Brendel, K., *Diabetes* **18**, 262 (1969).
147. Chiumello, G., Del Guercio, M. J., and Bidone, G., *Diabetes* **17**, 133 (1968).
148. Watkins, D., Cooperstein, S. J., Dixit, C. K., and Lazaarow, A., *Science* **162**, 283 (1968).
149. Matschinsky, F. N., Kauffman, F. C., and Ellerman, G. E., *Diabetes* **17**, 475 (1968).
150. Chlouverakis, C., *Metab. Clin. Exptl.* **17**, 708 (1968).
151. Askari, A., and Rao, S. N., *Biochim. Biophys. Acta* **151**, 198 (1968).
152. Heinz, F., Lamprecht, W., and Kirsch, G., *J. Clin. Invest.* **47**, 1826 (1968).
153. White, A., Handler, P., and Smith, E. F., "Principles of Biochemistry". McGraw-Hill, New York, 1964.
154. Williamson, G. R., Wright, P. H., Malaisse, W. J., and Ashmore, J., *Biochem. Biophys. Res. Commun.* **24**, 765 (1966).
155. Sutherland, E. W., and Robison, G. A., *Pharmacol. Rev.* **18**, 145 (1966).
156. Sutherland, E. W., Robison, G. A., and Butcher, R. W., *Circulation* **37**, 279 (1968).
157. Robison, G. A., Butcher, R. W., and Sutherland, E. W., *Ann. Rev. Biochem.* **37**, 149 (1968).
158. Sutherland, E. W., *Recent Progr. Hormone Res.* **21**, 623 (1965).
159. Haynes, R. C., Jr., *J. Biol. Chem.* **233**, 1220 (1958).
160. Vilchey, I., and Cholvarojian, A. N., *Metab. Clin. Exptl.* **17**, 725 (1968).
161. Butcher, R. W., Ho, R. J., Mengz, H. C., and Sutherland, E. W., *J. Biol. Chem.* **240**, 4515 (1965).
162. Butcher, R. W., and Sutherland, E. W., *J. Biol. Chem.* **237**, 1244 (1962).
163. Breckenridge, B. N., Burn, J. H., and Matschinsky, F. N., *Proc. Natl. Acad. Sci. U.S.* **57**, 1893 (1967).
164. Turtle, J. R., and Kipnis, B. N., *Biochem. Biophys. Res. Commun.* **48**, 797 (1967).
165. Huijing, F., and Larner, J., *Proc. Natl. Acad. Sci. U.S.* **56**, 647 (1966).
166. Ozawa, E., *J. Biochem.* (*Tokyo*) **62**, 285 (1967).
167. Mansour, T. E., *Pharmacol. Rev.* **18**, 173 (1966).
168. Rasmussen, H., and Tennenhouse, A., *Proc. Natl. Acad. Sci. U.S.* **59**, 1364 (1968).
169. Kirshner, N., Sage, H. J., and Smith, W. J., *Mol. Pharmacol.* **3**, 254 (1967).
170. Kirshner, N., and Smith, W. J., *Science* **159**, 422 (1966).
171. Colomo, F., and Rahamimoff, R., *J. Physiol.* (*London*) **198**, 203 (1968).
172. Hubbard, J. I., Jones, S. F., and Landau, E. M., *J. Physiol.* (*London*) **194**, 355 (1968).
173. Douglas, W. W., and Rubin, R. P., *J. Physiol.* (*London*) **167**, 288 (1963).
174. Baker, P. F., and Blaustein, N. P., *Biochim. Biophys. Acta* **150**, 167 (1968).
175. Scales, B., and McIntosh, D., Jr., *Pharmacol. Exptl. Therap.* **160**, 249 (1968).
176. Martonosi, A., and Feretos, R., *J. Biol. Chem.* **239**, 648 (1964).
177. Kadota, K., Mori, S., and Imaizumi, R., *J. Biol. Chem.* **61**, 424 (1964).
178. Woodin, H. N., and Wieneke, A. A., *Biochem. J.* **90**, 498 (1964).

179. Blioch, Z., Glagoleva, I., Liberman, E., and Nenaschev, V., *J. Physiol.* (*London*) **199**, 11 (1968).
180. Schatzman, H. J., *Experientia* **22**, 364 (1966).
181. Fanburg, B. L., *J. Clin. Invest.* **47**, 2499 (1968).
182. Karnovsky, M. L., and Wallach, D. F. H., *J. Biol. Chem.* **236**, 1895 (1961).
183. Dean, P. M., and Matthews, E. K., *Nature* **219**, 389 (1968).
184. Mohri, T., Dynashiki, T., Furuno, I., and Kitayawa, H., *Biochim. Biophys. Acta* **150**, 537 (1968).

Antineoplastic Principles in Plants: Recent Developments in the Field

JONATHAN L. HARTWELL AND BETTY J. ABBOTT

Cancer Chemotherapy National Service Center, National Cancer Institute, National Institutes of Health, U.S. Public Health Service, Bethesda, Maryland

I. Introduction

The earliest record, known to the writers, of plants being recommended for what is believed to be cancer is the Ebers papyrus of Egypt (Joachim, 1890; Ebbell, 1937) dating from about 1550 B.C. but representing an already high development of medicine from far earlier times. Since that time there has been a constantly expanding use, both popular and iatric, of plants for the treatment of cancer throughout the ages, until at the present time there is hardly an area of the world where plants in some form are not administered for this disease. According to a recent survey (Hartwell, 1967, 1968) the list of plant species so used has grown to a total of over 3000.

Beginning about 25 years ago organic chemists undertook seriously to investigate this branch of natural products as a source of useful anticancer drugs.

The effort has since come to embrace groups of investigators in several different countries. The persistence of popular healers and medical practitioners, and more recently of modern researchers in different disciplines of science, documented for three and one-half millenia, was finally rewarded by the development of the first clinically useful drug of plant origin, vincaleukoblastine (vinblastine; velban), in 1958 (cf. Neuss *et al.*, 1964). Beside vincaleukoblastine there are now four other drugs of plant origin rated (Goldin *et al.*, 1966) as having established clinical antitumor activity: demecolcine (*N*-deacetyl-*N*-methylcolchicine; omain), leurocristine (vincristine; oncovin), colchicine, and *N*-deacetylcolchicine (trimethylcolchicinic acid methyl ether).

The only recent reviews of the present subject known to the writer are Balitskii *et al.* (1966, written in Russian), valuable for its emphasis on Slavic and Chinese work, and Neuss *et al.* (1967) which also discusses antitumor agents from microorganisms and from animal sources. A recent symposium on tumor inhibitors from plant sources is available in abstract form (American Chemical Society, 1966). A valuable review on the biological and phytochemical screening of plants gives a table listing some 400 species of plants from which antineoplastic activity has been reported (Farnsworth, 1966).

II. Scope of the Present Report

A. Definitions

In reviewing recent progress in this field it is necessary to define the limits. By "plants" will be meant those that are commonly called higher plants and ferns or, more properly, spermatophytes (phanerogams) and pteridophytes. Lower forms, including algae, fungi, mosses, bacteria, etc., will be excluded, except in a few cases where appropriate substances obtained from these forms serve to contribute to the discussion. Antineoplastic activity will imply activity in experimental tumors only; clinical studies will not be included. Finally, only the work fostered by the Cancer Chemotherapy National Service Center (CCNSC) will be considered. While this may seem to be an unnatural and undesirable restriction on the scope implied in the title of this review, it has a certain advantage, namely, that all the screening results reported were obtained under generally uniform experimental procedures.

B. Some Characteristics of the Plant Program

Since the mass screening of synthetic compounds and of microbial filtrates against selected experimental tumor systems had already been set up at CCNSC, the plant program was designed to fit in with these other programs. Since antitumor activity did not appear to be limited to any single class or even to a few classes of compounds, and since many compounds of unusual structure were known to reside in plants, this natural source appeared to offer a good opportunity for obtaining new active compounds, and a program of random plant collecting was initiated. Any plants whose extracts showed reproducible activity in the antitumor screen were to be re-collected in quantity and fractionated for the active agent(s). The active agents would then be evaluated like the "synthetics." If they satisfied certain criteria for antitumor activity and chemical structural novelty they would enter preclinical pharmacology; if, again, they passed certain further requirements they would go into clinical study. It has been the justification of this program that several agents have already progressed into clinical study while many more are in the various preliminary stages. Many of these agents have proved to be of novel chemical types. Many would have been otherwise unavailable for study by virtue not only of difficulty of synthesis but also for lack of any particular reason for attempting synthesis in the absence of prior knowledge of antitumor activity.

The isolation of these compounds illustrates the usefulness of fractionation guidance by means of a biological test as contrasted with the classic phytochemical procedure of isolating the constituents first and studying biological properties later. Many of the compounds being isolated would have remained unknown if their presence in crude plant extracts had not been indicated by their antitumor properties.

It was the original belief that this mass fractionation effort would turn up a large number of active compounds of novel chemical structure. This hope is being realized. Additionally, there are being isolated many "old" compounds already in the "synthetic" program whose activity against certain tumors had never been ascertained; these are now being evaluated in the tumor systems used in their isolation. Some of these compounds are found to be useless for our purposes; others are useful. Many plants are found to owe their antitumor activity in our tests to either of two ubiquitous constituents, tannin and β-sitosterol. Once evaluated, it is no longer important to develop new sources for them. Methods have been developed for detecting and eliminating these substances from plants, in order to reveal the possible presence of other active agents without investing time in tedious fractionations. An important outgrowth of this work has been the continuous provision of leads for the synthesis of related compounds of hopefully improved properties. Also, it has been possible to make a reexamination of some of the compounds already in the CCNSC collection. Our results with these related compounds (both natural and synthetic) will be considered here along with the actual plant constituents in order to derive as meaningful generalizations as possible.

Besides the production of actual agents of interest, recent progress can be expressed in terms of certain generalizations which can now be attempted and which are possible only because of the enormous amount of raw data of different kinds provided by a mass screening program. As an indication of the extent of such data it will be useful to give some basic statistics. In the 9 years since the CCNSC let its first contracts for plant collection, extraction, and fractionation, over 40,000 crude extracts have been prepared from plants collected randomly from around the world. About 3.5% of these have shown reproducible activity in one or another of the tumor systems employed. Because activity in many cases was shown in more than one part of a plant and by more than one type of extract, a corrected figure of 2.5% for the yield of active species (rather than extracts) may be cited. In the course of fractionating several hundred of these plants, over 150 (excluding duplicates) of the responsible active agents have been isolated to date. These agents presently run the gamut from well-characterized to poorly characterized, structure known to structure unknown, and available in large amount to available in negligible amount. A continuing effort is being put into supplying more plant source material for the production of these agents in sufficient quantity for characterization, structure determination, and pharmacology.

Finally, some background should be presented regarding the experimental tumor systems used to evaluate the plant extracts and their constituents—our "screen." Since our goal is the production of useful drugs for the treatment of human cancer, a screen should be as predictive as possible. In fact, a program of this kind is no better than the screen. In practice, our screen has been and is under constant modification and development as feedback from the clinic has become available. Originally, following recommendations of the Gellhorn report which were based upon a consideration of clinically active drugs known at the time (Gellhorn and Hirschberg, 1955), a battery of three mouse tumors was used: sarcoma 180 (SA), adenocarcinoma 755 (CA), and lymphoid leukemia L-1210 (LE). Early in the program (about 1958) the Ehrlich ascites tumor system (EA) in the mouse host was added as an alternate to CA because of the considerable interest and usage by laboratories outside the CCNSC program. However, the Ehrlich ascites system proved to be highly sensitive to a wide spectrum of drugs and was phased out of the screen early in 1960 because of this insufficient selectivity. Cell culture (KB) was made a routine part of the screen shortly thereafter and in the same year. In 1962, a broad spectrum of tumor systems, utilizing the mouse, rat, and hamster hosts, was introduced to diversify the screen even further. This was intended to make it possible to develop experience in a wide variety of experimental tumor systems which might lead to better screening tools. Within the last 3 years, and based on a new evaluation of experimental results with the growing number of clinically useful drugs (Goldin *et al.*, 1966), the screen was sharply altered to comprise only LE, the Walker-256 intramuscular rat carcinosarcoma (WM), and KB cell culture. The latter system is in the nature of a prescreen for natural products only, which has been retained because it appears to be useful in detecting certain crude extracts that on fractionation may yield agents active in LE or WM. At the present time additional improvements in the screen are under way. With a sufficient number of drugs under development toward clinical trial which have been selected for activity in the WM system, further use of this system has been postponed until clinical evaluation of the compounds gives a better indication of the system's potential in selecting useful drugs. Following a growing recognition that clinically slow-growing tumors are less drug-sensitive than rapidly growing tumors, attention is now being given to the development of a screening system which will utilize a slower-growing tumor. It is felt that such a system may simulate more closely the clinical problem with solid tumors where the doubling time of the tumor is slower, probably because a larger portion of the tumor consists of a pool of nonproliferating cells. A more detailed discussion of some of the factors involved in screening and of modifications in experimental design of screening systems for special purposes has been given by Venditti and Abbott (1967).

III. Classes of Active Agents

Experimental screening results are presented in Tables II–XV and XVIII; they show, for each material tested, the CCNSC accession number (NSC number), the supplier, the compound name, the molecular formula, the tumor systems used for screening, the vehicle used for administration, the doses or range of doses at which the compound was screened, the maximum tolerated dose (MTD), the minimum effective dose (MED), and the response to treatment.

Supplier. The suppliers are coded as follows:

Code	*Source*
1	Abbott Laboratories North Chicago, Illinois
2	Aldrich Chemical Co. Milwaukee, Wisconsin
3	Allied Chemical Corporation Buffalo, New York
4	Dr. Jack L. Beal Ohio State University Columbus, Ohio
5	Prof. Werner Bergman (dec.) Yale University New Haven, Connecticut
6	Dr. I. R. C. Bick University of Tasmania Hobart, Tas., Australia
7	Dr. F. Thomas Bond Oregon State University Corvallis, Oregon
8	Bose Institute Calcutta, India
9	Prof. Albert J. Castro San Jose State College San Jose, California
10	Prof. Michael P. Cava Wayne State University Detroit, Michigan
11	Central Drug Research Inst. Lucknow, India
12	Chemical-Biological Coordination Center National Research Council Washington, D.C.
13	Prof. Wesley Cocker University of Dublin Trinity College Dublin, Ireland

Code	*Source*
14	Dr. Jack R. Cole University of Arizona Tucson, Arizona
15	Columbia University New York, New York
16	Commonwealth Scientific and Industrial Research Organization Melbourne, Australia
17	Dr. Carl Djerassi Stanford University Stanford, California
18	Dr. Raymond W. Doskotch Ohio State University Columbus, Ohio
19	Dr. Norman R. Farnsworth University of Pittsburgh Pittsburgh, Pennsylvania
20	Prof. Louis F. Fieser Harvard University Cambridge, Massachusetts
21	Dr. Benjamin Gilbert Faculdade Nacional de Farmacia Rio de Janeiro, Brazil
22	Dr. V. Herout Czechoslovak Academy of Science Prague, Czechoslovakia
23	Prof. Werner Herz Florida State University Tallahassee, Florida
24	Dr. D. Ilse Univ. of New South Wales Sydney, Australia
25	Istituto Carlo Erba per Ricerche Terapeutiche Milano, Italy
26	Dr. P. R. Jefferies University of Western Australia Nedlands, Australia
27	Dr. Govind J. Kapadia Howard University Washington, D.C.
28	Dr. Jerzy Konopa Politechnika Gdanska Gdansk, Poland
29	Dr. S. Morris Kupchan University of Wisconsin Madison, Wisconsin
30	Laroche Navarron Laboratories Levallois (Seine), France
31	Prof. Nelson J. Leonard University of Illinois Urbana, Illinois
32	Leo Pharmaceutical Products Ballerup, Denmark
33	L. Light & Co., Ltd. Colnbrook, Bucks. England
34	Arthur D. Little, Inc. Cambridge, Massachusetts
35	Dr. Tom J. Mabry The University of Texas Austin, Texas
36	Dr. H. George Mandel The George Washington Univ. Washington, D.C.
37	Mann Research Labs. New York, New York
38	McNeil Laboratories, Inc. Fort Washington, Pennsylvania
39	Merck, Sharp, and Dohme Research Laboratories Rahway, New Jersey
40	Dr. Albert I. Meyers Louisiana State Univ. in New Orleans New Orleans, Louisiana
41	Midwest Research Inst. Kansas City, Missouri
42	Dr. Walter B. Mors Universidade Federal do Rio de Janeiro Rio de Janeiro, Brazil
43	Dr. Koji Nakanishi Tohoku University Sendai, Japan
44	National Cancer Institute Bethesda, Maryland
45	National Heart Institute Bethesda, Maryland
46	National Institute of Arthritis and Metabolic Diseases Bethesda, Maryland
47	Prof. Carl R. Noller Stanford University Stanford, California

Code	*Source*
48	Prof. Thomas S. Oakwood Pennsylvania State Univ. University Park, Pennsylvania
49	Parke Davis and Co. Ann Arbor, Michigan
50	Prof. George R. Pettit Arizona State University Tempe, Arizona
51	Chas. Pfizer & Co. Maywood, New Jersey
52	Pierce Chemical Co. Rockford, Illinois
53	Dr. Frank D. Popp Clarkson College of Technology Potsdam, New York
54	Dr. Yolanda T. Pratt University of Maryland College Park, Maryland
55	Research Triangle Institute Research Triangle Park North Carolina
56	Dr. E. Ritchie The University of Sydney Sydney, Australia
57	Prof. David Rittenberg Columbia University College of Physicians and Surgeons New York, New York
58	Sandoz Ltd. Basle, Switzerland
59	Schering Corporation Bloomfield, New Jersey
60	Dr. Edward E. Schweizer University of Delaware Newark, Delaware
61	Dr. Harold M. Sell Michigan State University East Lansing, Michigan
62	Sloan-Kettering Institute for Cancer Research Rye, New York
63	South African Council for Scientific and Industrial Research Pretoria, South Africa

Code	*Source*
64	Southern Research Institute Birmingham, Alabama
65	Squibb Institute for Medical Research New Brunswick, New Jersey
66	Stanford Research Institute Menlo Park, California
67	Sterling-Winthrop Research Institute Rensselaer, New York
68	Syntex Laboratories, Inc. Palo Alto, California
69	Union Carbide Chemicals Co. South Charleston, West Virginia
70	U.S. Dept. of Agriculture Beltsville, Maryland
71	The Upjohn Co. Kalamazoo, Michigan
72	Dr. Wyman R. Vaughan University of Connecticut Storrs, Connecticut
73	Dr. A. Wander S. A. Berne, Switzerland
74	Prof. Stanley Wawzonek State University of Iowa Iowa City, Iowa
75	Prof. Desmond M. S. Wheeler University of Nebraska Lincoln, Nebraska
76	The Worcester Foundation for Experimental Biology Shrewsbury, Massachusetts
77	Dr. Gunter Wulff Organisch-Chemisches Institut der Universität Bonn Bonn, West Germany
78	Dr. Kenneth H. Dudley University of North Carolina Chapel Hill, North Carolina
79	Prof. J. W. Clark-Lewis University of Adelaide Adelaide (S.A.), Australia
80	Smith Kline & French Laboratories Philadelphia, Pennsylvania.

*Tumor System.** The host-tumor assays used for screening are coded as follows:

A3. Lieberman plasma cell No. 1. Mouse
CA. Adenocarcinoma 755. Mouse
DA. Dunning leukemia (ascites). Rat
DL. Dunning leukemia (solid). Rat
EA. Ehrlich ascites. Mouse
FV. Friend virus leukemia. Mouse
5H1. HS1 human sarcoma. Rat
8H1 HS1 human sarcoma. Egg
HE. Hepatoma 129. Mouse
KB. Human epidermoid carcinoma of the nasopharynx. Cell culture
3L8. L-5178Y lymphatic leukemia. Mouse
LE. Leukemia L-1210. Mouse (intraperitoneal)
LL. Lewis lung carcinoma. Mouse
LZ. Leukemia L-1210. Mouse (subcutaneous). Delayed treatment
MM. Melanotic melanoma. Hamster
MS. Murphy Sturm lymphosarcoma. Rat
OS. Osteogenic sarcoma He 10734. Mouse
P1. Plasmacytoma No. 1. Hamster
P4. P-1534 leukemia. Mouse
8P. P-1798 lymphosarcoma. Mouse
PS. P-388 lymphocytic leukemia. Mouse
SA. Sarcoma 180. Mouse
WA. Walker carcinosarcoma 256. Rat (subcutaneous)
WI. Walker carcinosarcoma 256 ascites. Rat
WM. Walker carcinosarcoma 256. Rat (intramuscular)
91. S-91 Cloudman melanoma. Mouse

Vehicle. The following abbreviations are used:

CMC. Carboxymethylcellulose
DMF. Dimethylformamide
DMSO. 5% Dimethylsulfoxide in water
MC. Methylcellulose
Oil. Olive oil, sesame oil, or peanut oil
PG. Propylene glycol
SSS. Steroid suspending solution

Dose Range Tested. Individual levels are separated by commas. A dose response test is indicated by a range.

MTD. Maximum tolerated dose at approximately the LD_{10}. A comparison of this figure with the dose range tested indicates whether doses were used that were as high as possible.

* Detailed protocols for many of the tumors may be found in *Cancer Chemotherapy Repts.* No. 25, Dec., 1962. Protocols for other tumors and for recent revisions may be obtained by writing Chief, Drug Evaluation Branch, Cancer Chemotherapy National Service Center, Bethesda, Maryland 20014.

MED. Minimum effective dose, i.e., minimal dose level resulting in a TWI $\geqq 58\%$ or ILS $\geqq 25\%$.

Response. TWI. Tumor weight inhibition. A reproducible TWI in drug treated animals vs untreated control animals $\geqq 58\%$ is considered significant.

ILS. Increase in life span. A reproducible ILS $\geqq 25\%$ for treated vs control animals is considered significant.

ED_{50}. Dose level in μg/ml at which 50% inhibition of growth of cells (*in vitro*) is noted vs untreated controls. A value $\leqq 1.0$ is considered significant.

It should be emphasized that the values for the TWI, ILS, and ED_{50} considered significant, as well as the value for the TI (below), are cut-off figures in current use at CCNSC. They are arrived at statistically and are set arbitrarily to assure a percentage of "passes" low enough to be quite selective and to keep subsequent work-up within our practical means.

Abbreviations:

Alk. Alkali
BID. Twice daily
$LD_{10(50)}$. Dose level producing 10% (50%) lethality
P.O. Per os
QNS. Quantity not sufficient
S.C. Subcutaneous
TI. Therapeutic index, MTD/MED, or effective therapeutic range. A TI of at least 2.0 in solid tumors is one of the factors currently considered necessary for qualification for additional studies leading to clinical trial. A more detailed discussion of current criteria for evaluating responses to treatment has been given by Venditti and Abbott (1967).

A. Alkaloids

1. *Tylocrebrine and related alkaloids from Tylophora crebriflora*

A recent review of the chemistry of these phenanthroindolizidine alkaloids is to be found in Govindachari (1967). Six new alkaloids have been isolated from the plant (Rao *et al.*, 1966, 1967) and the structures determined as in formula (I) and Table I.

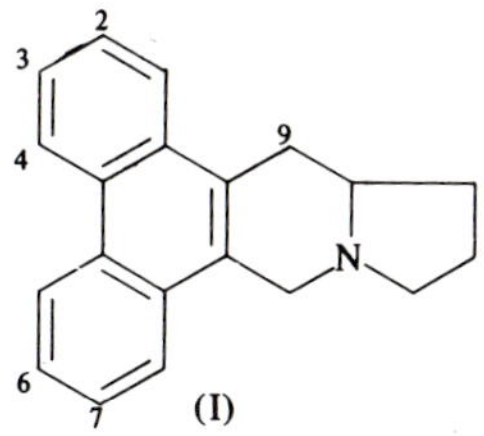

(I)

In addition, the parent substance [(I); NSC-101,644] has been synthesized by Zee-Cheng and Cheng (1969) and has been included in Table II for comparison.

TABLE I

STRUCTURE OF ALKALOIDS FROM *Tylophora crebriflora*

Alkaloid	Substituents at C-atom					
	2	3	4	6	7	9
Tylocrebrine	—	OCH_3	OCH_3	OCH_3	OCH_3	—
Tylophorine	OCH_3	OCH_3	—	OCH_3	OCH_3	—
Tylophorinine	—	OCH_3	—	OCH_3	OCH_3	OH
Compound A	—	OCH_3	OCH_3	OCH_3	OCH_3	OH
Compound B	—	OCH_3	OH	OCH_3	OCH_3	—
Compound C	—	OCH_3	OH	OCH_3	OCH_3	OH
Compound D	OCH_3	OCH_3	OCH_3	OCH_3	OCH_3	OH
Compound E	OCH_3	OCH_3	OCH_3	OCH_3	OCH_3	—
Compound F	Structure unknown					

The test results are listed in Table II.

It is apparent that significant activity is shown by tylocrebrine against CA, MS, PS, and LE; by tylophorine against LE; by compound A against SA, WM, LE, and P4; by compound B against CA and WM; by compound C against SA, CA, WM, LE, and P4; by compound D against LE; by compound E against WM; and by tylophorinine against LE. Erratic results, reducing the significance of some of the data, are noted in the table. This group of alkaloids is exceptional in that antitumor activity is retained throughout the series of analogs. The more usual situation, as will be evident later on, is for slight changes in chemical structure to destroy antitumor activity. It is notable that the unsubstituted parent compound (NSC-101,644) is inactive in all tests.

Tylocrebrine was chosen for pharmacological work-up and clinical study. Unexpected irreversible central nervous system toxicity, shown in the clinic, resulted in the drug's withdrawal from test pending further laboratory study.

2. *Ellipticine and Related Compounds*

The chemistry of these alkaloids has been recently reviewed by Gilbert (1965). The structure of the parent 6*H*-pyrido[4,3-*b*]carbazole is given in formula (II) and the analogs, both natural and synthetic, that have been tested for antitumor activity are listed in Table III.

(II)

TABLE II

ALKALOIDS FROM *Tylophora crebriflora*

NSC No.	Supplier	Compound name	Tumor system	Vehicle	Dose range tested (mg/kg)	Response (mg/kg)		Evaluation		
						MTD	MED	TWI(%)	ILS(%)	ED_{50}
60387	16; 51	Tylocrebrine	SA	CMC	12, 50	< 12	—	38		
			CA	H_2O	5–20	~20	~15	79		
			OS	H_2O	5–20	< 20	—	24		
			HE	H_2O	5–20	~20	—	33		
			8P	Saline	1.25–10	> 10	—	22		
			MS	H_2O	4.4–22.5	< 15	15	80		
			5H1	H_2O	4–10	< 10	—	41		
			WM	H_2O	5–45	~20	20	59		
			LL	H_2O	1.7–15	~7	—	50		
			MM	H_2O	7.5–60	< 15	—	26		
			PS	Saline	1.25–12.5	~8	6		70	
			P4	Saline	1.25–20	~1.25	—		7	
			DA	Saline	1.25–10	~10	—		0	
			LE	CMC	1.25–30	~15	10		51	
			LZ	CMC	3–180	~108	—		15	
76387	16: 51	Tylophorine	SA	H_2O	12–20	18	18	58		
			CA	H_2O	8.8–20	~20	—	50		
			WM	H_2O	6–24	~15	—	44		
			LE	H_2O	4–500	< 30,500	—		50[a]	
			P4	Saline	3.9–250	7.8	—		15	

TABLE II—*continued*

NSC No.	Supplier	Compound name	Tumor system	Vehicle	Dose range tested (mg/kg)	Response (mg/kg) MTD	MED	Evaluation TWI(%)	ILS(%)	ED_{50}
85706	51	Compound A	SA	H_2O	2.2–8	~5	5	90		
			CA	H_2O	2.2–20	~5	3.7	81		
			WM	H_2O	2.5–15	7.5	6	75		
			LE	H_2O	3–15	~9	6		40[b]	
			P4	H_2O	2.7–12	~7.5	6		40	
85707	51	Compound B	SA	H_2O	8–24	~12	—	28		
			CA	H_2O	6–15	~12	—	62		
			WM	H_2O	6–15	~12	12	70		
			LE	H_2O	3–18	~12	—		20	
85708	51	Compound C	SA	H_2O-saline	2.2–15	7	5	82		
			CA	H_2O	2.2–15	6	5	69		
			WM	H_2O	2.8–15	~3.5	—	60[a]		
			LE	H_2O	0.2–20	~9	~6		30[a]	
			P4	H_2O	2.0–12	~9	~6		36	

85709	51	Compound D	LE	H_2O	6–36	20	~16		45
92070	51	Compound E	SA	H_2O + T-80	10–40	~40	—	28	
			CA	H_2O + T-80	5–20	~10	—	0	
			LE	H_2O	5–30	10	—		11
			P4	H_2O	5–15	> 15	—		0
			WM	H_2O + T-80	10–80	~60	~60	65	
94738	51	Compound F	WM	H_2O	30	> 30	—	0	
100,055	51	Tylophorinine	LE	H_2O	0.57–20	~12	—		30
101,644	41	Dibenzo[*f*,*h*]pyrrolo-[1,2-*b*]-isoquinoline-9,11,12,13,-13a,14-hexahydro-	LE	CMC	50–400	400	—		5
			WM	CMC	400	> 400	—	30	

[a] Results erratic.
[b] Results not reproducible.

Again, activity in one tumor system or another is shown by a number of analogs. Substitution on (II) of 5-methyl, 6-methyl, 1,5-dimethyl, 5,11-dimethyl, 9-methoxy-5,11-dimethyl, and 9-methoxy-5,6,11-trimethyl, does not destroy activity. However, activity is destroyed by substitution of 3-methyl, 9-methyl, 5,7,10,11-tetramethyl, and 9-bromo. Hydrogenation plays a mixed role. 3,4-Dihydroolivacine has lost its activity against LE but retained it against SA. Of three 1,2,3,4-tetrahydro derivatives, one (*d*-guatambuine) is active against LE while two (*dl*-guatambuine and 1,2,3,4-tetrahydro-9-methoxy-2-methylellipticine) are inactive. Movement of the hetero atom in the pyridine nucleus from the 2 to the 3 position (as in isoellipticine and 3,4-dihydroisoellipticine) destroys activity against LE.

Ellipticine, 9-methoxyellipticine, and 11-demethylellipticine are all suitable for further pharmacological work-up. Ellipticine has been selected for further work on the basis of better activity by the oral route. A good method has been developed for its large-scale synthesis (Dalton *et al.*, 1967).

3. *Bisbenzylisoquinoline and Related Alkaloids*

A recent review of this class of alkaloids is given by Curcumelli-Rodostamo and Kulka (1967). Some structures too recently elucidated to be given in this review are to be found elsewhere as, for instance, thalidasine (Kupchan *et al.*, 1967d) and dehydrothalicarpine (Kupchan *et al.*, 1968b). Examples of the general structure of this class of alkaloids are provided by that of tetrandrine (III) and thalicarpine (IV). Representatives are listed in Table IV containing one diphenyl ether linkage and two diphenyl ether linkages, but not three such linkages.

Cytotoxic activity (in KB) is shown by many in this group. Of those tested in *in vivo* tumor systems, however, significant activity (in WM) is shown only by thalicarpine (IV), *d*-, *l*-(pheanthine), *dl*-tetrandrine (III) and by thalidasine; dehydrothalicarpine shows marginal activity. While these compounds are all fully methylated, even to the tertiary nitrogen atoms, and these (except for isotetrandrine) are the only ones in the list so characterized, too few compounds have been tested and the data are too scanty to enable it to be said with assurance that methylation is necessary for activity. Also, in the only cases where *N*-methylation has been carried still further to quaternization—*d*-tubocurarine (NSC-36387) and its *O,O'*-dimethyl derivative (NSC-36388)—data are even more scanty. The incompletely methylated compound (NSC-36387) is inactive against WM, but the completely methylated compound (NSC-36388) was not tested against WM.

Thalicarpine is undergoing preclinical pharmacology, while *dl*-tetrandrine is scheduled for this work.

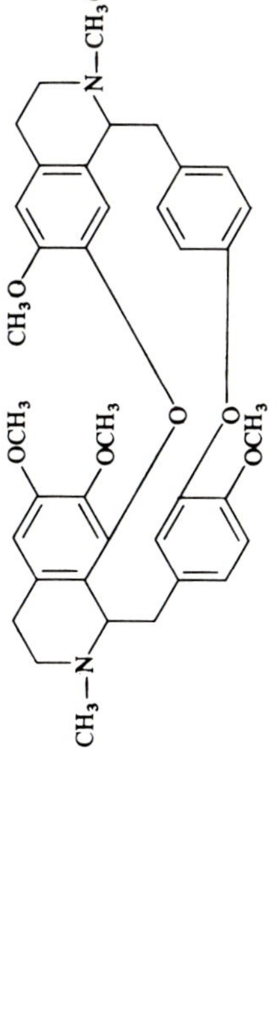

Tetrandrine
(III)

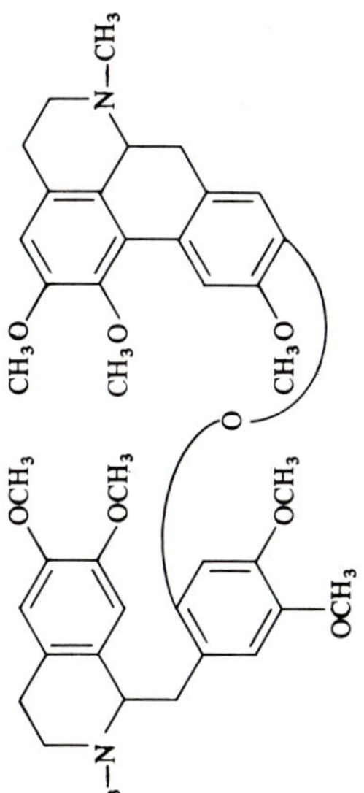

Thalicarpine
(IV)

TABLE III

ELLIPTICINE AND RELATED COMPOUNDS

NSC No.	Supplier	Name	Molecular formula	Tumor system	Vehicle	Dose range tested (mg/kg)	Response (mg/kg) MTD	Response (mg/kg) MED	Evaluation TWI(%)	Evaluation ILS(%)	Evaluation ED_{50}
69187	16	9-Methoxyellipticine	$N_2OC_{18}H_{16}$	SA	CMC-saline	3–300	~150	90	75		
				8P	Saline	0.39–100	25	25	58		
				LE	Saline	6–255	~75	~25		70	
				P4	Saline	2.5–160	~40	—		20	
				KB	PG						<1.0
70133	73; 66	3,4-Dihydroolivacine	$N_2C_{17}H_{16}$	SA	H_2O	25–250	~200	200	72		
				LE	CMC	14–112	112	—		23	
				KB	Alcohol						2.6
70134	73; 42	Olivacine (6 *H*- pyrido[4,3*b*]-carbazole,1,5-dimethyl-)	$N_2C_{17}H_{14}$	SA	H_2O	25–300	200	200	58		
				LE	Saline	2.5–250	84	10		51	
				KB	DMF						0.4
71795	16	Ellipticine (6 *H*-pyrido[4,3-*b*]-carbazole,5,11-dimethyl-)	$N_2C_{17}H_{14}$	LE	Saline	6.2–75	~75	6.2		88[a]	
				PS	Saline	2.5–160	40	2.5		79	
74432	42	*d*-Guatambuine (6 *H*-pyrido [4,3*b*]carbazole,1,2,3,4-tetrahydro-1,2,5-trimethyl-)	$N_2C_{18}H_{20}$	LE	Saline or CMC	15–300	150	50		45[b]	

87206	66	11-Demethylellipticine	$N_2C_{16}H_{12}$	LE	Saline	11–210	140	11		70
				P4	Saline	3.13–200	50	—		17
				WM	Saline	140	>140	—	40	
98927	16	9-Bromoellipticine	$N_2BrC_{17}H_{13}$	LE	Saline + T-80	100,400	400	—		8
98949	16	9-Methylellipticine	$N_2C_{18}H_{16}$	LE	Saline	125–340	340	—		5
100,594	16	Ellipticine, 1,2,3,4-tetrahydro-9-methoxy-2-methyl-	$N_2OC_{19}H_{22}$	LE	Saline	29–150	~150	—		2
100,596	16	6-Methylellipticine	$N_2C_{18}H_{16}$	LE	Saline	29–150	>150	~150		34[c]
101,152	66	Isoellipticine (10 *H*-pyrido-[3,4-*b*]carbazole,5,11-dimethyl-]	$N_2C_{17}H_{14}$	LE	Saline	25–500	>500	—		13
101,976	42	*dl*-Guatambuine	$N_2C_{18}H_{20}$	LE	CMC	50–400	400	—		9
102,726	16	7,10-Dimethylellipticine	$N_2C_{19}H_{18}$	LE	Saline	25–400	100	—		12
102,822	16	3-Methylellipticine	$N_2C_{18}H_{16}$	LE	Saline	400	400	—		5
				WM	Saline	400	400	—	14	
102,981	16	3,4-Dihydroisoellipticine	$N_2C_{17}H_{16}$	LE	CMC	400	400	—		10
109,442	16	9-Methoxy-6-methylellipticine	$N_2OC_{19}H_{18}$	LE	Saline	25–400[d]	400	—		52

[a] P.O. = >100.
[b] Results not reproducible.
[c] P.O. = 71.
[d] Single injection procedure only.

TABLE IV

Bisbenzylisoquinoline and Related Alkaloids

NSC No.	Supplier	Compound name	Molecular formula	Tumor system	Vehicle	Dose range tested (mg/kg)	Response (mg/kg)		Evaluation		
							MTD	MED	TWI(%)	ILS(%)	ED_{50}
21075	49; 55	Pilocereine	$N_2O_4C_{30}H_{44}$	SA	—	85, 170	85	—	29		
				CA	—	38, 76	38	—	44		
				LE	—	85	>85	—		0	
				PS	Saline	12.5–100	50	—		0	
				P4	Saline	25–200	100	—		15	
				DA	Saline	12.5–100	>100	—		0	
				WM	Saline	12.5–100	>100	—	35		
				KB	PG						0.26
					DMF						0.69
27255	1	Bebeerine iodide, *O*-dimethyl-, trihydrate	$N_2O_6C_{40}H_{48}{++}$ 2I- $\cdot 3H_2O$	SA	Saline	0.25–500	~0.25	—	4		
				CA	Saline	0.12, 0.23	~0.12	—	1		
				LE	Saline	0.23	~0.23			3	
36387	44	*d*-Tubocurarine, dichloride	$N_2O_6C_{38}H_{44}{++}$ 2Cl-	SA	MC	0.15	>0.15	—	0		
				CA	MC	0.07–0.14	~0.07	—	39		
				WM	CMC	0.25–0.50	~0.25	—	24		
				LE	MC	0.07	>0.07	—		0	
36388	44	*d*-Tubocurarine, *O,O′*-dimethyl-, diiodide	$N_2O_6C_{40}H_{48}{++}$ 2I-	SA	MC	0.20	0.20	—	1		
				CA	MC	0.14	>0.14	—	3		
				LE	MC	0.14	>0.14	—		0	
36413	44	Dauricine	$N_2O_6C_{38}H_{44}$	SA	MC	125	>125	—	32		
				CA	MC	55–110	~55	—	0		
				LE	MC	55	~55	—		0	
				WM	Saline	75	~75		19		
68075	29	Thalicarpine	$N_2O_8C_{41}H_{48}$	SA	Saline	7.8–500	~100	—	40		
				CA	Saline + T-80	40	~40	—	0		
				LL	CMC	50–200	~100	~100	74		
				WM	CMC	40–320	>320	~75[a]	90		
				PS	CMC	37.5–400	~400	—		10	
				LE	CMC	80–320	~160	—		0	
				KB	PG						2.1

77304	29	*l*-Curine (*l*-bebeerine)	$N_2O_6C_{36}H_{38}$	KB	Acidified saline						<0.14 2.9
77035	29	*d*-Isochondrodendrine (Isobebeerine)	$N_2O_6C_{36}H_{38}$	KB	Acidified saline						0.17 2.6
77036	29	Fangchinoline	$N_2O_6C_{37}H_{40}$	KB	Acidified saline						0.12 0.93 0.20
77037	29	D-Tetrandrine	$N_2O_6C_{38}H_{42}$	LE	Saline	200–400	~400	—		0	
				WM	CMC	100–400	>400	~200[b]	60		
				KB	Acidified saline						0.091 0.17
79640	29	Cissampareine	$N_2O_6C_{37}H_{38}$	KB	PG						2.0
90285	29	Thalidasine	$N_2O_7C_{39}H_{44}$	WM	CMC	200–300	>300	<200[c]	80		
				KB	PG						12
90601	17	Piloceredine	$N_2O_4C_{30}H_{44}$	KB	PG						7.8
91771	29	DL-Tetrandrine	$N_2O_6C_{38}H_{42}$	LE	Saline	400	~400	—		0	
				WM	CMC & saline	20–450	>450	~200[d]	78		
93135	33; 4; 29	Oxyacanthine	$N_2O_6C_{37}H_{40}$	SA	CMC	125–400	~125	—	17		
				LE	CMC	50–100	~50	—		1	
				WM	CMC	>200	200	—	0		
				KB	Alcohol						1.2; .76
93673	6	Daphnoline	$N_2O_6C_{35}H_{36}$	KB	Dioxane						20.0
93674	6	Aromoline	$N_2O_6C_{36}H_{38}$	KB	Dioxane						6.4

TABLE IV—*continued*

NSC No.	Supplier	Compound name	Molecular formula	Tumor system	Vehicle	Dose range tested (mg/kg)	Response (mg/kg)		Evaluation		
							MTD	MED	TWI(%)	ILS(%)	ED_{50}
97338	6; 29	Isotetrandrine	$N_2O_6C_{38}H_{42}$	KB	PG						1.5
104,944	29	Thalmethine	$N_2O_6C_{36}H_{36}$	WM	CMC	45–180	>180	—	0		
104,946	29	Dehydrothalicarpine	$N_2O_8C_{41}H_{46}$	WM	CMC	80–160	>160	—	57		
105,130	29	Pheanthine (L-Tetrandrine)	$N_2O_6C_{38}H_{42}$	WM	Saline	25–400	~400	~400[e]	75		
123,123	4	Obamegin	$N_2O_6C_{36}H_{38}$	KB	H_2O						4.1
409,664	44	Berbamine, dihydrochloride, hydrate	$N_2O_6C_{37}H_{40} \cdot 2HCl \cdot H_2O$	LE	Saline	65–500	~65	—		4	
				LL	Saline	65	>65	—	0		
				WM	Saline	100–300	~100	—	13		
				KB	—						5.5

[a] TI ≅ 4. [b] TI ≅ 2. [c] TI > 1.5. [d] TI > 2. [e] TI ≧ 1.

4. *Camptothecin*

A group of alkaloids of a novel type has been isolated by Wall and co-workers (1966a,b, 1968) in small amounts from different parts of a tree, *Camptotheca acuminata* Decne. (fam. Nyssaceae). These alkaloids are camptothecin (V), its hydroxy derivative, and its methoxy derivative (see Table V).

The preparation of the derivatives listed in Table V has made it possible to draw some broad preliminary conclusions with regard to structure-activity relationships. Nuclear substitution in the benzene ring has little effect on antitumor activity (*cf.* NSC-107,124 and NSC-111,533). Oxidation of the quinoline-N to the N-oxide reduces but does not destroy activity (*cf.* NSC-106,748). The lactone group appears to be essential for activity since activity is lost after reduction to the lactol (NSC-102,621). However, the α-hydroxy group does not appear to be always essential to activity since, although replacing the hydroxyl group with other groups (NSC-95382 and NSC-101,833) destroys activity, replacing it with hydrogen (NSC-105,132) causes no great reduction in activity. The activity of the "open" compounds (VI) is believed to be due to their subsequent cyclization to the lactone after administration to the animal. The mechanism of action of camptothecin is of great interest and is being actively studied.

The fact that the open compound, "camptothecin sodium salt" (NSC-100,880) is active against LE and is active orally is of practical importance. This compound has been carried through preclinical pharmacology and is in clinical trial.

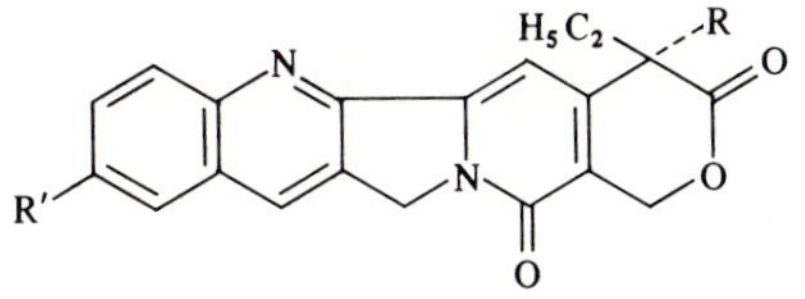

H_5C_2 R O N N O O R′

Camptothecin R = OH, R′ = H

(V)

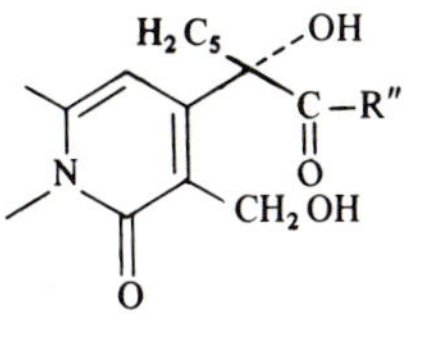

H_2C_5 OH C—R″ O N CH_2OH O

(VI)

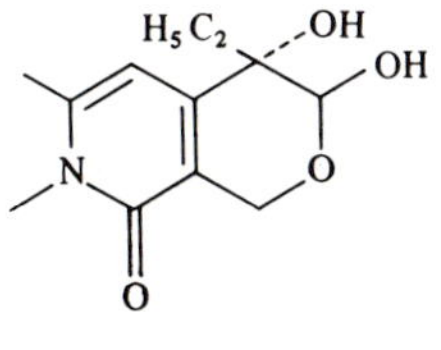

H_5C_2 OH OH N O O

Camptothecin lactol

(VII)

5. *Pyrrolizidine Alkaloids and Related Compounds*

Recent reviews of the chemistry of the pyrrolizidine alkaloids are to be found in Leonard (1960) and Boit (1961). An example of the general structure

TABLE V

Camptothecin and Derivatives

NSC No.	Supplier	name	R	R′	R″	Tumor system	Vehicle	Dose range tested (mg/kg)	Response (mg/kg) MTD	Response (mg/kg) MED	Evaluation TWI(%)	Evaluation ILS(%)	Evaluation ED_{50}
94600	55	Camptothecin (V)	OH	H	—	WM	Saline	0.63–16	~16	~1.25[a]	100		
						LE	Saline or CMC	0.22–100	~3.2	~1.0		122	
						KB	DMF						0.74
95382	55	Camptothecin acetate (V)	$OCOCH_3$	H	—	WM	CMC	0.38–3	>3	—	11		
						LE	H_2O	0.13–1	~0.6	0.6		28	
100,880	55	"Camptothecin, sodium salt" (VI)	—	H	ONa	LE	Saline	0.50–16	~3.0	~0.60		109[b]	
101,833	55	Chlorocamptothecin (V)	Cl	H	—	LE	Saline	1–6	≧6	—		3	
102,621	55	Camptothecin lactol (VII)	—	H	—	LE	Saline	0.5–16	≧16	—		~20	
105,132	55	Desoxycamptothecin (V)	H	H	—	LE	Saline	7.5, 15	~7.5	<7.5		95[c]	
106,609	55	Camptothecin methylamide (VI)	—	H	$NHCH_3$	LE	Saline	1–12	~3.5	~1		72	
106,748	55	Camptothecin *N*-oxide	OH	H	—	WM	Saline	1–16	~16	~16	85		
						LE	Saline	1–16	~4	2		44	
107,124	55	Hydroxycamptothecin (V)	OH	OH	—	LE	Saline	0.044–5.8	~4	~0.044		129	
						PS	CMC	0.87–7.0	~1.75	<0.87		168	
						WM	Saline	1.90–15.6[d]	<7.8	7.8	84		
111,533	55	Methoxycamptothecin (V)	OH	OCH_3	—	LE	Saline	0.127–3.3	1.4	0.191		125	

[a] TI > 10.
[b] Also active P.O. and by various treatment schedules.
[c] Tested only once.
[d] Toxicity erratic.

of this class of alkaloids is illustrated by that of monocrotaline (VIII). Natural alkaloids and related synthetic compounds tested in the CCNSC program are listed in Table VI.

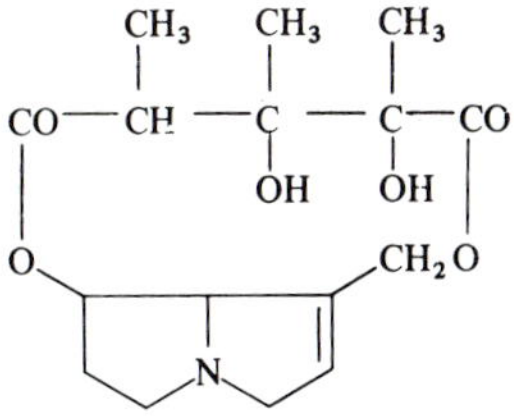

(VIII)

Antitumor activity, notably against WM, is exhibited by monocrotaline, heliotrine, heliotrine *N*-oxide, lasiocarpine, fulvine, spectabiline, senecionine, senecionine *N*-oxide, and monocrotaline diacetate. While it appears that the active alkaloids include representatives of both the mono esters of monobasic acids and the cyclic diesters of dibasic acids, none of the unesterified amino alcohols shows activity. However, while one of the amino alcohols (retronecine) gives rise to six active cyclic diesters (monocrotaline and its diacetate, fulvine, spectabiline, and senecionine and its *N*-oxide), it is also the base for four other cyclic diesters which are inactive (seneciphylline, jaconine, crispatine, and jacobine). Similarly, while two monoesters of heliotridine are active against WM (heliotrine and lasiocarpine), two others (echinatine and europine) are inactive. Oxidation to the *N*-oxide does not destroy activity against WM in two cases (senecionine and heliotrine), but does destroy it in two other cases (monocrotaline and lasiocarpine). None of the pyrrolizidine compounds tested shows significant cytotoxicity. It must be said, therefore, that structure-activity relationships in this class of compounds are obscure at this time.

Monocrotaline and spectabiline both have high therapeutic indexes against WM and would be considered for further studies if it were not for the reported hepatotoxicity of pyrrolizidine alkaloids. Studies are being done further to evaluate this factor.

6. *Alkaloids of Solanum tripartitum*

In the course of seeking the antitumor agents in active plant extracts arising out of the CCNSC program's routine screen, Kupchan *et al.* (1967a) isolated two members of a new class of alkaloids. This fact is the more remarkable when it is considered that, of more than 200 species of *Solanum* in which the alkaloids have been identified, all have yielded only members of the large class of steroid alkaloids except for rare instances where atropine, 5-hydroxytryptamine,

TABLE VI

Pyrrolizidine Alkaloids and Related Compounds

NSC No.	Supplier	Compound name	Molecular formula	Tumor system	Vehicle	Dose range tested (mg/kg)	Response (mg/kg)		Evaluation		
							MTD	MED	TWI(%)	ILS(%)	ED_{50}
27683	38	3 *H*-Pyrrolo[1,2-a]pyrrole, hexahydro-2-methyl-	NC_8H_{15}	SA	—	23	~23	—	10		
				CA	—	16	~16	—	14		
				LE	—	16	~16	—		0	
28693	1	Monocrotaline	$NO_6H_{16}H_{23}$	SA	CMC	50, 100	~100	~100	60		
				CA	MC	22.5–200	~150	50[a]	85		
				LL	MC	90	>90	—	29		
				EA	MC	100	~100	?	80		
				FV	CMC	31–500	250	250	62		
				8P	CMC	3.75–60	~30	~30	70		
				WM	Saline	6.25–100	>100	~6.25[b]	100		
				MM	CMC	25–200	~80	~80	66		
				P1	CMC	3.75–84	>84	~15[c]	97		
				LE	Saline	3.13–90	~90	—		0	
				PS	Saline	3.13–25	~25	—		4	
				P4	Saline	3.13–25	~25	—		7	
				DA	Saline	1.57–25	>25	25		40	
				8H1	Alkali saline	0.30–5	>5	—	30		
				KB	H_2O						>100
30618	16	Retronecine, hydrochloride	$NO_2C_8H_{13} \cdot HCl$	SA	Saline	125	~125	—	21		
				EA	Saline	125	>125	—	0		
				LL	CMC	25–450	>450	—	10		
				WM	Saline	50–400	>400	—	11		
				LE	Saline	112	~112			12	
41156	1	Retronecine, hydrochloride	$NO_2C_8H_{13} \cdot HCl$	SA	MC	500	>500	—	6		
				CA	MC	450	>450	—	0		
				LE	MC	450	>450	—		0	

30620	16	Heliotrine	$NO_5C_{16}H_{27}$	SA	MC	125	~125	—	13		
				EA	MC	125	~125	—	27		
				WM	Saline	50–188	~125	85[d]	100		
				LE	MC	112	>112	—		8	
				KB	H_2O						15
30621	16	Heliotrine, *N*-oxide	$NO_6C_{16}H_{27}$	SA	MC	125	~124		35		
				EA	MC	125	~125		0		
				WM	Saline	100	>100	?	60		
				KB	—						>100
30622	16	Seneciphylline	$NO_5C_{18}H_{23}$	SA	MC	62, 125	62	—	34		
				EA	MC	62	62	—	26		
				WM	Saline	50	>50	—	44		
				LE	MC	50	~50	—		0	
				KB	PG						>100
30623	16	Sarracine, *N*-oxide	$NO_6C_{18}H_{27}$	SA	MC	125	>125	—	0		
				EA	MC	125	~125	—	2		
				WM	Saline	50–400	>400	—	13		
				LE	MC	112	>112	—		0	
30624	16	Jaconine, hydrochloride	$NO_6ClC_{18}H_{26} \cdot HCl$	SA	MC	25–200	~25	—	39		
				EA	MC	25	~25	—	0		
				WM	Saline	25	>25	—	0		
				LE	Saline	3–24	24	—		7	
30625	16	Lasiocarpine	$NO_7C_{21}H_{33}$	SA	CMC	12–150	~40	40	60		
				EA	MC	31	~31	—	33		
				WM	CMC	5–40	~20	20	60		
				LE	H_2O + T-80	28, 45	~45	—		0	
				PS	Saline	12.5–100	~25	—		0	
				KB	PG						>100
35046	44	Lasiocarpine, *N*-oxide	$NO_8C_{21}H_{33}$	CA	MC	110	110	—	6		
				WM	Saline	31.3, 110	>31.3	—	8		
				LE	MC	110	>110	—		0	
				KB	—						>100
54838	40	1 *H*-Pyrrolizine, hexahydro-1-isopropylidene-3,3-dimethyl-	$NC_{12}H_{21}$	SA	MC	125, 30, 8	~8	—	2		
				CA	CMC	8	8	—	0		
				LE	CMC	8	8	—		1	

TABLE VI—*continued*

NSC No.	Supplier	Compound name	Molecular formula	Tumor system	Vehicle	Dose range tested (mg/kg)	Response (mg/kg) MTD	Response (mg/kg) MED	Evaluation TWI(%)	Evaluation ILS(%)	Evaluation ED_{40}
62958	1	Retronecanol (1 *H*-pyrrolizin-1 β-ol, 2,3,5,6,7,7a-α-hexahydro-7β-methyl-)	NOC_8H_{15}	SA	CMC	70	>70	—	9		
				CA	CMC	7–450	~56	—	0		
				LE	CMC	28	>28	—		12	
62959	1	1 *H*-pyrrolizin-1-ol, 2,3,5,7a-tetrahydro-7-methyl-	NOC_8H_{13}	SA	CMC	188	~188	—	26		
				CA	CMC	38–300	~150	—	25		
				LE	CMC	132	~132	—		3	
76020	33	Platyphylline, tartrate	$NO_5C_{18}H_{27} \cdot O_6C_4H_6$	SA	H_2O	62, 250	~62	—	12		
				91	H_2O	50	>50	—	9		
				WM	Saline	100	>100	—	0		
				LE	H_2O	50	>50	—		1	
				KB	H_2O						>100
79540	42	Integerrimine	$NO_5C_{18}H_{25}$	KB	Acidified saline						>100
89241	60	3 *H*-Pyrrolizine	NC_7H_7	SA	CMC	125, 500	>125	—	21		
				WM	Saline	125	>125	—	8		
				LE	CMC	100	>100	—		0	
				KB	PG						45
89242	60	1 *H*-Pyrrolizine, 2,3-dihydro-	NC_7H_9	LE	CMC	80, 400	~80	—		4	
				KB	PG						>100
89932	16	Fulvine	$NO_5C_{16}H_{23}$	WM	Saline	45–200	~100	~100	71[e]		
				LE	Saline	50	~50	—		12	
				KB	PG						>100
89933	16	Crispatine	$NO_5C_{16}H_{23}$	WM	Saline	1.56–75	20	—	38		
				LE	Saline	20	20	—		0	
				KB	PG						>100

89934	16	Spectabiline	$NO_7C_{18}H_{25}$	WM	Saline, CMC	2.5–100	75	~ 10^f	96		
				LE	Saline	50	50			12	
				KB	PG						>100
89935	16	Senecionine	$NO_5C_{18}H_{25}$	WM	Saline, CMC	6.25–150	50	35	60		
				LE	Saline	10–50	~ 50	—		0	
				PS	SSS	7.5–120	60	—		9	
				KB	PG						>100
89936	16	Jacobine	$NO_6C_{18}H_{25}$	WM	Saline	25–100	>100	—	8		
				LE	Saline	25, 100	~ 25	—		0	
				KB	PG						>100
89937	16	Echinatine	$NO_5C_{15}H_{25}$	WM	Saline	50–400	200	—	50		
				LE	Saline	200	200	—		0	
				KB	PG						>100
89938	16	Supinine	$NO_4C_{15}H_{25}$	WM	Saline	200–400	>400	—	2		
				LE	Saline	200	200			0	
				KB	PG						>100
89939	16	Europine	$NO_6C_{16}H_{27}$	WA	Saline	25	>25	—	0		
				KB	PG						21
89940	16	Heleurine	$NO_4C_{16}H_{27}$	WM	Saline	40–200	~ 200	—	11		
				LE	Saline	40	40	—		2	
				KB	PG						33
89941	16	1 *H*-Pyrrolizine, hexahydro-1-methylene-	NC_8H_{13}	WM	Saline	25–100	50	—	45		
				LE	Saline	25, 100	25			0	
89942	16	1 *H*-Pyrrolizin-1β-ol, 2,3,5,7a-α-tetrahydro-7-(methoxymethyl)-	$NO_2C_9H_{15}$	KB	DMF						>100
89944	16	2 *H*-Oxireno[*a*]pyrrolizine, hexahydro-6 b-(methoxy-methyl)-	$NO_2C_9H_{15}$	KB	DMF						76
89945	16	Renardine; (senkirkine)	$NO_6C_{19}H_{27}$	KB	DMF						110
90874	60	1 *H*-Pyrrolizine, hexahydro-	NC_7H_{13}	KB	DMF						110

TABLE VI—*continued*

NSC No.	Supplier	Compound name	Molecular formula	Tumor system	Vehicle	Dose range tested (mg/kg)	Response (mg/kg)		Evaluation		
							MTD	MED	TWI(%)	ILS(%)	ED_{40}
100,218	31	1 *H*-Pyrrolizinium, 4-benzyl-hexahydro-7a-hydroxy-, perchlorate	$NOC_{14}H_{20}^{+}ClO_4^{-}$	LE	Saline	40, 80, 400	40	—		2	
				WM	Saline	40	>40	—	0		
106,677	29	Senecionine *N*-oxide	$NO_6C_{18}H_{25}$	WM	Saline	10–100	~100	~50[g]	70		
				LE	Saline	20–40	>40	—		2	
				PS	Saline	10–80	~40	—		13	
108,378	16	Monocrotaline *N*-oxide	$NO_7C_{16}H_{23}$	LE	Saline	400	~400	—		22	
109,445	16	Monocrotaline diacetate (ester)	$NO_8C_{20}H_{27}$	WM	Saline	15–240	30	15	95		
				LE	Saline	60	60	—		22	
				KB	—						30
113,087	16	Monocrotaline α-epoxide	$NO_7C_{16}H_{23}$	WM	Saline	400	>400	—	7		
113,088	16	Monocrotaline α-epoxide, *N*-oxide, trifluoroacetate (ester)	$NO_9F_3C_{18}H_{22}$	LE	DMSO	400	~400	—		0	
				WM	DMSO	400	400	—	28		
114,571	16	Anacrotine	$NO_6C_{18}H_{23}$	LE	CMC	70	<70	—		19	
116,334	16	Monocrotaline β-epoxide	$NO_7C_{16}H_{23}$	KB							>100
117,181	63	Cyclopiazonic acid	$N_2O_3C_{20}H_{20}$	LE	Saline	2	>2	—		0	

[a] TI ≧ 3. [b] TI ≧ 16. [c] TI ≧ 5. [d] TI > 1. [e] Results erratic. [f] TI ≅ 7. [g] TI ≦ 2.

tyramine, and trigonelline have also been found. These two alkaloids are relatively simple aliphatic diamino amides, whose structures are shown in (IX) and (X) (see Table VII).

$$\begin{matrix} (CH_3)_2N(CH_2)_4 \\ (CH_3)_2N(CH_2)_4 \end{matrix} \rangle N{-}R$$

(IX) Solapalmitine: $R{=}CO(CH_2)_{14}CH_3$

(X) Solapalmitenine: $R{=}\textit{trans}{-}COCH{=}CH(CH_2)_{12}CH_3$

While the therapeutic indexes of these alkaloids do not justify further pharmacological work designed to develop them into useful drugs, the real interest in these alkaloids lies in their representing a new class of active compounds and the fact that their structure is such as to encourage the synthesis of series of analogs designed to explore spatial, solubility, and other factors in structure-activity relationships.

B. Sesquiterpene Lactones

The cytotoxicity shown by several of the sesquiterpene lactones isolated from members of the plant family Compositae submitted by Kupchan (Table VIII, supplier 29) and by Herz (Table VIII, supplier 23), followed later by demonstration of *in vivo* antitumor activity (WM) in other related compounds submitted by Kupchan, created interest in this whole class of substances. A summary of the results obtained with all these compounds in the CCNSC collection is given in Table VIII.

Chemically, these compounds fall naturally into three well-defined types—those derived from decahydronaphthalene (XI) including the eudalene type, those from cyclopentanocycloheptane (XII) including the guaianolides, and those from cyclodecane (XIII) including the germacranolides—along with a miscellaneous group of diverse structures with too few members of any one type to justify segregation, and a small group with unknown structure.

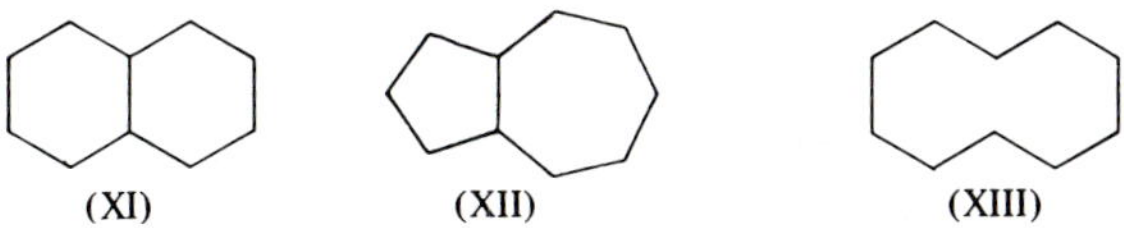

(XI) (XII) (XIII)

These types are listed in Table VIII as I, II, III, Misc. and Unk., respectively. Recent reviews of the chemistry of most of these compounds are to be found in de Mayo (1959a), Dean (1963), Šorm and Dolejš (1966), and Romo and Romo de Vivar (1967).

In an attempt to elucidate structure-activity relationships, the possible effects of various functional groups present have been considered. These relate to the presence and location of an ethylenic linkage, the presence of an epoxy

TABLE VII

ALKALOIDS OF *Solanum tripartitum*

NSC No.	Supplier	Compound name	Molecular formula	Tumor system	Vehicle	Dose range tested (mg/kg)	Response (mg/kg)		Evaluation		
							MTD	MED	TWI(%)	ILS(%)	ED_{50}
123,124	29	Solapalmitine (VIII)	$N_3OC_{28}H_{59}$	WM	Saline or CMC	6.6–20	~8.5	>8.5	70[a]		
				KB	PG						0.22
123,125	29	Solapalmitenine (IX)	$N_3OC_{28}H_{57}$	WM	CMC	6–30	~11	>11	85[a]		
				KB	PG						0.14

[a] Results erratic—based on plotted data.

TABLE VIII

SESQUITERPENE AND RELATED LACTONES

NSC No.	Supplier	Compound name	Molecular formula	Type	Tumor system	Vehicle	Dose range tested (mg/kg)	Response (mg/kg)		Evaluation		
								MTD	MED	TWI(%)	ILS(%)	ED_{50}
4900	44	Santonin	$O_3C_{15}H_{18}$	ld	SA	Saline + T-80	250–500	250	—	18		
					CA	Saline + T-80	125	>125	—	~25		
					LE	Saline + T-80	125	>125	—		0	
					KB	—						140
14190	61	Gibberellin	$O_{5-7}C_{19}H_{22-26}$	Misc.	SA	MC	125, 250	>250	—	~25		

16037	10	Isocolumbin	$O_6C_{20}H_{22}$	Misc., f	SA	MC	125, 500	>125	—	0		
					CA	MC	112	>112	—	21		
					LE	MC	125	>125	—		7	
19450	1	Gibberellic acid	$O_6C_{19}H_{22}$	II	LL	Saline	400	>400	—	0		
					WM	Saline	25–200	>200	—	0		
					LE	Saline	400	~400	—		0	
					KB	PG						>100
19942	23	Tenulin	$O_5C_{17}H_{22}$	IId	SA	MC	500	<500	—	17		
					CA	MC	350	>350	—	8		
					WM	CMC	100	>100	—	0		
					LE	MC	250, 500	~250			1	
22070	23; 54	Pyrethrosin	$O_5C_{17}H_{22}$	IIIabc	SA	CMC	50, 100, 500	50	—	6		
					CA	CMC	45	45	—	0		
					WA	CMC	16–125	62	—	28		
					LE	CMC	45	~45	—		15	
					DL	CMC	10–100	50	—		0	
35037	44	Lactone from *Arctium minus*	$O_6C_{18}H_{24}$	Unk., ab	CA	MC	70	70	—	0		
					LE	MC	30	~30	—		0	
35044	44	Lactone from *Centaurea maculosa*	$O_7C_{20}H_{26}$	Unk.	SA	MC	10	>10	—	0		
					CA	MC	9	<9	—	22		
					LE	MC	9	~9	—		0	
35419	44	Pulvinic acid di-γ-lactone (pulvic anhydride)	$O_4C_{18}H_{10}$	Misc., ae	SA	Saline	125	>125	—	2		
					LE	Saline	115	>115	—		20	
41306	13	1-β-Desmotroposantonin	$O_3C_{15}H_{18}$	I	SA	MC	125	~125		13		
					LE	MC	125	>125			0	
					KB	—						>100
41307	13	1-β-Desmotroposantonin acetate	$O_4C_{17}H_{20}$	I	SA	MC	125	>125	—	15		
					CA	MC	112	112	—	10		
					LE	MC	125	>125			0	
41308	13	1-α-Desmotroposantonin	$O_3C_{15}H_{18}$	I	SA	MC	125	>125	—	0		
					CA	MC	112	>112		2		
					LE	MC	125	>125			0	

TABLE VIII—*continued*

NSC No.	Supplier	Compound name	Molecular formula	Type	Tumor system	Vehicle	Dose range tested (mg/kg)	Response (mg/kg) MTD	Response (mg/kg) MED	Evaluation TWI(%)	Evaluation ILS(%)	Evaluation ED_{50}
41311	13	β-Santonin	$O_3C_{15}H_{18}$	Id	SA	MC	125	>125	—	25		
					CA	MC	112	112	—	43		
					LE	MC	125	>125	—		0	
					KB	—						>100
42037	13	Eudesma-3,5,7(11)-trien-6,13-olide, **3-hydroxy,** acetate	$O_4C_{17}H_{20}$	Ia	SA	MC	125	125	—	0		
					CA	MC	100	>100	—	0		
					LE	MC	100	>100	—		0	
42038	13	Santonin oxime	$NO_3C_{15}H_{19}$	Id	SA	MC	62.5, 125	~62.5	—	9		
					CA	MC	28, 56	28	—	25		
					LE	MC	56	56			0	
85234	23	Pinnatifidin	$O_3C_{15}H_{18}$	Iabd	SA	Saline	500	<500	—	10		
					LL	Saline	400	~400	—	9		
					8P	Saline	100	>100	—	13		
					LE	Saline	100	>100	—		4	
					DA	Saline	50	>50	—		0	
					KB	PG						1.7
85235	23	Ambrosin	$O_3C_{15}H_{18}$	IIabd	SA	Saline	500, 100	>100	—	13		
					8P	Saline	100	>100	—	7		
					LE	Saline	100	>100	—		0	
					DA	Saline	50	>50	—		0	
					KB	PG						0.040
85236	23	Helenalin	$O_4C_{15}H_{18}$	IIabd	SA	Saline	4	>4	—	0		
					LL	Saline	3.2	>3.2	—	33		
					8P	Saline	1.56–100	~1.56	—	23		
					H1	DMF	0.31–20	<0.31	—	0		
					WM	Saline	0.5–4	>4	—	0		
					LE	Saline	1.56	1.56	—		4	
					DA	Saline	0.78	>0.78	—		0	
					KB	PG						0.22

85237	23	Ivalin	$O_3C_{15}H_{20}$	Iab	SA	Saline	250, 500	~250	—	20		
					8P	Saline	100	>100	—	0		
					LE	Saline	100	>100	—		10	
					DA	Saline	50	>50	—		0	
					KB	PG						0.72
85238	23	Asperilin	$O_3C_{15}H_{20}$	Iab	8P	Saline	100	>100	—	12		
					LE	Saline	100	>100	—		20	
					DA	Saline	50	>50	—		4	
					KB	PG						1
85239	23	Parthenin	$O_3C_{15}H_{20}$	IIab	SA	Saline	12.5, 50	>12.5	—	0		
					LL	Saline	10	>10	—	21		
					8P	Saline	25, 100	>25	—	26		
					WM	Saline	1.56–12.5	>12.5	—	0		
					KB	PG						0.025
85240	23	Neotenulin, deacetyl-	$O_4C_{15}H_{20}$	IId	8P	Saline	100	>100	—	0		
					LE	Saline	100	>100	—		17	
					DA	Saline	50	>50	—		0	
					KB	PG						100
85241	23	Ivasperin	$O_4C_{15}H_{20}$	Iab	SA	Saline	125, 500	125	—	30		
					8P	Saline	100	100	—	36		
					LE	Saline	100	100	—		22	
					DA	Saline	50	50	—		0	
					H1	DMF	0.31–20	<0.31	—	35		
					KB	PG						1.6
85242	23	Coronopilin	$O_4C_{15}H_{20}$	IIab	SA	Saline	125, 500	~125	—	17		
					8P	Saline	100	>100	—	0		
					LE	Saline	100	>100	—		6	
					DA	Saline	50	>50	—		0	
					KB	PG						1.4
85243	23	Pseudoivalin	$O_4C_{15}H_{20}$	IIab	SA	Saline	500	<500	—	17		
					LL	Saline	400	400	—	24		
					8P	Saline	100	>100	—		2	
					DA	Saline	50	>50	—		0	
					KB	PG						1.8
85244	23	Pulchellin	$O_4C_{15}H_{22}$	IIab	SA	Saline	500	500	—	5		
					8P	Saline	100	>100	—	0		
					LE	Saline	100	>100	—		18	
					DA	Saline	50	>50	—		0	
					KB	PG						1.8

TABLE VIII—*continued*

NSC No.	Supplier	Compound name	Molecular formula	Type	Tumor system	Vehicle	Dose range tested (mg/kg)	Response (mg/kg)		Evaluation		
								MTD	MED	TWI(%)	ILS(%)	ED_{50}
85245	23	Microcephalin	$O_4C_{15}H_{22}$	Iab	8P	Saline	100	>100	—	0		
					LE	Saline	100	<100	—		3	
					DA	Saline	50	>50	—		13	
					KB	PG						22
85246	23	Gaillardilin	$O_6C_{17}H_{22}$	IIabc	8H1	DMF	2, 5, 10, 20	<10	—	0		
					KB	PG						2.2
85247	23	Isotenulin	$O_5C_{17}H_{24}$	II	8P	Saline	100	>100	—	36		
					LE	Saline	100	>100	—		0	
					DA	Saline	50	>50	—		0	
					KB	PG						16
85248	23	Flexuosin B	$O_6C_{17}H_{24}$	II	8P	Saline	100	<100	—	0		
					KB	PG						26
85249	23; 18	Damsin	$O_3C_{15}H_{20}$	IIab	KB	PG						0.58
85250	23	Spathulin	$O_8C_{19}H_{26}$	IIab	KB	PG						4.5
93131	33	Alantolactone	$O_2C_{15}H_{20}$	Iab	SA	Saline	125, 500	<125	—	28		
					LL	Saline	100	~100	—	29		
					WM	Saline	100	>100	—	0		
					LE	Saline	100	~100	—		0	
					KB	PG						1.4
94032	23	Pulchellin B	$O_5C_{17}H_{22}$	IIab	KB	PG						7.
94033	23	Pulchellin C	$O_4C_{15}H_{20}$	IIab	KB	PG						>100
94034	23	Pulchellin E	$O_5C_{17}H_{22}$	IIab	KB	PG						~1.0
94035	23	Fastigilin B	$O_6C_{17}H_{22}$	IId	KB	PG						1.9
94036	23	Fastigilin C	$O_6C_{20}H_{24}$	IIabd	KB	PG						0.34

94037	23	Mikanolide	$O_6C_{15}H_{14}$	IIIabce	WM	Saline	6, 10, 50	>50	—	55[a]		
					LE	CMC	5–400	~5	—		12	
					KB	PG						<1
100,046	29	Elephantopin	$O_7C_{19}H_{20}$	IIIabcde	SA	Saline	2.5–10	>10	—	0		
					LL	Saline	2–8	>8	—	0		
					8P	Saline	2.5–10	>10	—	6		
					WM	CMC	2.5–150	~75	75	78[a]		
					LE	CMC	2.5–40	~2.5	—		28	
					PS	Saline or CMC	5–60	~40	5		71	
					DA	Saline	2.5–10	>10	—		8	
					KB	PG						0.32
102,817	29	Elephantin	$O_7C_{20}H_{22}$	IIIabcde	WM	CMC	25–100	<100	—	70		
					KB	Alcohol						1.6
104,942	29	Euparotin	$O_7C_{20}H_{24}$	IIabc	KB	DMF						0.21
104,943	29	Euparotin acetate	$O_8C_{22}H_{26}$	IIabc	WM	CMC	20–200	~75	75	77[b]		
					PS	SSS	10–80	40	—		18	
					KB	DMF						0.22
106,390	35; 16	Psilostachyin A	$O_5C_{15}H_{20}$	Misc., abe	WM	Saline	200	>200	—	0		
					KB	PG						5.4
106,391	35	Psilostachyin B	$O_4C_{15}H_{18}$	Misc., abi	WM	Saline	100	>100	—	11		
106,392	35	Psilostachyin C	$O_4C_{15}H_{20}$	Misc., abi	WM	Saline	50	>50	—	25		
106,394	29	Gaillardin	$O_5C_{17}H_{22}$	IIab	WM	CMC	15–300	~40	—	9		
					LE	CMC	50–200	<50	—		0	
					KB	PG						0.80
106,395	29	Isogaillardin	$O_5C_{17}H_{22}$	Unk., ab	KB	PG						1.6
106,397	29	Vernolepin methanol adduct	$O_6C_{16}H_{20}$	Misc., abdg	WM	CMC	6.3–100	>100	—	7		
					PS	SSS	0.5–10	~8	~4		40	
					KB	PG						25
106,398	29	Vernolepin	$O_5C_{15}H_{16}$	Misc., abi	WM	Saline	6–100	~10	~10	70		
					KB	PG						2.0
106,404	18	Costunolide	$O_2C_{15}H_{20}$	IIIab	WM	Saline	25–100	>100	—	11		
					LE	Saline	50–100	~200	—		0	
					KB	PG						0.26

TABLE VIII—*continued*

NSC No.	Supplier	Compound name	Molecular formula	Type	Tumor system	Vehicle	Dose range tested (mg/kg)	Response (mg/kg)		Evaluation		
								MTD	MED	TWI(%)	ILS(%)	ED_{50}
106,405	18	Tulipinolide	$O_4C_{10}H_{22}$	IIIab	WM	Saline	31.3–125	>62.5	—	20		
					LE	Saline	50–400	~100	—		2	
					KB	PG						0.52
106,908	55	Fomannosin	$O_4C_{15}H_{18}$	Misc., ag	WM	Saline	20	<20	—	35		
					LE	Saline	5–400	~20	—		5	
109,433	22	Laserolide	$O_6C_{22}H_{30}$	IIId	WM	Saline	350	>350	—	43		
109,435	22	Scabiolide	$O_8C_{21}H_{28}$	IIIab	WM	Saline	8.5–350	<17	—	0		
109,436	23	Pulchellin C epoxide	$O_5C_{15}H_{20}$	IIabc	WM	Saline	200	>200	—	49		
110,257	49	Gingko lactone	$O_{10}C_{20}H_{24}$	Misc., h	KB	DMF						>100
112,152	21	Plumericine	$O_6C_{15}H_{14}$	Misc., abd	LE	Saline	100–400[c]	~400	—		4	
112,153	21	Isoplumericine	$O_6C_{15}H_{14}$	Misc., abd	LE	Saline	5–200[c]	40	—		6	
113,091	16	Dihydroparthenolide	$O_3C_{15}H_{22}$	IIIabc	KB	PG						>100
116,070	29	Vernomenin	$O_5C_{15}H_{16}$	Misc., abi	WM	Saline	20–80	~40	40	56[d]		
					KB	PG						20
403,139	44	Picrotoxin	$O_6C_{15}H_{16}$	Misc., ci	SA	CMC	3,12, 60	~3	—	43		
					CA	CMC	2.4	<2.4	—	0		
					LE	CMC	2.4	<2.4	—		0	
					KB	—						40

[a] Results erratic.
[b] Results not reproducible.
[c] Single injection procedure only.
[d] Erratic toxicity.

group, and the presence and size of a lactone group. These structural functions are indicated in Table VIII in the column headed "Type," as follows: (*a*) An ethylenic linkage α,β- to the lactone carbonyl group; (*b*) the double bond in (*a*) is *exo*; (*c*) one or more epoxy groups; (*d*) an additional α,β-unsaturated ketone group (or ester or oxime); (*e*) 2 γ-lactone groups; (*f*) 2 δ-lactone groups; (*g*) 1 δ-lactone group; (*h*) 3 γ-lactone groups; and (*i*) 1 γ- and 1 δ-lactone group.

Unless otherwise noted as above, the lactone is assumed to be a saturated γ-lactone. While structure-activity relationships are complicated by such factors as solubility in the solvent used in the tests, biological variation in the responses, and statistically small numbers of examples, it is difficult not to try to make some judgments. These may have some value in guiding future work although their limited basis must always be borne in mind. Cytotoxicity (in KB) is commonly shown by these lactones. In every case the active compounds are α,β-unsaturated lactones; the same applies to all but one (NSC-94035) of the compounds with borderline activity in KB. The fact that the α,β-ethylenic linkage is *exo* in every case is of doubtful significance as there are only two compounds in the whole list (NSC-42037 and NSC-106,908) for comparison where the double bond is *endo* and these have not been tested in KB. While the α,β-unsaturated lactone grouping appears to be important for cytotoxicity, it does not always confer this activity as 8 out of 17 of the least active compounds also possess this grouping. The additional α,β-unsaturated ketone grouping seems to be of little significance because although one borderline KB-active compound (NSC-94035) contains it as has been noted, three other compounds that contain it (NSC-4900, 41311 and 85240) are inactive. Cytotoxicity also appears to be independent of the type of compound (many examples of types I, II, and III being active and others being inactive), the size and number of the lactone rings, and the presence or absence of an epoxy group.

In the sesquiterpene lactones, *in vivo* activity is shown by five compounds (NSC-100,046, 102,817, 104,943, 106,397 and 106,398; NSC-116,070 is marginal) in WM, and marginal activity in LE is shown only by NSC-100,046 and NSC-106,397. Again, all the active compounds are α,β-unsaturated lactones while many of the inactive ones also have this structural feature. As before, little discernible influence is shown by the type of compound, the size of the lactone ring, and the presence or absence of the α,β-unsaturated ketone system, and the epoxy group. It may have some significance that the most interesting compound of the group, elephantopin (XIV; NSC-100,046), showing activity in WM, LE (marginal), PS, and KB, has the largest number of structural features—an α,β-unsaturated lactone group with an exocyclic double bond, an α,β-unsaturated ester group, an epoxy group, and a second α,β-unsaturated γ-lactone group. The other compound with all these characteristics, elephantin (NSC-102,817), is active against WM and KB but has not been tested against any other *in vivo* tumor.

While elephantopin and elephantin do not have therapeutic indexes in the range that would justify further pharmacological study, the sesquiterpene lactones are a group that should certainly be more completely investigated as a source of practical antitumor drugs.

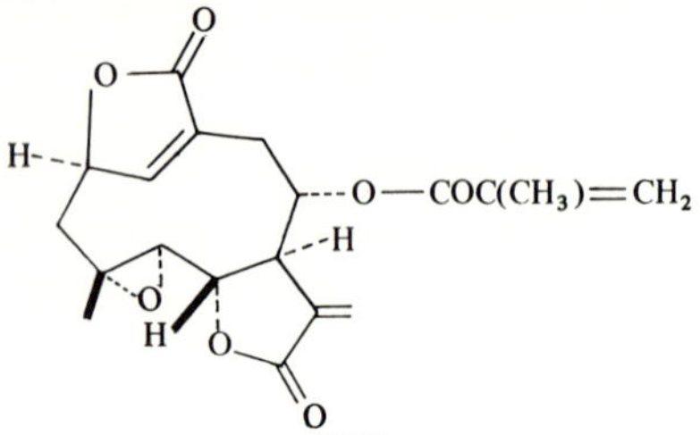

(XIV)

C. Sterols

Early in the plant fractionation work, β-sitosterol appeared frequently as a constituent active against WM. Further work showed it to have some activity against LL and MS and marginal activity against CA. A survey of the other sterols in the CCNSC program (Table IX) showed that no other "simple" sterol (i.e., excluding those with a lactone function) possesses *in vivo* or *in vitro* antitumor activity with the exception of estrone which is only marginally active against SA. Attempts to utilize β-sitosterol by converting it into a more soluble derivative resulted in the half-esters, NSC-99628 and NSC-110,372. While these derivatives had better solubility than the original sterol and activity against WM was retained, the therapeutic indexes were not sufficiently high to justify development as a useful drug. However, the finding is of interest because of β-sitosterol being the first simple sterol to show activity against WM and the possibility that more suitable derivatives will be prepared. A list of plants whose activity is due solely to β-sitosterol and other plant sterols is given in Table XVII.

In this connection it is important to qualify the meaning of β-sitosterol as used here. It has been found* that the samples of β-sitosterol, commercial and otherwise, used in these tests and used to prepare the two soluble half esters, are not pure but contain substantial amounts of campesterol and sometimes also stigmasterol and/or stigmastanol. Since the latter two sterols are inactive in WM and since campesterol-enriched mixtures are less active than impure β-sitosterol, it would appear that the activity should be ascribed to β-sitosterol.

D. Saponins

Saponins are a heterogeneous group of glycosides found widely dispersed in the plant kingdom. The aglycones, or sapogenins, belong either to the class of

* Private communication from Chas. Pfizer and Co., Inc., Maywood, N.J.

TABLE IX

PLANT STEROLS AND RELATED COMPOUNDS

NSC No.	Supplier	Compound name	Molecular formula	Tumor system	Vehicle	Dose range tested (mg/kg)	Response (mg/kg)		Evaluation		
							MTD	MED	TWI(%)	ILS(%)	ED_{50}
1610	64	Lanosterol (isocholesterol)	$OC_{30}H_{50}$	SA	SSS	125, 500	500	—	0		
60677	2			CA	SSS	60, 450	450	—	13		
				LE	SSS	125, 400	400	—		3	
				KB							35
1611	64; 16	8-Lanostene-7,11-dione, 3 β-hydroxy-	$O_3C_{30}H_{48}$	SA	—	62.5	>62.5	—	11		
				CA	—	30	~30		34		
				LE	—	60	>60	—		3	
4920	12	24-Bromolanosterol	$BrOC_{30}H_{49}$	SA	SSS	62–500	>500	—	0		
				8P	SSS	50–400	>400	—	0		
				LE	SSS	62–500	~500	—		2	
8095	39	Stigmasterol	$OC_{29}H_{48}$	SA	MC	300, 500	~300	—	25		
				CA	MC	55, 270	~55	—	0		
				WM	CMC	400	400	—	21		
				LE	CMC	400	400	—		0	
8096	39	β-Sitosterol	$OC_{29}H_{50}$	SA	H_2O	200–500	400	—	53		
18173	57			CA	H_2O	100–300	~200	~200[a]	58		
49083	71			LL	H_2O	15–450	~200	~150[b]	68		
86199	51			MS	H_2O	100–200	~200	200[b]	62		
				WM	H_2O	2.9–450	~100	~40[c]	97		
				LE	H_2O	100–300	~300	—		0	
				P4	H_2O	50–300	~300	—		8	
8798	45	Cholesterol	$OC_{27}H_{46}$	SA	MC	150–500	~500	—	14		
				CA	MC	135	>135	—	4		
				LE	MC	150	~150	—		0	
9699	68	Estrone	$O_2C_{18}H_{22}$	SA	MC	250–500	250	—	62		
				CA	MC	225	225	—	6		
				LE	MC	250	250	—		2	
				WM	SSS	400 —	>400		17		

TABLE IX—*continued*

NSC No.	Supplier	Compound name	Molecular formula	Tumor system	Vehicle	Dose range tested (mg/kg)	Response (mg/kg) MTD	Response (mg/kg) MED	Evaluation TWI(%)	Evaluation ILS(%)	Evaluation ED_{50}
14329	24	5 α-Lanost-8-ene-7 β-hydroperoxide, 3 β-hydroxy-, 3-acetate	$O_4C_{32}H_{54}$	SA	MC	500	500	—	17		
				EA	MC	500	500	—	31		
16347	24	3 β-Hydroxy-8-lanostene-7,11-dione, acetate	$O_4C_{32}H_{50}$	SA	MC	125	125	—	10		
				CA	MC	115	115	—	0		
				LE	MC	125	125	—		0	
34201	50	5 α-Chol-8-en-24-oic acid, 3 β-hydroxy-4,4,14-trimethyl-7,11-dioxo-, methyl ester, acetate	$O_6C_{30}H_{44}$	CA	—	450	450	—	0		
				KB	—						>100
34202	50	5 α-Cholan-24-oic acid, 3 β-hydroxy-4,4,14-trimethyl-7,11-dioxo-, methyl ester, acetate	$O_6C_{30}H_{46}$	CA	—	400	~400	—	0		
34203	50	5 α-Lanost-8-en-3 β-ol, 24,25-dibromo-, acetate	$Br_2O_2C_{32}H_{52}$	CA	—	300	>300		0		
36571	44	Euphol	$OC_{30}H_{50}$	SA	MC	65, 125	~65	—	34		
				KB	—						19
41969	65	Eburicolic acid	$O_3C_{31}H_{50}$	SA	MC	500	500	—	37		
				CA	MC	450	450	—	29		
				LE	MC	222–500	333			0	
49081	71	5 α-Stigmastan-3 β-ol hydrate	$OC_{29}H_{52}\cdot H_2O$	SA	MC	350	~350	—	3		
				CA	MC	70	>70	—	36		
				LE	MC	245	~245	—		0	
				WM	SSS	350	>350	—	21		
					H_2O	100–800	~800	400	75		
				KB	—						40
49082	71	Stigmast-4-en-3-one	$OC_{29}H_{48}$	SA	MC	350	<350	—	0		
				CA	MC	250	>250	—	23		
				LE	MC	245	~245	—		0	

62791	44	Ergosterol	$OC_{28}H_{44}$	SA	CMC	188, 375	~188	—	0		
				CA	CMC	169	<169	—	0		
				LE	CMC	169	~169	—		0	
				WM	Saline	400	400	—	10		
				KB	Dioxane						31
67783	76	Lanosta-1,8,24-trien-3-one, 2-hydroxy-	$O_2C_{30}H_{46}$	SA	CMC	250	250	—	0		
				FV	SSS	200	200	—	0		
				KB	Acetone						27
72255	65	Lanosta-8,20(22),23-trien-21-oic acid, 3 β,24-dihydroxy-, δ-lactone, acetate	$O_4C_{32}H_{46}$	SA	SSS	250	>250	—	3		
				91	SSS	200	>200	—	0		
				LE	SSS	200	>200			12	
76475	75	Cholest-5-en-3-one, 4,4-dimethyl-	$OC_{29}H_{48}$	SA	SSS	125	>125	—	8		
				LE	SSS	100	>100	—		0	
				KB	DMF						>100
82135	65	5 α-Lanosta-8,20-dien-3 β-ol, 24-methyl-21,21-diphenyl-, acetate	$O_2C_{45}H_{62}$	SA	SSS	125	>125	—	0		
				CA	SSS	100	>100	—	15		
				KB	Dioxane						28
93683	63	19-Nor-9 β,10 α-lanosta-5,23-diene-3,11-dione, 2 β,16 α-20,25-tetrahydroxy-9-methyl-, mixture with 3, 16α,20,25-tetrahydroxy-9-methyl-19-nor-9β,10α-lanosta-5,23-diene-2,-11-dione	$O_6C_{30}H_{46}$	LE	Oil	200	<200	—		6	
				KB	DMF						5.3
99628	51	β-Sitosterol hemisuccinate	$O_4C_{33}H_{54}$	A_3	H_2O	50–400	~100	—		2[d]	
				LL	H_2O	200–800	600	400	~60[d]		
				WM	H_2O	100–600	400	200[e]	~75		
104,467	7	Echinodol	$O_4C_{32}H_{50}$	LE	SSS	325 —	325	—		3	
104,468	7	Echinodiol	$O_3C_{30}H_{48}$	LE	SSS	120 —	>120	—		0	
110,372	51	β-Sitosterol carboxymethyl-thiohemisuccinate	$O_6SC_{35}H_{56}$	LE	H_2O	25–200	100	—		3	
				PS	H_2O	25–200	25	—		0	
				P_4	H_2O	12–200	25	—		9	
				WM	H_2O	25–200	~100	40[f]	85		
				WI	H_2O + T-80	6.25–50	~50	—		20	

TABLE IX—*continued*

NSC No.	Supplier	Compound name	Molecular formula	Tumor system	Vehicle	Dose range tested (mg/kg)	Response (mg/kg)		Evaluation		
							MTD	MED	TWI(%)	ILS(%)	ED_{50}
403,164	44	Tirucallol	$OC_{30}H_{50}$	KB	—						12
403,182	44	5 α-Lanost-8-en-26-oic acid, 3 α,12 α-dihydroxy-24-methyl-ene-	$O_4C_{31}H_{50}$	KB	—						28
404,567	8	5 ξ-Lanosta-7,24-dien-26-oic acid, 3-oxo-, methyl ester	$O_3C_{31}H_{48}$	KB	PG						>100
404,568	8	Cholesta-7,24-dien-26-oic acid, 4,4,14-trimethyl-3-oxo-	$O_3C_{30}H_{46}$	KB	PG						27
404,569	8	5 ξ-Lanosta-8,24-dien-24-oic acid, 3-oxo-, methyl ester	$O_3C_{31}H_{48}$	KB	PG						43
407,136	44	Cycloartenone	$OC_{30}H_{48}$	KB	Dioxane						26

[a] TI ≦ 1.
[b] TI ~ 1.
[c] TI ~ 2.5 (erratic).
[d] Erratic toxicity.
[e] TI ~ 2.
[f] TI ~ 2.2.

steroids (XV) or pentacyclic triterpenes including the α- and β-amyrin and the friedelin types based on (XVI), and the lupeol type based on (XVII) (cf. Karrer, 1958).

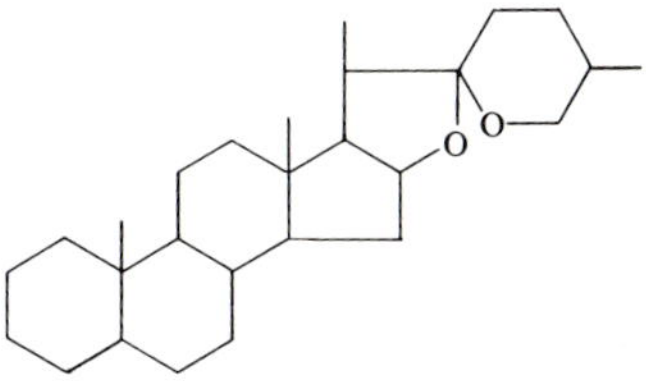

(XV) 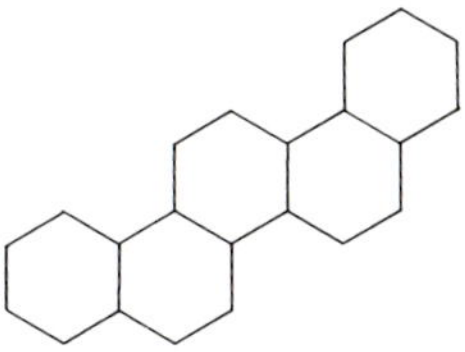 (XVI) 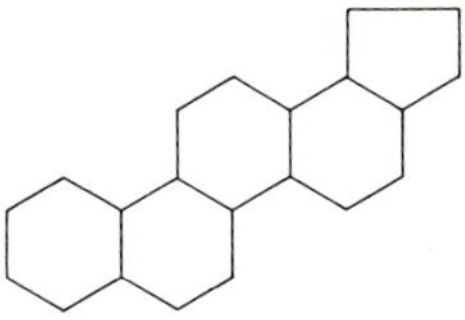 (XVII)

Recent reviews of the chemistry of these substances are to be found in Fieser and Fieser (1959; steroids only), de Mayo (1959b), and Dean (1963).

In the following table, these classes are indicated in the column headed "Type," structures (XV)–(XVII) being indicated as types I–III, respectively. In this column, also, a glycoside is indicated by the letter G, while a and b indicate respectively the presence of a COOH group and a quinonoid group.

Among the compounds listed, cytotoxicity is conspicuously absent. *In vivo* antitumor activity is frequently found, notably in WM. No meaningful structure-activity relationships can be found with the small numbers of compounds involved. Of the 13 active compounds (in WM) there are representatives of all these types, while all three types are also represented among the 21 inactive compounds. There are glycosides as well as aglycones among both the active and inactive compounds. Activity also appears to be independent of the presence or absence of a COOH group. Only two compounds contain a quinonoid group and one was not tested in WM; consideration of this group is meaningless at this point.

Of the active compounds, the most interesting is *Acer* saponin P (NSC-100,045) a saponin from *Acer negundo** of unknown structure, because it has the largest TI in WM of any of the active compounds of this group. This compound is being investigated further, chemically and pharmacologically. In the meantime, the lead provided by this agent is being developed to include the testing of others of this large class of compounds.

E. Cucurbitacins

This is a group of higher terpenoids whose chemistry has been recently reviewed by Ourisson *et al.* (1964). Members of this group had been found only in many species of the plant family Cucurbitaceae until recently when members were found in the families Cruciferae and Scrophulariaceae (cf. Moss, 1966). Most recently, one of them has been found in the Begoniaceae (Doskotch *et al.*,

* Kupchan *et al.* (1967e).

TABLE X

SAPONINS, THEIR AGLYCONES, AND RELATED SUBSTANCES

NSC No.	Supplier	Compound name	Molecular formula	Type	Tumor system	Vehicle	Dose range tested (mg/kg)	Response (mg/kg) MTD	MED	Evaluation TWI(%)	ILS(%)	ED_{50}
1151	48	Lupeol, benzoate	$O_2C_{37}H_{54}$	III	SA	MC	125, 500	500	—	48		
43869	48				CA	MC	113	~113	—	22		
					LE	MC	113	~113	—		0	
1615	64	Sarsasapogenin	$O_3C_{27}H_{44}$	I	SA	—	125	~125	—	0		
					CA	—	30, 60	30	—	0		
					LE	—	125	~125	—		4	
2800	12	Glycyrrizic acid,	$O_{16}C_{42}H_{62}\cdot$	II	SA	Saline	500	~500	—	8		
35348	44	NH_4 salt	NH_3		CA	Saline	250, 450	450	—	2		
					WM	Saline	75–1200	1000	—	33		
					LE	Saline	450, 500	450			5	
4060	44	Ursolic acid	$O_3C_{30}H_{48}$	II	LE	Saline	400	400			0	
					WM	Saline	400	400		9		
4644	48	Betulin (betulinol)	$O_2C_{30}H_{50}$	III	SA	MC	150–500	300	—	15		
					CA	MC	105	>105	—	42		
					EA	MC	400	<400	—	0		
					LL	CMC	50–200	~200	—	32		
15308	15	Amyrin (mixture of α and β)	$OC_{30}H_{50}$	II	SA	MC	125, 500	125	—	27		
					CA	MC	100	~100	—	60[a]		
					LE	MC	125	125	—		2	
22071	23	Lantadene A + B	$O_5C_{35}H_{52}$	II	SA	MC	500	<500	—	41		
					CA	MC	400	400	—	3		
					LE	MC	250, 500	250	—		0	
					KB	—						30

23471	44	Digitonin	$O_{29}C_{56}H_{92}$	G I	SA	SSS	90, 350	90	—	13		
					CA	SSS	80	80	—	2		
					LL	CMC	6.2–200	12.5	—	42		
					WM	SSS	12.5–200	100	—	34		
					LE	SSS	80	~80	—		0	
					KB	—						30
23919	25	18 α-Olean-12-en-30-oic acid, 3,11-dioxo-	$O_4C_{30}H_{44}$	II	SA	MC	500	500	—	3		
					CA	MC	400	400	—	10		
					LE	MC	50–400	50	—		0	
23920	25	18 β-Olean-12-en-3,11,30-trione, 30-(hydroxymethyl)-, acetate	$O_5C_{33}H_{48}$	II	SA	—	125	>125	—	17		
					CA	—	110	>110	—	6		
					LE	—	110	>110	—		2	
24954	70	Hederagenin	$O_4C_{30}H_{48}$	II	SA	—	400	400	—	30		
					CA	—	360	360	—	0		
33395	46	Saponin of diosgenin	Unk.	G I	SA	MC	500	<500	—	34		
					KB	Dioxane						3.4
33396	46	Diosgenin	$O_3C_{27}H_{42}$	I	SA	MC	500	>500	—	0		
					CA	MC	450	>450	—	0		
					LE	MC	450	~450	—		5	
					KB	—						17
35347	44	Glycyrrhetinic acid	$O_4C_{30}H_{46}$	II	SA	H_2O	125, 500	125	—	22		
					CA	H_2O	67, 113	67	—	24		
					HE	CMC	75	75	—	0		
					WM	Saline	50–200	>200	—	29		
					LE	H_2O	56, 113	~56	—		1	
35349	44	Glycyrrhetinic acid, acetate	$O_5C_{32}H_{48}$	II	SA	H_2O	500	>500	—	35		
					EA	H_2O	450	>450	—	18		
					LE	H_2O	450	>450	—		3	
35350	44	18 α-Glycyrrhetinic acid	$O_4C_{30}H_{36}$	II	SA	H_2O	500	>500	—	23		
					EA	H_2O	450	>450	—	21		
					LE	H_2O	450	>450	—		3	
35351	44	18 α-Glycyrrhetinic acid, acetate	$O_5C_{32}H_{48}$	II	SA	H_2O	500	>500	—	34		
					EA	H_2O	450	>450	—	0		
					LE	H_2O	450	>450	—		2	
					KB	—						24

TABLE X—*continued*

NSC No.	Supplier	Compound name	Molecular formula	Type	Tumor system	Vehicle	Dose range tested (mg/kg)	Response (mg/kg) MTD	Response (mg/kg) MED	Evaluation TWI(%)	Evaluation ILS(%)	Evaluation ED_{50}
36002	30	Asiaticoside	$O_{19}C_{48}H_{78}$	G II	SA	SSS	375	>375	—	0		
					CA	SSS	338	338	—	31		
					LE	SSS	169, 338	169	—		0	
					KB	PG						85
38876	50	Betulin diacetate	$O_4C_{34}H_{54}$	III	SA	MC	500	~500	—	41		
					CA	MC	400	<400	—	19		
					LE	MC	400	~400	—		0	
38945	49	Lupenol I, benzoate	$O_2C_{37}H_{54}$	II	SA	MC	375	>375	—	22		
					CA	MC	337	>337	—	19		
					LE	MC	375	375	—		0	
40898	49	Sarsasapogenin, acetate	$O_4C_{29}H_{46}$	I	SA	MC	375	375	—	40		
					CA	MC	300	300	—	23		
					LE	MC	300	300	—		0	
53993	54	Norfriedelene	$C_{29}H_{48}$	III	SA	MC	125	>125	—	6		
					CA	MC	110	>110	—	0		
					LE	MC	55, 110	55	—		0	
53994	54	Friedelin oxime	$NOC_{30}H_{51}$	II	SA	MC	500	>500	—	35		
					CA	MC	450	450	—	40		
					LE	MC	450	450	—		0	
					WM	Saline	50–400	>400	—	18		
53997	54	Friedelin, enol benzoate	$O_2C_{37}H_{54}$	II	SA	MC	125	125	—	38		
					CA	MC	100	~100	—	29		
					WM	Saline	400	>400		10		
					LE	MC	100	100	—		0	
55141	54	Friedelin	$OC_{30}H_{50}$	II	SA	CMC	500	<500	—	15		
					CA	CMC	450	450	—	31		
					WM	Saline	50–400	>400	—	36		
					LE	CMC	450	450	—		0	

56594	54	Friedelin iodoacetate	$O_2IC_{32}H_{53}$	II	SA	MC	125	>125	—	0		
					CA	CMC	60, 115	60	—	0		
					LE	MC	115	115	—		0	
57737	54	3-Methoxyfriedelane	$OC_{31}H_{54}$	II	SA	CMC	500	>500	—	21		
					CA	CMC	450	>450	—	0		
					WM	Saline	50–400	>400	—	20		
					LE	CMC	450	>450	—		0	
70931	59	Celastrol	$O_4C_{29}H_{38}$	IIab	SA	CMC	0.06–250	0.06	—	29		
					91	CMC	0.06	0.06	—	21		
					WM	CMC + Saline	1.97–15	~10	~7[b]	80		
					LE	CMC	2–20	2	—		2	
74511	2	Tigogenin, 11-oxo-	$O_4C_{27}H_{42}$	I	SA	SSS	500	500	—	0		
					LL	SSS	400	400	—	0		
					WM	SSS	50–400	>400	—	22		
					LE	SSS	400	400	—		0	
77472	51	*Saponaria* saponin	ca. $O_{30}C_{57}H_{96}$	G I	SA	H_2O	0.5–9	~6	~6	70[a]		
					CA	H_2O	0.5–2	2	—	28		
					LL	H_2O	1.5	~1.5	—	42		
					WM	H_2O	0.5–9	~3	2	86[a]		
					LE	H_2O	0.5–2	~1	—		0	
					PS	H_2O	0.125–1.5	~0.125	—		0	
80698	2	Tigogenin, 23-bromo-3 β,12 β-dihydroxy-11-oxo-	$O_5BrC_{27}H_{41}$	I	8P	SSS	400	400	—	51		
					LE	SSS	400	400	—		0	
					DA	SSS	200	~200	—		10	
					KB	PG						28
80699	2	Tigogenin, 3 β, 12 β-dihydroxy-11-oxo-, diacetate	$O_7C_{31}H_{46}$	I	8P	SSS	400	400	—	11		
					LE	SSS	400	400	—		0	
					DA	Saline	200	>200	—		0	
					KB	PG						>100
87530	2	α-Hederagenin	$O_{11}C_{41}H_{64}$	IIa	KB	DMF						100
90487	53	Lupeol	$OC_{30}H_{50}$	III	SA	Saline	125	125	—	15		
					WM	Saline	50–500	~330	200	71		
					KB	PG						28

TABLE X—*continued*

NSC No.	Supplier	Compound name	Molecular formula	Type	Tumor system	Vehicle	Dose range tested (mg/kg)	Response (mg/kg) MTD	Response (mg/kg) MED	Evaluation TWI(%)	Evaluation ILS(%)	Evaluation ED_{50}
92227	26	Lup-20(30)-ene-3 β, 16 β-diol	$O_2C_{30}H_{50}$	III	SA	SSS	500 —	500	—	18		
					LL	SSS	400	400	—	11		
					LE	SSS	400	400	—		2	
94656	56	Ifflaionic acid	$O_3C_{30}H_{46}$	II	SA	SSS	300	>300	—	12		
					WM	SSS	240	>240	—	5		
					LE	SSS	240	>240	—		0	
					KB	DMF						47
99281	43	Pristimerin	$O_4C_{30}H_{40}$	IIab	LE	SSS	37.5–300[c]	~300	—		4	
100,045	29	*Acer* saponin P	—	G IIba	WM	Saline	1–24	6	2.5[d]	80		
104,793	77	Desgluco-parillin	$O_{17}C_{45}H_{74}$	G I	WM	SSS	3–120	>120	—	23		
104,794	77	Desgluco-desrhamno-parillin	$O_{13}C_{39}H_{64}$	G I	WM	SSS	3–120	>120	—	12		
104,795	77	Cyclamin	$O_{27}C_{58}H_{94}$	G II	WM	SSS	3–60	~15	10	64[e]		
104,796	77	Hederasaponin C	$O_{26}C_{59}H_{96}$	G II	WM	SSS	3–60	<60	60	72[f]		
104,797	77	Escin	$O_{24}C_{55}H_{86}$	G II	WM	SSS	3–60	<30	30	67[f]		
104,798	77	Primulasaponin	$O_{23}C_{54}H_{88}$	G II	WM	SSS	3–60	~60	—	52		
104,799	77	Lanatonin	$O_{27}C_{56}H_{92}$	G I	WM	SSS	3–120	120	120	79		
106,552	77	Parillin	$O_{22}C_{51}H_{84}$	G I	WM	Saline	15–60	<60	60	63[f]		
106,553	77	α-Hederin	$O_{12}C_{41}H_{66}$	G IIa	WM	Saline	15–60	15	—	40		
106,554	77	Musennin	$O_{21}C_{51}H_{82}$	G IIa	WM	Saline	2–60	8	—	0		
106,555	77	Desglucomusennin	$O_{16}C_{45}H_{72}$	G IIa	WM	Saline	1–60	4	4	58		
106,556	77	Avenacoside A	$O_{23}C_{51}H_{82}$	G I	WM	Saline	15–120	60	—	4		

106,557	77	*Digitalis lanata* saponin	$O_{27}C_{56}H_{92}$ (chiefly)	G I	WM	Saline	15–120	60	—	11		
109,440	77	*Thea sinensis* saponin	$O_{26}C_{57}H_{90}$	G II	WM	SSS	5.5–175	~5.5	—	44		
113,090	11	Betulic acid	$O_3C_{30}H_{48}$	IIIa	WM	CMC	50–400	>400	—	24		
114,787	52	α-Amyrin	$OC_{30}H_{50}$	II	WM	SSS	50–400	~400	400	63		
118,342	77	Senegasaponin A	Unknown	G IIa	WM	Saline	1.88–30	1.88	1.88	59		
122,753	77	Quillajoside	Unknown	G IIa	WM	Saline	1.56–400	~1.56	—	48		
123,126	29	Saponin from *Myrsine africana*	$O_{27}C_{60}H_{98}$	G II	WM	Saline	1–16	8	7	74[e]		
123,429	29	*Acer* saponin Q	Unknown	G IIba	SA WM	Saline Saline	1–6 1.5–12	4 8	<1 —	78 14		
401,399	44	Taraxerol	$OC_{30}H_{50}$	II	KB	—						>100
401,400	44	Taraxasterol acetate	$O_2C_{32}H_{52}$	II	KB	—						>10
403,165	44	Olean-18-en-3-ol, acetate	$O_2C_{32}H_{52}$	II	KB	—						8.5
403,166	44	β-Amyrin acetate	$O_2C_{32}H_{52}$	II	KB	—						11
404,866	54	Bromofriedelin	$OBrC_{30}H_{49}$	II	KB	—						43
404,867	54	Friedelinol chloro-acetate	$O_2ClC_{32}H_{53}$	II	KB	—						>100
404,869	54	Friedelin, (2,4-dinitro-phenyl)-hydrazone	$N_4O_4C_{36}H_{54}$	II	KB	—						29
404,870	54	Friedelin-3-enol, phenyl-acetate	$O_2C_{38}H_{56}$	II	LE KB	Saline —	100–400[c]	>400	—		4	 46
404,871	54	Friedelin-3-enol, hydrocinnamate	$O_2C_{39}H_{58}$	II	LE KB	Saline —	50–200[c]	~200	—		2	 39
407,035	54	A-Norfriedelanone	$OC_{29}H_{48}$	III	KB	Dioxane						>100
407,037	54	Norfriedelane	$C_{29}H_{50}$	III	KB	Dioxane						>100

TABLE X—*continued*

NSC No.	Supplier	Compound name	Molecular formula	Type	Tumor system	Vehicle	Dose range tested (mg/kg)	Response (mg/kg)		Evaluation		
								MTD	MED	TWI(%)	ILS(%)	ED_{50}
407,041	54	Friedelan-3 α-ol	$OC_{30}H_{52}$	III	SA	CMC	375	375	—	7		
					CA	CMC	263	<263		0		
					WM	Saline	400	>400	—	12		
					LE	CMC	263	263	—		0	
					KB	—						>100
407,042	54	Norfriedelan-3-ol, acetate	$O_2C_{31}H_{52}$	III	KB	Dioxane						120
407,045	54	Isofriedelan-2-one (2,4-dinitrophenyl)hydrazone	$N_4O_4C_{36}H_{54}$	II	KB	Dioxane						69

[a] Results erratic.
[b] TI ~ 1.4 (erratic).
[c] Single injection procedure only.
[d] TI > 2.
[e] Erratic toxicity.
[f] Activity at $>LD_{10}$.

1969) on the basis of cytotoxicity of the crude extract. An example of the structure of this type of compound is given for cucurbitacin C (XVIII).

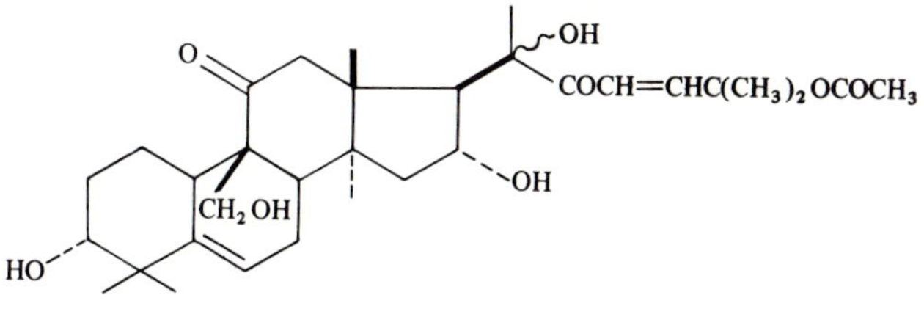

(XVIII)

The cucurbitacins (Table XI) are characterized by generally high cytotoxicity (in KB) but little activity in the *in vivo* tumor systems tried. Cucurbitacin C is active in WM while cucurbitacin E (α-elaterin) is active in LL and has borderline activity in WM. Little chemical reason can be advanced for the remarkably high toxicity—among the lowest known values—of some of the compounds. While all the natural compounds have the α,β-unsaturated ketone group in the side chain at sterol position 17, in the highly cytotoxic compound dihydrocucurbitacin B (NSC-106,401), the ethylenic linkage in this group has been reduced. However, such high cytotoxicity may have some general significance for other *in vivo* tumor systems not considered here and for this reason the cucurbitacins are an interesting new development (see also Table XX).

F. Digitaloid Glycosides and Their Aglycones

The large group of compounds considered here and listed in Table XII can be divided into cardenolides (XIX), bufadienolides (XX), a group related to withaferin A (XXI), and a small group of those members in which the steroid group is attached to the lactone ring at a different position on the latter.

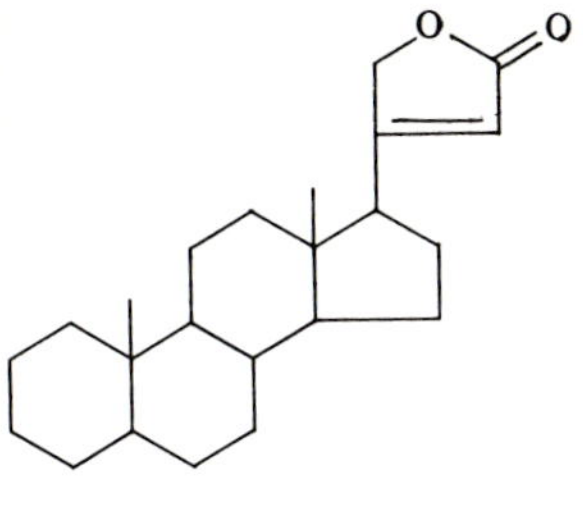

Cardenolides (XIX)

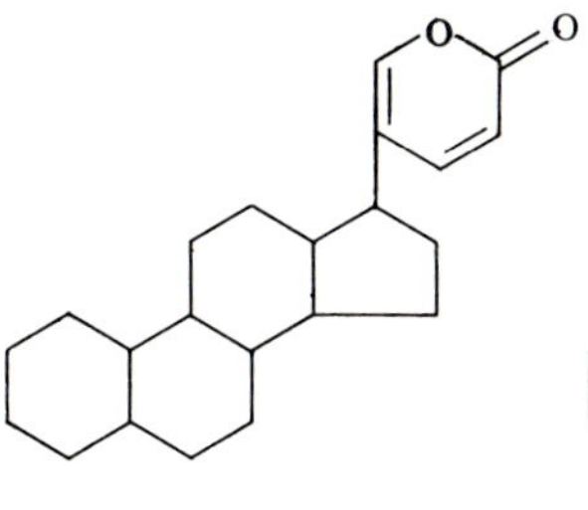

Bufadienolides (XX)

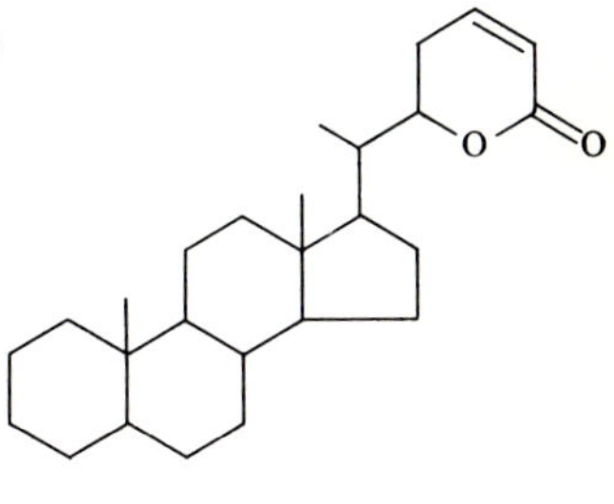

Withaferins (XXI)

TABLE XI
CUCURBITACINS

NSC No.	Supplier	Compound name	Molecular formula	Tumor system	Vehicle	Dose range tested (mg/kg)	Response (mg/kg)		Evaluation		
							MTD	MED	TWI(%)	ILS(%)	ED_{50}
49451	47	Cucurbitacin B	$O_8C_{32}H_{46}$	SA	MC	1–500	~1	—	32		
				CA	MC	0.9	>0.9	—	0		
				LE	CMC	0.4–3.20	~0.8	—		8	
				P4	Saline	0.57–0.16	0.38	—		3	
				LL	Saline	0.16–3.20	~0.80	—	50		
				8P	CMC	0.20–3.20	~0.57	—	40		
				DA	Saline	0.16–0.57	~0.38	—		0	
				WM	CMC	0.40–3.20	~0.80	—	45		
				KB	PG						0.0000025
49452	47	Fabacein	$O_9C_{34}H_{48}$	SA	MC	30–500	~30	—	28		
				WM	Saline	5–50	~18	—	30		
				LE	MC	27	~27	—		8	
				KB	Alcohol						~1.0
94743	63	Cucurbitacin A	$O_9C_{32}H_{46}$	SA	Saline	0.16–2.0	~0.57	—	43		
				LL	Saline	0.57–2.0	~0.57	—	7		
				8P	Saline	0.16–0.57	~0.38	—	8		
				WM	Saline	0.57–2.00	~1.30	—	35		
				LE	Saline	0.57–2.00	~0.86	—		14	
				P4	Saline	0.16–0.57	~0.25	—		7	
				DA	Saline	0.16–0.57	~0.25	—		0	
				KB	PG						0.0014
94744	63	Cucurbitacin C	$O_8C_{32}H_{50}$	SA	Saline	0.16–2.0	~0.57	—	43		
				LL	Saline	0.57–2.0	~0.57	—	33		
				8P	Saline	0.16–0.57	>0.57	—	0		
				WM	Saline	0.57–6.70	~3.00	~3.00	66		
				LE	Saline	0.57–2.00	~1.30	—		12	
				P4	Saline	0.16–0.57	>0.57	—		3	
				DA	Saline	0.16–0.57	~0.25	—		0	
				KB	PG						0.001

106,399 521,775	29	Cucurbitacin E (α-elaterin)	$O_8C_{32}H_{44}$	SA	CMC	0.40–3.20	~3.20	—	12		
				LL	CMC	0.40–12.8	~3.20	—	67		
				8P	CMC	0.40–3.20	~3.20	—	53		
				WM	CMC	2.50–150	~75	—	55		
				LE	CMC	0.40–3.20	~1.60	—		5	
				DA	CMC	0.40–3.20	~3.20	—		0	
				KB	PG						0.00000045
106,400	29	Isocucurbitacin B (2-Epicucurbitacin B)	$O_8C_{32}H_{46}$	KB	PG						0.40
106,401	29	Dihydrocucurbitacin B	$O_8C_{32}H_{48}$	WM	Saline	1–4	>4	—	0		
				KB	PG						0.0017
112,164	28	Tetrahydrocucurbitacin I	$O_7C_{30}H_{46}$	WM	Saline or CMC	0.25–8	4	24	71		
112,165	28	Cucurbitacin J	$O_8C_{30}H_{44}$	WM	Saline or CMC	0.25–36	>36	—	12		
112,166	28	Cucurbitacin K	—	WM	Saline or CMC	0.25–36	>36	—	9		
112,167	28	Cucurbitacin L	$O_7C_{30}H_{46}$	WM	Saline or CMC	0.25–12	>12	—	0		
				KB	DMF						0.34
521,776	62	Cucurbitacin D (Elatericin A)	$O_7C_{30}H_{44}$	LE	SSS	0.50–8	~0.70	—		9	
				WM	SSS	0.70	0.70	—	30		
521,777	62	Cucurbitacin I (Elatericin B)	$O_7C_{30}H_{42}$	LE	SSS	0.10–0.80	~0.40	—		0	

These four groups are referred to as types I–IV, respectively, in Table XII. In addition, the symbol G indicates that the compound is a glycoside.

The chemistry of these compounds, except for withaferin A, has been recently reviewed in Karrer (1958) and Fieser and Fieser (1959). The structure of withaferin A has been elucidated by Lavie *et al.* (1965) and by Kupchan *et al.* (1965a).

In this group, cytotoxicity (in KB) is shown by about 70% of the compounds on which this test was carried out. Structure-activity relationships within the group of compounds on which cytotoxicity is available are not clear since not only are a substantial majority of both type I and type II compounds cytotoxic but also both glycosides and aglycones. The numbers of compounds of types III and IV are too small for statistical consideration. While all of the compounds showing cytotoxic activity are α,β-unsaturated lactones, all but one (NSC-87319) of those inactive against KB also contain this group. Data on more compounds containing the saturated lactone ring would permit better evaluation of the effects of α,β-unsaturation.

Of the compounds tested, a few show activity in *in vivo* tumor systems. Lanatoside A (NSC-7532) and lanatoside C (NSC-7533) are active against CA. Lanatoside A is also active against LL. Withaferin A (NSC-101,088) is active against SA. Withaferin A and hellebrigenin 3-acetate (NSC-106,676) are active against WM. While the latter two compounds have too small a TI to justify further pharmacological evaluation, it is possible that other digitaloid compounds, which are so widely distributed in nature and of which so few have been studied, will have properties that will recommend them as antitumor agents.

G. Lapachol

The chemical investigation of plant extracts showing activity against *in vivo* tumors revealed that the activity against WM of one of the plants, *Stereospermum suaveolens* (fam. Bignoniaceae), was due to the well-known quinone, lapachol (NSC-11905) (XXII). This compound had been submitted to the

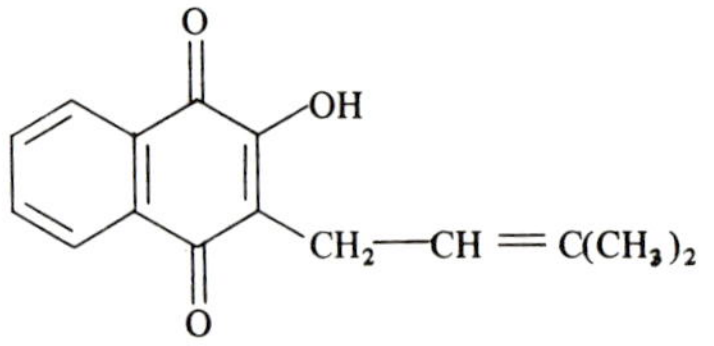

O, OH, CH_2—CH = $C(CH_3)_2$, O

(XXII)

program several years earlier, before WM was added to the antitumor screen, and was found to be inactive. It is interesting to note that lapachol is a known constituent of the wood of several species of tree of the family Bignoniaceae

TABLE XII
DIGITALOID GLYCOSIDES AND THEIR AGLYCONES

NSC No.	Supplier	Compound name	Molecular formula	Type	Tumor system	Vehicle	Dose range tested (mg/kg)	Response (mg/kg) MTD	Response (mg/kg) MED	Evaluation TWI(%)	Evaluation ILS(%)	Evaluation ED_{50}
4320	46; 44;	Strophanthin	$O_{14}C_{36}H_{54}$	G I	SA	MC	12.5, 50, 250	12.5	—	45		
7670	58	(*k*-Strophanthin-β)			CA	MC	1, 8	>1	—	14		
					WM	CMC	0.25–64	8	—	2		
					LE	CMC	0.25–10	2	—		13	
					KB	DMF						0.003
7521	58	Proscillaridin A	$O_8C_{30}H_{42}$	G II	SA	MC	10–170	10	—	16		
					EA	MC	10–20	10	—	5		
					LL	Saline	1.25–10	10	—	17		
					WM	CMC	2.5–20	10	—	31		
					LE	MC	5–20	5	—		4	
					KB	DMF						0.001
7522	58; 29	Cymarin	$O_9C_{30}H_{44}$	G I	SA	MC	2.5–170	10	—	38		
					CA	MC	4–60	4	—	43		
					LL	SSS	2.6–9	4	—	22		
					WM	SSS	2–128	32	—	37		
					LE	SSS	0.62–10	1.25	—		0	
					PS	SSS	0.62–20	5	—		0	
					P4	Saline	1.25–10	5	—		3	
					KB	Alcohol						0.013
7523	58	Scilliroside	$O_{12}C_{32}H_{44}$	G II	SA	MC	0.10–170	0.10	—	8		
					EA	MC	0.10	0.10	—	8		
					WM	CMC	0.25–2	0.50	—	47		
					LE	SSS	0.10–2.56	0.16	—		6	
					KB	DMF						0.023
7525	58	Scillaren A	$O_{13}C_{36}H_{52}$	G II	SA	—	10–170	~10	—	13		
					CA	—	7	7	—	0		
					LL	CMC	1.2–40	5	—	20		
					WM	CMC	0.50–40	~40	—	27		
					LE	SSS	1–32	~4	—		0	
					KB	DMF						0.012

TABLE XII—*continued*

NSC No.	Supplier	Compound name	Molecular formula	Type	Tumor system	Vehicle	Dose range tested (mg/kg)	Response (mg/kg) MTD	Response (mg/kg) MED	Evaluation TWI(%)	Evaluation ILS(%)	Evaluation ED_{50}
7529	58	Digitoxin	$O_{13}C_{41}H_{64}$	G I	SA	CMC	3.75–350	3.75	—	39		
					CA	MC	6	6	—	53		
					WM	Saline	2.5–20	10	—	9		
					LE	SSS	1–64	16	—		5	
					PS	Saline	0.63–10	2.5	—		18	
					KB	DMF						0.078
7530	58	*k*-Strophanthoside	$O_{19}C_{42}H_{64}$	G I	SA	—	3.5–350	3.5	—	4		
					EA	—	3.5	3.5	—	21		
					WM	SSS	0.075–16	8	—	18		
					LE	—	0.38–3.5	1	—		10	
					KB							0.032
7531	58	Desacetyl lanatoside C (desacetyldigilanid C)	$O_{19}C_{47}H_{74}$	G I	SA	MC	8–350	8	—	36		
					CA	MC	5.6	5.6	—	21		
					WM	Saline S/SSS	2–128	64	—	17		
					LE	SSS	4–256	64	—		14	
					KB	DMF						<1.0
7532	58	Lanatoside A (digilanid A)	$O_{19}C_{49}H_{76}$	G I	SA	—	11–350	11	—	0		
					CA	—	1.25–80	10	—	68[a]		
					LL	CMC	1.2–40	5	—	58		
					WM	CMC	2.5–20	10		0		
					LE	—	11	11			4	
					KB	—						<1.0
7533	58	Lanatoside C (digilanid C)	$O_{20}C_{49}H_{76}$	G I	SA	—	350	350	—	50		
					CA	CMC	122, 245	~122	<122	68		
					WM	SSS	162	>162	—	0		
					LE	SSS	162, 325	162	—		10	
					KB							0.024
7534	58	Scillirosidine	$O_7C_{26}H_{34}$	II	SA	—	0.5–17	0.5	—	0		
					EA	MC	0.5	>0.5	—	0		
					LE	MC	0.012–0.05	0.012	—		3	
					WM	Saline	0.05	>0.05	—	0		

7535	58	Lanatoside B (digilanid B)	$O_{20}C_{49}H_{76}$	G I	SA	MC	4.25–350	4.25	—	1		
					CA	CMC	3.8	~3.8	—	33		
					WM	CMC	1.25–40	>40	—	3		
					LE	SSS	4.25–80	20	—		1	
					PS	CMC	12.5–100	25	—		9	
					KB	DMF						0.38
25485	46	Ouabain (strophanthin G)	$O_{12}C_{29}H_{44}$	G I	SA	—	6.25, 25	6.25	—	45		
					CA	—	1.10–4.38	1.10	—	32		
					LE	—	4.38	4.38	—		11	
					KB	DMF						<0.13
61812	44	Digitalin	$O_{14}C_{36}H_{56}$	G I	SA	MC	500	500	—	24		
					CA	MC	225, 450	225	—	42		
					LL	CMC	100–400	100	—	33		
					LE	MC	450	450	—		0	
					KB	DMF						>100
65944	44	Carda-4,20(22)-dienolide-11 β,19-epoxy-14-hydroxy-11-methoxy-3-oxo-	$O_6C_{24}H_{30}$	I	SA	SSS	250	>250	—	0		
					CA	SSS	200	>200	—	28		
					LE	SSS	200	~200	—		2	
					KB	PG						>100
					WM	Saline	400	>400	—	17		
72255	44	5 α-Cholesta-8,20(22),23-trien-21-oic acid, 3 β,24-dihydroxy-4,4,14-trimethyl-, δ-lactone, acetate	$O_4C_{32}H_{46}$	IV	SA	SSS	250	>250	—	3		
					91	SSS	200	>200	—	0		
					LE	SSS	200	>200	—		12	
83216	29	Apocannoside	$O_8C_{30}H_{44}$	G I	SA	SSS	3.13–100	~25	—	49		
					WM	SSS	1.88–75	~9	—	23		
					LE	CMC	5–20	10	—		0	
					PS	SSS	5–40	10	—		0	
					KB	PG						0.098
86078	29	Strophanthidin	$O_6C_{23}H_{32}$	I	KB	PG						0.24
87314	29	Strophanthidol	$O_6C_{23}H_{34}$	I	KB	DMF						0.78
87315	29	Strophanthidin, 5-anhydro-, 3-acetate	$O_6C_{25}H_{32}$	I	KB	DMF						16
87316	29	Strophanthidin, 14-anhydro-, 3-acetate	$O_6C_{25}H_{32}$	I	KB	DMF						>100

TABLE XII—*continued*

NSC No.	Supplier	Compound name	Molecular formula	Type	Tumor system	Vehicle	Dose range tested (mg/kg)	Response (mg/kg)		Evaluation		
								MTD	MED	TWI(%)	ILS(%)	ED_{50}
87317	29	Strophanthidin, 5,4-dianhydro-, acetate	$O_4C_{25}H_{32}$	I	KB	DMF						>100
87318	29	5 α-Card-20(22)-enolide, 5,6 α-epoxy-3 β,14-dihydroxy-1-oxo, 3-acetate	$O_7C_{25}H_{32}$	I	KB	DMF						15
87319	29	5 β-Cardanolide, 3 β,5,14-trihydroxy-19-oxo-	$O_6C_{23}H_{34}$	I	KB	DMF						14
87320	29	Strophanthidinic acid, 3-acetate	$O_8C_{25}H_{34}$	I	KB	DMF						32
87321	29	Strophanthidinic acid, methyl-ester, 3-acetate	$O_8C_{26}H_{36}$	I	KB	DMF						34
89594	2	Bufotalidin	$O_6C_{24}H_{32}$	II	LE	Saline	5–400[b]	80	—		4	
					KB	DMF						<0.001
89595	2	Bufalin	$O_4C_{24}H_{34}$	II	KB	DMF						<0.1
89596	2	Bufotalin	$O_6C_{26}H_{36}$	II	WM	SSS	400, 800	400	—	51		
					LE	SSS	400	400	—		1	
					KB	DMF						0.026
90325	2	Cinobufagin	$O_6C_{26}H_{34}$	II	WM	Saline + T-80	20	>20	—	18		
					LE	Saline + T-80	5–400	20	—		0	
					KB	Dioxane						0.011
90326	2	Cinobufotalin	$O_7C_{26}H_{34}$	II	KB	Dioxane						0.24
90384	2	Gamabufotalin	$O_5C_{24}H_{34}$	II	KB	DMF						>100
90782	2	Telocinobufagin	$O_5C_{23}H_{34}$	II	KB	DMF						0.033

90783	2	Resibufogenin	$O_4C_{24}H_{32}$	II	LE	SSS	50–400	400	—		5	
					KB	DMF						0.34
91580	2	α(and β)-Digoxin acetate	$O_{15}C_{43}H_{66}$	I	KB	DMF						0.30
92954	29	Strophanthidin, 3-acetate	$O_7C_{25}H_{34}$	I	WM	CMC	5–50	>50	—	14		
					KB	DMF						0.089
92955	29	5 β-Card-20(22)-enolide, 5,6 β:14,15 α-diepoxy-3 β-hydroxy-19-oxo-, acetate	$O_7C_{25}H_{30}$	I	KB	DMF						2.7
92956	29	5 α-Card-2)(22)-enolide, 5,6 α:14,15 α-diepoxy-3 β-hydroxy-19-oxo-, acetate	$O_7C_{25}H_{30}$	I	KB	DMF						>100
93069	29	5 α-Card-20(22)-enolide, 6 β-chloro-3 β,5,14-tri-hydroxy-19-oxo, 3-acetate	$O_7ClC_{25}H_{33}$	I	KB	DMF						0.23
93070	29	5 α-Card-20(22)-enolide, 5-chloro-6 β,19-epoxy-3 β, 14,19-trihydroxy-, 3-acetate	$O_7ClC_{25}H_{33}$	I	KB	DMF						1.4
93134	33	Hellebrin	$O_{15}C_{36}H_{52}$	G II	SA	CMC	6–500	~6	—	22		
					WM	CMC	2.5–100	~40	—	18		
					LE	CMC	2.5–20	2.5	—		0	
					PS	CMC	0.6–20	5	—		20	
					KB	DMF						0.017
93373	29	Strophanthidin-oxime	$O_6C_{23}H_{33}N$	I	KB	PG						0.10
93374	29	5 β-Card-20(22)-enolide, 5,6 β-epoxy-3 β,14-di-hydroxy-19-oxo-, 3-acetate	$O_7C_{25}H_{32}$	I	KB	PG						>100
93446	29	Carda-5,14,20(22)-trienolide, 3 β-hydroxy-19-oxo-, acetate	$O_5C_{25}H_{30}$	I	KB	PG						50
95008	29	Strophanthidin, 3-iodoacetate	$O_7C_{23}H_{33}I$	I	KB	PG						0.0014
95009	29	Strophanthidol, 3-acetate, 19-iodoacetate	$O_8C_{27}H_{37}I$	I	KB	PG						0.022

TABLE XII—*continued*

NSC No.	Supplier	Compound name	Molecular formula	Type	Tumor system	Vehicle	Dose range tested (mg/kg)	Response (mg/kg)		Evaluation		
								MTD	MED	TWI(%)	ILS(%)	ED_{50}
95089	37	Oleandrin	$O_6C_{32}H_{48}$	G I	KB	PG						0.0018
95091	37	Gitalin (4-digitonin)	$O_{12}C_{35}H_{56}$	G I	WM	CMC	2–512	64	—	3		
					LE	CMC	11–450	11	—		5	
					KB	PG						0.032
95099	37	Gitoxin	$O_{14}C_{41}H_{64}$	I	KB	DMF						5.4
95100	37	Digoxin	$O_{14}C_{41}H_{64}$	I	KB	DMF						<1
97088	2	Ouabagenin	$O_8C_{23}G_{34}$	I	KB	DMF						2.5
101,088	29	Withaferin A	$O_6C_{28}H_{38}$	III	SA	CMC	10–40	20	~20	~60[b]		
					WM	CMC	10–60	~40	40	82		
					LE	CMC	10–40	20	—		1	
					PS	SSS	5–40	40	—		4	
					KB	DMF						0.15
106,393	29	Calotropin	$O_9C_{29}H_{40}$	G I	KB	PG						0.025
106,562	50	21-Norchola-5,20(22),23-triene-24-carboxylic acid, 3 β,20-dihydroxy-, δ-lactone, acetate	$O_4C_{26}H_{34}$	IV	WM	SSS	400	>400	—	12		
					LE	SSS	400	400	—		0	
106,676	29	Hellebrigenin 3-acetate	$O_7C_{26}H_{34}$	II	WM	CMC	0.5–16	8	6	75		
					KB	PG						0.0064
107,128	50	5 α-Cardanolide, 3 β-hydroxy-	$O_3C_{23}H_{36}$	I	LE	Saline	50–200[c]	>200	—		0	
107,129	50	5 α-Card-20(22)-enolide, 3 β-hydroxy-	$O_3C_{23}H_{34}$	I	LE	Saline	50–200[c]	>200	—		0	

109,330	29	5 β-Bufa-20,22-dienolide, 3 β-5,14-trihydroxy-19-oxo, 3,5-diacetate	$O_8C_{28}H_{36}$	II	WM	CMC	1.2–12	~1.8	—	53		
					KB	DMF						0.0019
109,437	77	Jaborosalactone A	$O_5C_{28}H_{38}$	II	WM	SSS	150	>150	—	49		
109,438	77	Jaborosalactone B	$O_5C_{28}H_{38}$	II	WM	SSS	110	>110	—	27		
109,439	77	Jaborosalactone D	$O_6C_{28}H_{40}$	II	WM	SSS	150	150	—	16		
113,569[d]	27	Acospectoside A	$O_{15}C_{38}H_{58}$	G I	KB	Alkali Saline						0.3
					LE	Saline	50–400[c]	~400	—		17	
116,787[d]	27	Acovenoside A	$O_9C_{30}H_{46}$	G I	KB	PG						0.031
116,788[d]	27	Acobioside A	$O_{14}C_{36}H_{56}$	G I	KB	PG						0.15
116,789[d]	27	Acovenoside B	$O_{10}C_{32}H_{48}$	G I	KB	PG						0.22
117,180	63	1 α,2 α-Epoxyscillirosidine	$O_8C_{26}H_{32}$	II	LE	SSS	1	1	—		0	
407,806	44	Digitoxigenin	$O_4C_{23}H_{34}$	I	SA	CMC	5–50	25	—	14		
					CA	CMC	5–50	~10	—	33		
					KB	Alcohol						20
407,807	44	Gitoxigenin	$O_5C_{23}H_{34}$	I	SA	SSS	3–50	>50	—	36		
					CA	SSS	3–50	~50	—	20		
					LL	Saline	10	>10	—	6		
					KB	Alcohol						36
407,808	44	Convallotoxin	$O_{10}C_{29}H_{42}$	G I	KB	Alcohol						34
407,809	44	Uzarine	$O_{14}C_{35}H_{54}$	G I	KB	H_2O						20

[a] Results not reproducible.
[b] Results erratic.
[c] Single injection procedure only.
[d] Kapadia and Zalucky (1968). These results are being separately reported by these authors.

from which a tea is prepared and used rather widely in Brazil, popularly and by physicians, for the treatment of cancer. A good characteristic of lapachol is that it is more active against WM when administered orally than intraperitoneally.

While several quinones of different types have shown activity in one or another of the tumor systems in use at CCNSC, the simplicity of the lapachol molecule and the presence of several sites for chemical alteration invited a special attempt to derive valid structure-activity relationships. For this purpose it was proposed to compare the antitumor activity of substituted 2-hydroxy-1,4-naphthoquinones, only, especially against WM. A list of such compounds is reproduced in Table XIII.

It is interesting to see that of 68 such compounds on which results with WM have been obtained, only one other compound (NSC-114,803) besides lapachol shows activity. It is noteworthy, however, that NSC-114,803 also possesses the rather unusual and desirable property of being more active by the oral route than by the intraperitoneal. This specificity is discouraging from the point of view of designing analogs for synthesis, but it illustrates a situation so often encountered in this type of work. Lack of sufficient numbers of compounds precluded investigating the effect of other alterations of the lapachol molecule. Finally, Table XIII shows that this class of compounds has a low incidence of activity in the cell culture test as well as against other *in vivo* tumor systems. Only two compounds (NSC-83430 and NSC-113,452) show even marginal cytotoxicity and only one (NSC-32079) has activity against DL. Lapachol, in addition to activity against WM, has activity against MS.

At present, preclinical pharmacology on lapachol has been completed and clinical studies have been initiated.

H. Diepoxy Compounds

The isolation of the unusual compound crotepoxide (NSC-106,396), (XXIII), by Kupchan *et al.* (1968a) as the active antitumor agent (LL) in the plant *Croton macrostachys* (fam. Euphorbiaceae) indicated a new type of diepoxide to be considered as a lead for further development. Good antitumor activity had

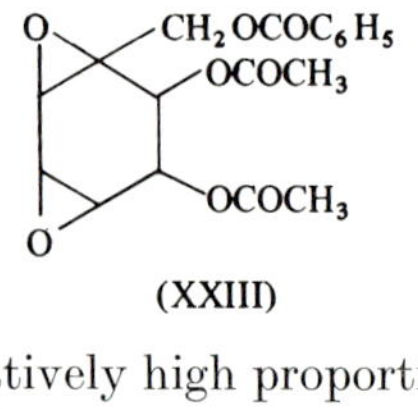

O

$CH_2OCOC_6H_5$

$OCOCH_3$

$OCOCH_3$

O

(XXIII)

already been found in a relatively high proportion of synthetic diepoxides of other types but this was the first compound with both epoxide groups attached to a single six-membered carbocyclic ring to show activity in any tumor system.

TABLE XIII
2-Hydroxy-1,4-Naphthoquinones

NSC No.	Supplier	Compound name	Molecular formula	Tumor system	Vehicle	Dose range tested (mg/kg)	Response (mg/kg)		Evaluation		
							MTD	MED	TWI(%)	ILS(%)	ED_{50}
278	46	1,4-Naphthoquinone, 2-cyclohexyl-3-hydroxy-	$O_3C_{16}H_{16}$	SA	—	42, 500	>42	—	30		
				CA	—	20	20	—	5		
				WM	Alkali saline	12.5–100	50	—	18		
				LE	—	42	~42	—		0	
377	46	1,4-Naphthoquinone, 2-hydroxy-3-[3-(*p*-phenoxyphenyl)-propyl]-	$O_4C_{25}H_{20}$	SA	—	8–250	8	—	32		
				CA	—	41	41	—	23		
				WM	CMC	6–50	6	—	8		
				LE	MC	5–40	5	—		0	
2035	46	1,4-Naphthoquinone, 2-[3-(decahydro-2-naphthyl)propyl]-3-hydroxy-	$O_3C_{23}H_{28}$	WM	Saline	200, 400	<200	—	28		
				KB	—						21
3578	12	1,4-Naphthoquinone, 2-hydroxy-3-(9-hydroxy-9-pentyltetradecyl)-	$O_4C_{29}H_{44}$	WM	CMC	31–250	250	—	42		
8625 27285	3 1	1,4-Naphthoquinone, 2-hydroxy-	$O_3C_{10}H_6$	SA	MC	100–500	100	—	15		
				CA	MC	100	>100	—	42		
				EA	MC	25, 100	>25	—	0		
				WM	Alkali saline	25–200	50	—	23		
				LE	MC	20, 80	~20	—		18	
10576 26606	12 1	1,4-Naphthoquinone, 2-hydroxy-3-(2-methyloctyl)-	$O_3C_{19}H_{24}$	SA	MC	100, 500	100	—	29		
				CA	MC	80	<80	—	0		
				LE	MC	100	<100	—		0	
11897	5	Phthiocol (1,4-naphthoquinone, 2-hydroxy-3-methyl-)	$O_3C_{11}H_8$	SA	MC	125, 500	>125	—	10		
				CA	MC	25–200	100	—	4		
				WM	Alkali saline	25–200	50	—	11		
				LE	MC	50–200	50	—		0	
				KB	—						20

TABLE XIII—*continued*

NSC No.	Supplier	Compound name	Molecular formula	Tumor system	Vehicle	Dose range tested (mg/kg)	Response (mg/kg) MTD	Response (mg/kg) MED	Evaluation TWI(%)	Evaluation ILS(%)	Evaluation ED_{50}
11905	5; 20; 51	Lapachol; 1,4-naphthoquinone, 2-hydroxy-3-(3-methyl-2-butenyl)-	$O_3C_{15}H_{14}$	SA	H_2O	30–150	~100	—	32		
				CA	MC	45–200	~50	—	28		
				LL	H_2O	45–150	100	—	29		
				MS	H_2O	45–150	>150	—	96		
				WM	H_2O	100–400	300	100[a]	73		
				PS	H_2O	50–200	150	—		20	
				P4	H_2O	20–600	400	—		15	
				LE	H_2O	0.5–400	200	—		37[b]	
				KB	—						7.5
24872	20	Lomatiol; 1,4-naphthoquinone, 2-hydroxy-3-(4-hydroxy-3-methyl-2-butenyl)-	$O_4C_{15}H_{14}$	SA	—	100, 500	~100	—	14		
				CA	—	90	~90	—	0		
				LE	—	90	~90	—		0	
				WM	H_2O	32–250	>250	250	58		
26654	44	1,4-Naphthoquinone, 2-hydroxy-3-isobutyl-	$O_3C_{14}H_{14}$	SA	—	250	250	—	5		
				WM	Saline	60, 250	~60	—	0		
26689	44	1,4-Naphthoquinone, 3-(diphenylmethyl)-2-hydroxy-	$O_3C_{23}H_{16}$	SA	MC	2–250	~2	—	3		
				WM	Saline	2, 4	2	—	45		
26694	44	1,4-Naphthoquinone, 2-hydroxy-3-isobutyl-, acetate	$O_4C_{16}H_{16}$	SA	—	250	>250	—	23		
26695	44	Hydrolapachol (1,4-naphthoquinone, 2-hydroxy-3-isopentyl-)	$O_3C_{15}H_{16}$	SA	—	65, 250	65	—	0		
				WM	H_2O	31–800	105	—	25		
				LE	H_2O	30–300	70	—		6	
26696	44	1,4-Naphthoquinone, 2-hydroxy-3-(2-methylpropenyl)-	$O_3C_{14}H_{12}$	SA	—	250	<250	—	26		
				WM	H_2O	200–400	400	—	38		
28845	1	1,4-Naphthoquinone, 2-(diethylaminomethyl)-3-hydroxy-	$NO_3C_{15}H_{17}$	SA	MC	500	500	—	20		
				EA	MC	500	500	—	0		
				LE	MC	450	450	—		15	

31435	1	1,4-Naphthoquinone, 2-(4-cyclohexylbutyl)-3-hydroxy-	$O_3C_{20}H_{24}$	SA	MC	125, 500	125	—	23		
				CA	MC	100	<100	—	0		
				WM	Saline + gum acacia	18.7–150	>150	—	2		
				LE	MC	100	100	—		0	
31458	1	1,4-Naphthoquinone, 2-decyl-3-hydroxy-	$O_3C_{20}H_{26}$	SA	MC	25–375	25	—	30		
				CA	MC	22	<22	—	0		
				WM	CMC	12.5–100	>100	—	0		
				LE	MC	21, 22	11	—		3	
31855	72	1,4-Naphthoquinone, 2-hydroxy-3-(morpholinomethyl)-	$NO_4C_{15}H_{15}$	SA	MC	500	500	—	28		
				CA	MC	75–450	75	—	41		
				WM	CMC	50–400	400	—	11		
				LE	MC	450	450	—		0	
31856	72	1,4-Naphthoquinone, 2-([bis-(2-hydroxyethyl)amino]-methyl)-3-hydroxy-, hydrate	$NO_5C_{15}H_{17}.H_2O$	SA	MC	500	500	—	38		
				CA	MC	450	<450	—	34		
				WM	CMC	250	>250	—	6		
				LE	MC	450	450	—		0	
				KB	—						>100
32079	72	1,4-Naphthoquinone, 2-[bis-(2-chloroethyl)aminomethyl]-3-hydroxy-	$NO_3Cl_2C_{15}H_{15}$	DL	Oil	5–100	10	5		53	
41233	1	1,4-Naphthoquinone, 2-hydroxy-3-(4-phenyl-1-cyclohexyl-methyl)-	$O_3C_{23}H_{22}$	SA	MC	4–500	4	—	0		
				CA	MC	0.9–3.6	0.9	—	0		
				LE	MC	3.6	3.6	—		0	
46847	1	1,4-Naphthoquinone, 2-[3-(2-cyclohexen-1-yl)propyl]-3-hydroxy-	$O_3C_{19}H_{20}$	SA	MC	63–500	63	—	0		
				CA	MC	25, 50	<25	—	0		
				WM	Saline	100	>100	—	20		
				LE	MC	25–50	25	—		0	
53562 98914	1 51	1,4-Naphthoquinone, 2-(3-chloro-3-methylbutyl)-3-hydroxy-	$O_3ClC_{15}H_{15}$	SA	MC	125, 500	~125	—	16		
				CA	MC	113	>113	—	3		
				WM	H_2O	125–500	125	—	0		
				LE	MC	113	113	—		0	
54932	1	1,4-Naphthoquinone, 2-(5-ethyl-2-methylnonyl)-3-hydroxy-	$O_3C_{22}H_{30}$	SA	MC	31–500	31	—	40		
				CA	CMC	6.2–24.8	<6.2	—	32		
				LE	CMC	24.8	24.8	—		5	

TABLE XIII—*continued*

NSC No.	Supplier	Compound name	Molecular formula	Tumor system	Vehicle	Dose range tested (mg/kg)	Response (mg/kg) MTD	Response (mg/kg) MED	Evaluation TWI(%)	Evaluation ILS(%)	Evaluation ED_{50}
65726	72	Carbamic acid, bis(2-chloroethyl)-, 10-(1,4-dihydro-3-hydroxy-1,4-dioxo-2-naphthyl)- decyl ester	$NO_5Cl_2C_{25}H_{33}$	WA	CMC	5.8–47	>47	—	12		
67451	1	Benzenesulfonamide, *p*-(1,4-dihydro-3-hydroxy-1,4-dioxo-2-naphthylazo)-	$N_3O_5SC_{16}H_{11}$	SA	CMC	500	500	[d]	61		
				KB	Acetone						>100
67462	1	1,4-Naphthoquinone, 2-(5-cyclohexylpentyl)-3-hydroxy-	$O_3C_{21}H_{26}$	KB	Acetone						10
74050	49	1,4-Naphthoquinone, 2,2′-methylenebis[3-hydroxy-	$O_6C_{21}H_{12}$	KB	DMF						>100
81054	51	Pyridinium, 1-(1,4-dihydro-3-hydroxy-1,4-dioxo-2-naphthyl)-hydroxide, inner salt	$NO_3C_{15}H_9$	CA	H_2O	60, 120	60	—	19		
				WM	H_2O	60–250	60	—	34		
83430	36	1,4-Naphthoquinone, 2-hydroxy-3-pentadecyl-	$O_3C_{25}H_{36}$	KB	PG						1.9
86268	51	1,4-Naphthoquinone, 2-hydroxy-3-nitro-	$NO_5C_{10}H_5$	SA	H_2O	125, 250	<125	—	31		
				WM	H_2O	125–500	125	—	42		
				LE	H_2O	150	150			0	
92074	51	1,4-Naphthoquinone, 2-hydroxy-3-styryl-	$O_3C_{18}H_{12}$	SA	H_2O	40, 80	40	—	17		
				WM	H_2O	4.7, 125, 250	4.7	—	31		
				LE	H_2O	40, 80	40	—		6	
92197	51	1,4-Naphthoquinone, 2-hydroxy-3-propenyl-	$O_3C_{13}H_{10}$	SA	H_2O	62, 125	<62	—	0		
				WM	H_2O	62, 125	62	—	2		
				LE	H_2O	100	100	—		0	

92198	51	1,4-Naphthoquinone, 2-allyl-3-hydroxy-	$O_3C_{13}H_{10}$	SA	H_2O	150	<150	—	17	
				WM	H_2O	125, 250	125	—	20	
				LE	H_2O	75, 150	75	—		0
92199	51	1,4-Naphthoquinone, 2-(1-butenyl)-3-hydroxy-	$O_3C_{14}H_{12}$	SA	H_2O	40, 80	40	—	38	
				WM	H_2O	62, 125, 250	62	—	21	
				LE	H_2O	40, 80	40	—		0
92200	51	1,4-Naphthoquinone, 2-hydroxy-3-(3-methyl-1-butenyl)-	$O_3C_{15}H_{14}$	SA	H_2O	25, 50	25	—	25	
				WM	H_2O	30–125	30	—	0	
				LE	H_2O	25, 50	25	—		1
92201	51	1,4-Naphthoquinone, 2,2′-(2-pyridylmethylene)bis[3-hydroxy-	$NO_6C_{26}H_{15}$	SA	H_2O	125, 250	125	—	0	
				WM	H_2O	125	125	—	14	
				LE	H_2O	125, 250	125	—		1
92202	51	1,4-Naphthoquinone, 2,2′-benzylidenebis[3-hydroxy-	$O_6C_{27}H_{16}$	SA	H_2O	1–125	1	—	23	
				WM	H_2O	0.5–125	0.5	—	33	
				LE	H_2O	30–250	30	—		0
92203	51	1,4-Naphthoquinone, 2,2′-[*p*-(dimethylamino)benzylidene]bis[3-hydroxy-	$NO_6C_{29}H_{21}$	SA	H_2O	60	60		14	
				WM	H_2O	62–250	62		17	
				LE	H_2O	30, 60	30			0
93072	51	1,4-Naphthoquinone, 2-(1-heptenyl)-3-hydroxy-	$O_3C_{17}H_{18}$	SA	H_2O	62.5–250	62.5	—	18	
				WM	H_2O	250	250	—	20	
				LE	H_2O	30–250	30	—		0
93074	51	1,4-Naphthoquinone, 2-chloro-3-hydroxy-	$O_3ClC_{10}H_5$	SA	H_2O	150	150	—	0	
				WM	H_2O	100, 250	100	—	23	
				LE	H_2O	125, 250	125	—		0
95400	51	1,4-Naphthoquinone, 2-(1,1-dimethylallyl)-3-hydroxy-	$O_3C_{15}H_{14}$	SA	H_2O	100, 200	100	—	43	
				WM	H_2O	125, 250	125	—	0	
				LE	H_2O	150	150	—		0
98019	51	1,4-Naphthoquinone, 2-benzyl-3-hydroxy-	$O_3C_{17}H_{12}$	SA	H_2O	125, 250	125	—	39	
				WM	H_2O	125–500	125	—	3	
				LE	H_2O	125, 250	125	—		0
98023	51	1,4-Naphthoquinone, 2-hydroxy-3-(1-hydroxy-2,2,2-trichloroethyl)-	$O_4Cl_3C_{12}H_7$	SA	H_2O	125, 250	125	—	15	
				WM	H_2O	125, 250	125	—	24	
				LE	H_2O	125	125	—		0

TABLE XIII—*continued*

NSC No.	Supplier	Compound name	Molecular formula	Tumor system	Vehicle	Dose range tested (mg/kg)	Response (mg/kg)		Evaluation		
							MTD	MED	TWI(%)	ILS(%)	ED_{50}
100,407	51	1,4-Naphthoquinone, 2-hydroxy-3-(2,3-dihydroxy-3-methylbutyl)-	$O_5C_{15}H_{16}$	WM LE	H_2O H_2O	250–500 100–400[a]	250 200	— —	20	 6	
100,414	51	1,4-Naphthoquinone, 2-hydroxy-3-(3-hydroxy-3-methylbutyl)-	$O_4C_{15}H_{16}$	LE WM	H_2O H_2O	250 125–433	<250 125	— —	 10	0	
102,530	2	1,4-Naphthoquinone, 2-hydroxy-3-(2-hydroxy-2-methylpropyl)-	$O_4C_{14}H_{14}$	LE	CMC	50–400[a]	400	—		5	
102,531	2	1,4-Naphthoquinone, 2-hydroxy-3-neopentyl-	$O_3C_{15}H_{16}$	LE	CMC	50–400[a]	400	—		14	
102,532	2	1,4-Naphthoquinone, 2-(*p*-bromophenyl)-3-hydroxy-	$O_3BrC_{16}H_9$	LE	CMC	50–400[a]	400	—		20	
102,533	2	1,4-Naphthoquinone, 2-hydroxy-3-phenyl-	$O_3C_{16}H_{10}$	LE	CMC	50–400[a]	400	—		14	
102,538	2	[2,2′-Binaphthalene]-1,4-dione, 3-hydroxy-	$O_3C_{20}H_{12}$	LE	Saline	400	400	—		0	
103,335	67	1,4-Naphthoquinone, 2-(7-cyclohexylheptyl)-3-hydroxy-	$O_3C_{23}H_{30}$	WM	Saline + gum acacia	100, 400	100	—	25		
103,336	67	1,4-Naphthoquinone, 2-(8-cyclohexyloctyl)-3-hydroxy-	$O_3C_{24}H_{32}$	WM	Saline + T-80	50–400	50	—	14		
108,019	2	1,4-Naphthoquinone, 2-(2,2-di-*p*-tolylethyl)-3-hydroxy-	$O_3C_{26}H_{22}$	WM	Saline	100	>100	—	5		
108,020	2	1,4-Naphthoquinone, 2-hydroxy-3-[3-(3,4-xylyl)-propyl]-	$O_3C_{21}H_{20}$	WM	Saline	40	>40	—	7		

108,021	2	1,4-Naphthoquinone, 2-hydroxy-3-[3-methyl-3-(*p*-tolylthio)-butyl]-	$O_3SC_{22}H_{22}$	WM	Saline	50	>50	—	44
108,022	2	1,4-Naphthoquinone, 2-ethyl-3-hydroxy-	$O_3C_{12}H_{10}$	WM	Saline	125	<125	—	44
108,024	2	1,4-Naphthoquinone, 2-hydroxy-6-isohexyl-3-isopentyl-	$O_3C_{21}H_{28}$	WM	Saline	125	>125	—	21
108,025	2	1,4-Naphthoquinone, 2-[3-(decylthio)-3-methylbutyl]-3-hydroxy-	$O_3SC_{25}H_{36}$	WM	Saline	40	>40	—	25
108,026	2	1,4-Naphthoquinone, 2-[1-(dodecylamino)ethyl]-3-hydroxy-	$NO_3C_{24}H_{35}$	WM	Saline	40	>40	—	0
108,027	2	1,4-Naphthoquinone, 2-hydroxy-3-(*p*-tolylthio)-	$O_3SC_{17}H_{12}$	WM	Saline	40	40	—	22
108,028	2	1,4-Naphthoquinone, 2-hydroxy-3-[(phenylthio)-methyl]-	$O_3SC_{17}H_{12}$	WM	Saline	40	>40	—	2
108,029	2	1,4-Naphthoquinone, 2-hydroxy-3-(phenylthio)-	$O_3SC_{16}H_{10}$	WM	Saline	40	>40	—	0
108,030	2	1,4-Naphthoquinone, 2-hydroxy-3-*p*-toluidino-	$NO_3C_{17}H_{13}$	WM	Saline	40	>40	—	0
108,700	2	1,4-Naphthoquinone, 2-[[(*p*-chlorophenyl)thio]methyl]-3-hydroxy-	$O_3SClC_{17}H_{11}$	WM	Saline	40	~40	—	42
108,701	2	1,4-Naphthoquinone, 2-[(dodecylamino)methyl]-3-hydroxy-	$NO_3C_{23}H_{33}$	WM	Saline	500	~500		53[d]
108,702	2	1,4-Naphthoquinone, 2-[α-(hexadecylamino)benzyl]-3-hydroxy-	$NO_3C_{33}H_{45}$	WM	Saline	400	400	—	0
108,703	2	1,4-Naphthoquinone, 2-hydroxy-3-[4-(*p*-tolylthio)-butyl]-	$O_3SC_{21}H_{20}$	WM	Saline	40	>40	—	30

TABLE XIII—*continued*

NSC No.	Supplier	Compound name	Molecular formula	Tumor system	Vehicle	Dose range tested (mg/kg)	Response (mg/kg) MTD	MED	Evaluation TWI(%)	ILS(%)	ED_{50}
109,542	2	1,4-Naphthoquinone, 2-(3-cyclohexylpropyl)-3-hydroxy-6-methoxy-	$O_4C_{20}H_{24}$	WM	Saline	100–300	>300	—	0		
109,543	2	1,4-Naphthoquinone, 2-hydroxy-3-[3-(5-indanyl)propyl]-	$O_3C_{22}H_{20}$	WM	Saline	100–300	100	—	0		
109,544	2	Peroxide, bis[1,4-dihydro-3-(3-methyl-2-butenyl)-1,4-dioxo-2-naphthyl]	$O_6C_{30}H_{26}$	WM	Saline	100–300	>300	—	16		
111,551	51	1,4-Naphthoquinone, 2-acetyl-3-hydroxy-	$O_4C_{12}H_8$	LE WM	H_2O H_2O	75 100–400	75 <100	— —	 35	0 	
112,151	51	1,4-Naphthoquinone, 2-hydroxy-3-(phenylazo)-	$N_2O_3C_{16}H_{10}$	LE WM	H_2O H_2O	400 400	~400 >400	— —	 25	0 	
112,829	67	1,4-Naphthoquinone, 2-(3,7-dimethyl-2,6-octadienyl)-3-hydroxy-, *trans*-	$O_3C_{20}H_{20}$	WM	CMC	25–200	~200	200	60		
113,452	34	1,4-Naphthoquinone, 2-[3-(*p*-cycloheptylphenyl)propyl]-3-hydroxy-	$O_3C_{26}H_{28}$	KB	PG						1.5
113,453	34	1,4-Naphthoquinone, 2-hydroxy-3-[3-[*p*-(phenylsulfonyl)-phenyl]propyl]-	$O_5S_2C_{25}H_{20}$	WM KB	Saline PG	100–300	100	—	5		 12
113,454	34	1,4-Naphthoquinone, 2-hydroxy-3-(4-morpholinobutyl)-, hydrochloride	$NO_4C_{18}H_{21} \cdot HCl$	WM KB	Saline PG	100	>100	—	7		 >100
113,455	34	1,4-Naphthoquinone, 2-[3-(*p*-cyclohexylphenyl)propyl]-3-hydroxy-	$O_3C_{25}H_{26}$	KB	PG						1.3
113,456	34	1,4-Naphthoquinone, 2-hydroxy-3-[3-(*p*-methoxyphenyl)-propyl]	$O_4C_{20}H_{18}$	KB	PG						12

113,457	34	1,4-Naphthoquinone, 2-(2-bromoethyl)-3-hydroxy-	$O_3BrC_{12}H_9$	WM	Saline	<800	800	—	15		
				KB	PG						6.0
113,458	34	1,4-Naphthoquinone, 2-hydroxy-3-[3-(*p*-hydroxyphenyl)-propyl]-, 3-acetate	$O_5C_{21}H_{18}$	WM	Saline	400	>400		0		
				KB	PG						>100
113,459	34	1,4-Naphthoquinone, 2-[3-[*p*-(benzyloxy)phenyl]-propyl]-2-hydroxy-	$O_4C_{26}H_{22}$	KB	PG						12
114,577	78	1,4-Naphthoquinone, 2-(2-bromo-3-methyl-1-butenyl)-3-hydroxy-	$O_3BrC_{15}H_{13}$	WM	Saline	25–200	50	—	34		
114,803	51	1,4-Naphthoquinone, 2-(3,7-dimethyl-2,6-octadienyl)-3-hydroxy-	$NO_3C_{20}H_{22}$	LE	H_2O	100–400	100	—		3	
				PS	H_2O	200	200	—		0	
				WM	H_2O	50–400	>400	~200[e]	75		
114,806	51	2-Naphthaleneacetic acid, 1,4-dihydro-3-hydroxy-1,4-dioxo-	$O_5C_{12}H_8$	LE	H_2O	400	400	—		1	
				WM	H_2O	400	400	—	0		
114,807	51	1,4-Naphthoquinone, 2-(2-butenyl)-3-hydroxy-	$O_3C_{14}H_{12}$	LE	H_2O	75	~75	—		4	
				WM	H_2O	50–400	~50	—	0		
114,930	41	1,4-Naphthoquinone, 2-(*p*-chloroanilino)-3-hydroxy-	$NO_3ClC_{16}H_{10}$	LE	Saline	400	400	—		2	
				WM	Saline	400	400	—	0		
400,568	44	1,4-Naphthoquinone, 2-hydroxy-3-isopropyl-	$O_3C_{13}H_{12}$	KB	—						6.5
400,858	44	1,4-Naphthoquinone, 6-bromo-2-hydroxy-, potassium deriv.	$O_3BrC_{10}H_5 \cdot K$	KB	—						32
401,100	44	1,4-Naphthoquinone, 2-bromo-3-hydroxy-	$O_3BrC_{10}H_5$	SA	MC	125	>125	—	32		
				CA	MC	112	>112	—	1		
				WM	Saline	150	>150	—	0		
				LE	MC	112	112	—		2	
				KB	DMF						46
401,107	44	1,4-Naphthoquinone, 2,3-dihydroxy-	$O_4C_{10}H_6$	KB	DMF						48
401,178	44	1,4-Naphthoquinone, 2-benzyl-6-bromo-3-hydroxy-	$O_3BrC_{17}H_{11}$	KB	—						>10

TABLE XIII—*continued*

NSC No.	Supplier	Compound name	Molecular formula	Tumor system	Vehicle	Dose range tested (mg/kg)	Response (mg/kg)		Evaluation		
							MTD	MED	TWI(%)	ILS(%)	ED_{50}
401,179	44	1,4-Naphthoquinone, 3-benzyl-6-bromo-2-hydroxy-	$O_3BrC_{17}H_{11}$	KB	—						30
401,185	44	1,4-Naphthoquinone, 6-bromo-2-hydroxy-3-styryl-	$O_3BrC_{18}H_{11}$	LE	Saline	50–200[c]	150	—		3	
				KB	—						6.0
401,186	44	1,4-Napththoquinone, 6-bromo-3-hydroxy-2-phenethyl-	$O_3BrC_{18}H_{13}$	KB	—						>100
401,187	44	1,4-Naphthoquinone, 6-bromo-2-hydroxy-3-phenethyl-	$O_3BrC_{18}H_{13}$	KB	—						22
401,193	44	1,4-Naphthoquinone, 6-bromo-2-hydroxy-3-(3-phenyl-propenyl)-	$O_3BrC_{19}H_{13}$	KB	—						26
401,194	44	1,4-Naphthoquinone, 6-bromo-3-hydrocinnamyl-2-hydroxy-	$O_3BrC_{19}H_{15}$	KB	—						>100
401,209	44	1,4-Naphthoquinone, 6-bromo-3-(diphenylmethyl)-2-hydroxy-	$O_3BrC_{23}H_{15}$	LE	Saline	100–400	400	—		6	
				KB	—						26
403,729	1	1,4-Naphthoquinone, 2-hydroxy-8-methoxy-3-(6-methoxy-*m*-tolyl)-5-methyl-	$O_5C_{20}H_{18}$	KB	Normal media						>100
403,747	1	1,4-Naphthoquinone, 2-hydroxy-3-(pentylaminomethyl)-	$NO_3C_{16}H_{19}$	KB	Normal media						26
403,788	1	1,4-Naphthoquinone, 2-(3-cyclo-hexylpropyl)-3-hydroxy-	$O_3C_{19}H_{22}$	KB	Normal media						15
407,503	46	1,4-Naphthoquinone, 2-[3-(*p*-chlorophenyl)propyl]-3-hydroxy-	$O_3ClC_{19}H_{15}$	SA	CMC	4–125	4		25		
				CA	CMC	1–4	1		0		
				LE	CMC	1–4	1			18	
				KB	Dioxane						40

[a] TI > 6 P.O.
[b] Results not reproducible.
[c] Single injection procedure only.
[d] Testing incomplete. QNS.
[e] P.O. TI ⩾ 2.

In fact, there is only one other compound (NSC-518,044) in the program with this structural feature and it was tested only in WM. While crotepoxide itself does not have sufficient activity to warrant further work with it, the fact that this type of compound is now known to occur in a plant augurs well for the isolation of other diepoxides. Recently, another compound, mikanolide (NSC-94037), isolated from *Mikania scandens* (fam. Compositae), has been shown by Herz *et al.* (1967) to be a diepoxide of the sesquiterpene dilactone group. It possesses cytotoxicity and is being studied for *in vivo* activity.

Table XIV summarizes the CCNSC screening results with three naturally occurring diepoxides as well as of those synthetic diepoxides which are derived from aliphatic straight-chain hydrocarbons of different chain lengths.

Of the naturally occurring diepoxides beside crotepoxide, only the antibiotic fumagillin (NSC-9168 and its cyclohexylamine salt NSC-58368) (XXIV), included here because of structural similarity, possesses *in vivo* antitumor activity. Mikanolide (NSC-94037) is active only against KB. It is interesting that fumagillin possesses the partial structure, XXIV, thus being related formally to 1,2:4,5-diepoxypentane (NSC-47545) while crotepoxide is related to 1,2:3,4-diepoxybutane (NSC-629, 32605, 32606, and 32607). Although 1,2:4,5-diepoxypentane does not show activity against SA as fumagillin does,

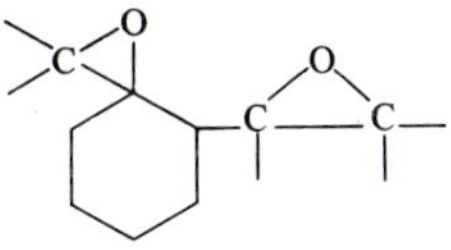

(XXIV)

all of the stereoisomers of 1,2:3,4-diepoxybutane are highly active against WM, unlike crotepoxide. Further separation of the two epoxy groups along the hydrocarbon chain does not necessarily result in loss of *in vivo* antitumor activity. The pentane (NSC-47545) and octane (NSC-109,888) derivatives are inactive in all tests tried, but the hexane derivative (NSC-47548) and the decane derivative (NSC-36649) are active against WM and the octadecane derivative (NSC-55269) is active against SA. It is unfortunate that data are missing on the effect of NSC-47545 and of NSC-48599 on WM as such data would make possible a more direct comparison of the effect of chain length and of chain branching.

I. Proteins and Polypeptides

Many materials that might be considered in this section have been tested in the CCNSC program. They form a very heterogeneous group of proteins, enzymes, hormones, simple polypeptides, antibiotics of a wholly or partly polypeptide nature, and synthetic polypeptides prepared from a single amino

TABLE XIV
DIEPOXY COMPOUNDS

NSC No.	Supplier	Compound name	Molecular formula	Tumor system	Vehicle	Dose range tested (mg/kg)	Response (mg/kg) MTD	MED	Evaluation TWI(%)	ILS(%)	ED_{50}
629	64	Butane, 1,2:3,4-diepoxy-	$O_2C_4H_6$	SA	CMC	4.5–500	~35	—	29[a]		
				CA	CMC	3–28	28	—	35		
				LE	CMC, Saline	3–96	48	—		26	
				FV	CMC	2.25–81	18	—	30		
				DL	CMC	2.5–500	25	—		78	
				WM	Saline	1.5–96	48	12	99		
				KB	—						9.0
9168	71	Fumagillin (2,4,6,8-Decatetraene-dioic acid, 4-(1,2-epoxy-1,5-dimethyl-4-hexenyl)-5-methoxy-1-oxaspiro[2.5]-oct-6-yl ester	$O_7C_{26}H_{34}$	SA	—	12–135	90	27[b]	80		
				CA	MC	10–160	80	80	63[c]		
				EA	—	2.5–10	~10	—	53		
				WM	Saline	125	>125	—	2		
				LE	—	72, 80	80	—		10	
				KB	—						24
58368	1	Fumagillin, compd. with dicyclohexylamine (1:1)	$O_7C_{26}H_{34}\cdot NC_{12}H_{23}$	SA	CMC	6–600	200	80[d]	81		
				CA	MC or saline	2.5–160	~40	40	78		
				LL	Saline	25–400	~50	~50	62		
				WA	CMC	25–200	200	50[e]	90		
				WM	Saline	18.8–300	150	—	30		
				LE	MC	2.5–160	160	—		23	
				DA	Saline	12.5–200	200	—		16	
				KB	H_2O						5.2
32605	32	Butane, *d*-1,2; 3,4-diepoxy-	$O_2C_4H_6$	WM	Saline	6–100	~75	15[f]	100		
				LE	Saline or H_2O	10–750	750	50		89	
				PS	H_2O	100–750	300	200		27	
32606	32	Butane, *l*-1,2; 3,4-diepoxy-	$O_2C_4H_6$	SA	Saline	18, 75	18	—	3		
				CA	Saline	16	>16	—	0		
				WM	Saline	22–100	50	[g]	100		
				KB	—						<1.0
32607	69	Butane, *meso*-1,2; 3,4-diepoxy-	$O_2C_4H_6$	WM	Saline	3.3–50	~25	17	100		

36649	69	Decane, 1,2: 9,10-diepoxy-	$O_2C_{10}H_{18}$	SA	Saline	500	500	—	2		
				EA	Saline	125–500	125	—	8		
				WM	CMC	400	400	[h]	94		
				LE	Saline	450	450	—		19	
47545	66	Pentane, 1,2: 4,5-diepoxy-	$O_2C_5H_8$	SA	MC	100, 500	100	—	48		
				CA	MC	45, 90	45	—	43		
				LE	MC	90	90	—		19	
47548	66	Hexane, 1,2:5,6-diepoxy-	$O_2C_6H_{10}$	SA	MC	50–500	50	—	1		
				CA	MC	40	40	—	46		
				WM	CMC	4–256	128	64	95[i]		
				LE	MC	9–90	~60	40		60[j]	
				KB	PG						5.0
48599	66	Butane, 1,2:3,4-diepoxy-2-methyl-	$O_2C_5H_8$	SA	MC	100, 500	100	—	0		
				CA	MC	40, 80	40	—	16		
				LE	MC	80	<80	—		10	
55269	74	Octadecane, 1,2:17, 18-diepoxy-	$O_2C_{18}H_{34}$	SA	MC	125, 250	125	—	75		
				CA	MC	125, 250	125	—	39		
				LE	MC	250	250	—		0	
94037	23	Mikanolide	$O_6C_{15}H_{14}$	WM	Saline	6, 10, 50	>50	—	55[a]		
				LE	CMC	5–400	~5	—		12	
				KB	PG						<1
106,396	29	Crotepoxide	$O_8C_{18}H_{18}$	LL	CMC	150–500	~200	200	64		
				WM	CMC	150–600	~450	450	50		
				LE	CMC	100–400	400	—		8	
				PS	SSS	50–400	~100	—		0	
109,888	2	4-Octene, 2,3:6,7-diepoxy-2,6-dimethyl- or 2-Octene, 4,5:6,7-diepoxy-3,7-dimethyl-	$O_2C_{10}H_{16}$	WM	Saline	400	>400	—	0		
				LE	Saline	400	>400	—		3	
518,044	62	Pseudoascaridole (*cis* form); *cis*-1,2:3,4-diepoxy-*p*-menthane	$O_2C_{10}H_{16}$	WM	CMC	400	>400	—	13		

[a] Results erratic.
[b] TI ~ 3.
[c] Activity not reproducible.
[d] TI ⩾ 2. Excessive animal weight loss.
[e] TI ~ 4.
[f] TI ≃ 5.
[g] Testing incomplete.
[h] Testing incomplete. QNS.
[i] TI ~ 2.
[j] Results erratic and not reproducible.

acid. Such materials have in common only a relatively high molecular weight and the presence of multiple peptide linkages. While several of the polypeptide antibiotics have been known for some time to have antitumor activity and are actually in clinical trial (for instance, actinomycin D is commercially available as an antitumor drug), these will not be dealt with here as they are of microbial origin. Similarly, most of the enzymes and the hormones are of animal origin and will not be discussed. The synthetic polypeptides prepared from a single amino acid are beginning to show antitumor activity in *in vivo* systems, but they are also outside the scope of this review. The value of mentioning these substances in the discussion is that they help to illustrate the generalization that high-molecular-weight materials composed of polypeptide linkages, whatever the origin, can possess the property of antitumor activity. Polypeptides and proteins, therefore, form a broad class of substances which should repay further investigation.

For some time, proteinaceous materials have been isolated as the active agents in several higher plants in the CCNSC program (Ulubelen *et al.*, 1965). The most interesting of these, NSC-110,435, isolated from the seeds of *Caesalpinia gilliesii* Wall. (fam. Leguminosae) (Ulubelen *et al.*, 1967), is scheduled for pharmacological study (Table XV).

Asparaginases are known to occur in certain higher plants, fungi, and bacteria as well as in animal tissues. One of these, an L-asparaginase (NSC-109,229), has recently become of great interest because of favorable clinical reports. A recent publication giving a good historical introduction is that of Oettgen *et al.* (1967). While the particular substance in use has been of bacterial origin, it is possible that an antitumor-active asparaginase may be found in higher plant forms. The special properties of L-asparaginase as an enzyme indicate the possibility of a mechanism of action different from that of other chemotherapeutic agents. The National Cancer Institute has supported the large-scale production of this drug and is engaged both in its clinical study and in supporting clinical studies elsewhere.

IV. Plants Showing Antitumor Activity but No Longer of Interest

Among the by-products of the plant program of the CCNSC is a rather substantial body of information relative to the constituents of certain plants found to be responsible for the antitumor activity of the plants but which is presently not being developed by CCNSC either because other plants are better sources of these constituents or because the compounds themselves do not meet the requirements for activity against *in vivo* tumor systems presently in effect. The presentation of this information in summary form is thought to be useful because other investigators using other criteria may find it of advantage.

TABLE XV
PROTEINS AND POLYPEPTIDES

NSC No.	Supplier	Name	Tumor system	Vehicle	Dose range tested (mg/kg)	Response (mg/kg)		Evaluation		
						MTD	MED	TWI(%)	ILS(%)	ED_{50}
109,229	—	L-Asparaginase from *Escherichia coli*	WM	H_2O	12.5–50	>50	—	44		
			3L8	Saline	1[a] 8[a]	>8[a]	<1[a]		38	
			LE	H_2O	1[b] 8[b]	>8[b]	—		0	
110,435	14	Protein from *Caesalpinia gilliesii*	WM	Saline	0.5–40	~20	~5[a]	88		
			LE	Saline	0.5–30	~10	—		0	
			PS	Saline	0.5–30	1	—		0	

[a] TI ~ 4.
[b] International units.

A. Plants Containing Tannin

The chemically heterogeneous group of polymeric compounds known as tannins is widely distributed in plants and is responsible for the antitumor activity shown by some crude extracts, especially against WM, SA, and LL. Tannins are notably inactive against KB. So far, all tannin samples have shown high toxicity and low TI in the antitumor tests. These characteristics, coupled with the difficulty of purification and the well-known chemical instability of tannins expressing itself in sensitivity to air oxidation and susceptibility to further polymerization, have caused tannins to be considered unpromising for development into practical useful drugs. Fortunately, methods exist for precipitating tannins from crude extracts, and when these methods are combined with bioassay of the tannin-free filtrates, a determination can be made as to whether tannins are the only active materials present or whether other active compounds are also present. Other methods, less definitive, qualitatively detect tannins; where a strong tannin test is given and the aqueous phase is either active against WM or toxic, experience has shown that tannins are the only active components. Table XVI lists those plants in which tannins are believed to be, for practical purposes, the only active constituents.

B. Plants Containing Phytosterols

Another widely distributed group of compounds, some of which show activity against WM, is the phytosterols. A substantial number of plants were showing activity against WM in the ligroin extract used to defat the plants prior to making the regular alcoholic or aqueous-alcoholic extracts. Chromatography showed that activity was concentrated frequently in the "β-sitosterol" fraction and sometimes in other sterol fractions. It was also found that β-sitosterol was never pure but contained large amounts of other sterols (see Section III,C). The usefulness of β-sitosterol as a practical antitumor agent has been discussed earlier (Section III,C). A list of plants in which β-sitosterol or a related sterol is believed to be the only active agent is given in Table XVII.

C. Plants Containing Cytotoxic Lignans

A few plants showing cytotoxicity (in KB) have been shown to owe their activity to the lactonic lignans podophyllotoxin or deoxypodophyllotoxin. The chemistry and sources of these and other lignans have been reviewed by Hartwell and Schrecker (1958). More recently, a new cytotoxic lignan, named burseran, nonlactonic in nature, has been isolated (Bianchi *et al.*, 1968; Cole *et al.*, 1969; Trumbull and Cole, 1969). In the course of the screening program of the CCNSC, several new sources have been noted. Both lactone compounds have been well tested (see Table XVII) and found to possess negative or

TABLE XVI

Plants Whose Antitumor Activity is Due to Tannin

Family	Genus and species	Plant part[a]	Origin of collection	Tumor	Supplier	Method of determination[b]
Amaranthaceae	*Celosia argentea* L.	Sd	Japan	SA	29[c]	I
Anacardiaceae	*Odina wodier* Roxb.	Wd	India	WM	51	V
Anacardiaceae	*Rhus typhina* L.	Ws, sb	Maryland	LL	29[c]	I
Apocynaceae	*Apocynum pumilum* Greene	Rt, st, lf, fl	California	SA	29[c]	I
Betulaceae	*Alnus arguta* (Schlecht.) Spach.	Fr, lf, st	Mexico	SA, FV	14	II
Bromeliaceae	*Tillandsia usneoides* L.	St, lf	Florida	SA	29[c]	I
Buxaceae	*Simmondsia chinensis*	Lf, st	Arizona	WM	29[c]	II
Caprifoliaceae	*Viburnum rafinesquianum* Schultes	St, lf, fr	Wisconsin	SA	29	I
Caryophyllaceae	*Siphonychia diffusa* Chapm.	St, lf, fl	Florida	SA	55[c]	I
Combretaceae	*Combretum molle* R. Br. ex G. Don	Ws	Ethiopia	SA	55[c]	II
Combretaceae	*Laguncularia racemosa* Gaertn. f.	Fr	Florida	SA	18[c]	I, II (a)
Cornaceae	*Cornus florida* L.	Ws, sb	Maryland	SA	29[c]	I
Cornaceae	*Cornus foemina* Mill.	St, lf, fl, fr	North Carolina	KB	55[c]	IV
Cornaceae	*Cornus nuttallii* Aud.	St, lf	California	SA	55[c]	II
Cornaceae	*Cornus racemosa* Lam.	Ws, sb	Connecticut	SA	55[c]	II

TABLE XVI—*continued*

Family	Genus and species	Plant part[a]	Origin of collection	Tumor	Supplier	Method of determination[b]
Cornaceae	*Cornus rugosa* Lam.	St, lf, inf (fr)	Michigan	WM	55[c]	II (a)
Cornaceae	*Cornus stolonifera* Michx.	Lf, st, fl	California	SA	55[c]	II
Cyrillaceae	*Cyrilla parvifolia* Raf.	St, lf, fr	Florida	SA	55[c]	II (a)
Ericaceae	*Chamaedaphne calyculata* (L.) Moen.	Pl	Wisconsin	SA	29	I
Ericaceae	*Lyonia ovalifolia* (Wall.) Drude	Px	India (U.P.)	WM	11	II
Ericaceae	*Xylococcus bicolor* (Nutt.)	Lf, st, fr	California	SA	55[d]	IV
Euphorbiaceae	*Euphorbia floridana* Chapm.	St, lf, fl, fr	Florida	SA	29[c]	I
Euphorbiaceae	*Glochidion obovatum*	Lf, st	Maryland	SA	29[c]	I
Fagaceae	*Castanea ashei* Sudw.	St, lf, fl	Florida	WM	55[c]	IV
Fagaceae	*Fagus grandifolia* Ehrh.	Rt	New York	FV (WM)	55[c]	II
Fagaceae	*Quercus kelloggii* Newb.	St, lf	California	WM	55[c]	II (a)
Geraniaceae	*Geranium maculatum* L.	Pl, fr	Wisconsin	SA	29	I
Gnetaceae	*Ephedra nebrodensis* Tineo var. *procera* Stapf.	St	Turkey	LL	29[c]	I
Gnetaceae	*Ephedra viridis* Cov.	St, lf	California	LL	55[c]	II
Guttiferae	*Hypericum revolutum* Vahl.	Lf, fl	Ethiopia	SA, LL	29[c]	I, II (a)

Lecythidaceae	*Careya arborea* Roxb.	Bk	India	SA	51	V
Lecythidaceae	*Planchonia papuana* R. Knuth	Sb	New Guinea	LL	16[f]	II
Leguminosae	*Acacia angustissima* Mill.	Lf, st, pods (fresh)	Arizona	SA, CA	14	III[e]
Leguminosae	*Acacia ixiophylla* Benth.	Lf	Australia (Qld.)	LL	79[f]	III[g]
Leguminosae	*Flemingia chappar* Ham.	Px	India (Bihàr)	WM	11	II
Leguminosae	*Hymenaea courbaril* L.	Lf	Costa Rica	LL	29[h]	I, II
Leguminosae	*Indigofera heterotricha* DC.	Pl	So. Africa (S.W.A.)	WM	80[d]	II (a)[m]
Leguminosae	*Krameria triandra* S.E. Rhatany root	Rt	—	SA	55[i]	II
Leguminosae	*Lespedeza cuneata* G. Don	Lf	Australia (Qld.)	LL	16[f]	II
Leguminosae	*Piliostigma thonningii* Milne-Redh.	Ws	Ethiopia	SA	29[c]	I
Liliaceae	*Yucca filamentosa* L.	Rt, st, lf	North Carolina	SA	29[c]	I
Liliaceae	*Yucca pallida* McKelvey	Lf	Texas	SA	29[c]	I
Melastomataceae	*Calycogonium squamulosum*	St, lf	Puerto Rico	WM	19[c]	II
Myrsinaceae	*Maesa lanceolata* Forsk.	Sb	Ethiopia	LL	29[c]	I
Onagraceae	*Ludwigia alternifolia*	Lf, st, rt	Georgia	SA	55[c]	II
Onagraceae	*Oenothera clavaeformis* Torr.	Rt, st, lf, fl, fr	California	SA (WM)	55[c]	II (a)
Palmae	*Cocos nucifera* L.	Rt, sb	Samoa	SA	55[c]	II (a)
Palmae	*Washingtonia robusta* Wendl.	Fr	California	SA	29[c]	I

TABLE XVI—*continued*

Family	Genus and species	Plant part[a]	Origin of collection	Tumor	Supplier	Method of determination[b]
Pinaceae	*Cedrus atlantica* Manetti	St, lf	Maryland	WM	55[c]	II (a)
Pinaceae	*Chamaecyparis nootkatensis* Spach.	Sb	Washington	LL	29[c]	I
Pinaceae	*Pinus australis* Michx. f.	St, bk	North Carolina	SA	55[c]	IV
Pinaceae	*Pinus elliottii* Engelm.	St, lf	Florida	SA	29[c]	I
Pinaceae	*Pinus glabra* Walt.	St, lf	Florida	LL	29[c]	I
Pinaceae	*Pinus lambertiana* Doug.	St, lf	California	WM	55[c]	II
Pinaceae	*Pinus virginiana* L.	St, bk	Ohio	KB	55[c]	IV
Polygonaceae	*Eriogonum alleni* S. Wats.	Rt, st, lf	Virginia	WM	29[c]	I, II
Polygonaceae	*Eriogonum tomentosum* Michx.	St, lf, fl	Florida	SA	29[c]	I
Polygonaceae	*Eriogonum umbellatum* Torr.	Rt, st, lf, fl	California	WM, LL	29[c]	II
Polygonaceae	*Polygonella americana*	Lf, st, fl, rt	Georgia	SA	55[j]	I, II
Polygonaceae	*Polygonum paronychia* (Cham. et Schlecht.)	Rt, st, lf, flr, fr	California	SA	55[c]	II
Polygonaceae	*Rumex hymenosepalus* Torr. var. Salt River Valley	Tu (fresh)	Arizona	SA	14[k]	III
Polygonaceae	*Rumex nervosus* Vahl.	Fl	Ethiopia	LL	55[c]	II (a)
Rhamnaceae	*Ceanothus americanus* L.	Rt (fresh)	North Carolina	SA	55[c]	IV

Rosaceae	*Amelanchier laevis* Wieg.	St, bk	North Carolina	KB	55[c]	IV
Rosaceae	*Amelanchier stolonifera* Wieg.	St, lf, fr	Michigan	WM	55[c]	II (a)
Rosaceae	*Cotoneaster marginatus* Schldl.	Px	India (H.P.)	WM	11	II
Rosaceae	*Eriobotrya japonica* Lindl.	Lf	Costa Rica	SA	29[h]	II
Rosaceae	*Heteromeles arbutifolia* M. Roem.	Sb	California	SA	29[c]	I, II
Rosaceae	*Potentilla recta* L.	Rt	North Carolina	MS	55[c]	IV
Rosaceae	*Rosa abyssinica* R. Br.	St, lf	Ethiopia	LL	55[c]	II
Rubiaceae	*Psychotria capensis* (Eckl.) Vatke	Pl	So. Africa (Natal)	SA	80[d]	II[l]
Salicaceae	*Salix exigua* Nutt.	St, lf	California	SA (WM)	55[c]	II
Sapindaceae	*Alectryon subcnereum* Radlk.	Lf	Florida	WM	55[c]	II
Sapindaceae	*Litchi chinensis* Sonner.	Rt	Maryland	SA	29[c]	II
Sapotaceae	*Manilkara hexandra* (Roxb.) Dub.	Px	India (M.P.)	WM	11	II
Sterculiaceae	*Argyrodendron peralatum*	Lf	Australia (Qld.)	SA	16[f]	II
Sterculiaceae	*Theobroma cacao*	Rt	Maryland	SA	29[c]	I
Symplocaceae	*Symplocos racemosa* Roxb.	Bk	India	WM	51	V
Tamaricaceae	*Tamarix gallica* L.	Ws, sb	Utah	SA, WM	55[c]	II
Taxaceae	*Podocarpus gracilior* Pilg.	St, lf	Ethiopia	LL	29[c]	I
Tiliaceae	*Carpodiptera ametiae* Lundell	Lf	Florida	WM	55[c]	II (a)

TABLE XVI—*continued*

Family	Genus and species	Plant part[a]	Origin of collection	Tumor	Supplier	Method of determination[b]
Ulmaceae	*Ulmus americana* L. var. *floridana* (Chapm.) Little	St, lf	Florida	SA	55[c]	II (a)

[a] Abbreviations: bk = bark, fl = flower, fr = fruit, inf = inflorescence, lf = leaf, pl = whole plant including root, px = whole plant excluding root, rt = root, sb = stem bark, sd = seed, st = stem, tu = tuber, wd = wood, ws = stem wood. Original plant material is assumed to be dried unless otherwise stated.

[b] I = Lead acetate precipitation. II = Caffeine precipitation (unpublished method of Dr. M. E. Wall); (a) caffeine filtrate not bioassayed. III = Isolation and identification. IV = Ferric chloride + salt-gelatin; aqueous phase either active against WM or toxic. V = Ferric chloride, salt-gelatin, and U.V. absorption at 280 mμ.

[c] Original plant material supplied by Dr. Robert E. Perdue, Jr., U.S. Department of Agriculture, Beltsville, Md.

[d] Original plant material supplied by Smith Kline & French Laboratories.

[e] Cole and Hammer (1965).

[f] Original plant material supplied by C.S.I.R.O., Australia.

[g] Clark-Lewis and Dainis (1968).

[h] Original plant material supplied by Prof. J. A. Sáenz Renauld, Univ. of Costa Rica.

[i] Original plant material supplied by Meer Corp., New York.

[j] Original plant material supplied by Eastern Utilization Research and Development Division, U.S.D.A.

[k] Cole and Buchalter (1965); Buchalter and Cole (1967).

[l] Unpublished work of Dr. M. E. Wall.

[m] Unpublished work Dr. A. Jordaan, C.S.I.R., South Africa.

TABLE XVII
PLANTS WHOSE ANTITUMOR ACTIVITY IS DUE TO PHYTOSTEROLS

Family	Genus and species	Plant part[a]	Origin of collection	Tumor	Supplier
Apocynaceae	*Plumeria acutifolia* Poir.	Bk	India	WM	51
Asclepiadaceae	*Calotropis gigantea* Linn.	Rt	India	WM	51
Capparidaceae	*Capparis decidua* Edgew.	Pl	India	WM	51
Combretaceae	*Quisqualis indica* L.	Lf	India	WM	51
Compositae	*Pericome caudata* Gray	Fl buds, lf, st (fresh)	Arizona	KB	51[b]
Cruciferae	*Brassica oleracea* L.	Lf	United States	WM	51
Cucurbitaceae	*Trichosanthes dioica* Roxb.	Pl	India	WM	51
Droseraceae	*Drosera rotundifolia* L.	Pl	United States	SA, WM	51
Euphorbiaceae	*Acalypha lanceolata* L.	Pl	India	WM	51
Geraniaceae	*Geranium robertianum* L.	Pl	United States	WM	51
Labiatae	*Scutellaria laterifolia* L.	Pl	United States	WM	51

TABLE XVII—*continued*

Family	Genus and species	Plant part[a]	Origin of collection	Tumor	Supplier
Leguminosae	*Cassia absus* L.	Pl	India	WM	51
Leguminosae	*Tephrosia purpurea* Pers.	Pl	India	WM	51
Malpighiaceae	*Thryallis glauca* O. Ktze.	Sb, lf, st	Mexico (Mex.)	SA	51[c]
Menispermaceae	*Tinospora cordifolia* Miers.	Pl	India	WM	51
Polygonaceae	*Rumex acetosella* L.	Rt	India	WM	51
Rubiaceae	*Galium aparine* L.	St, lf, fl	Texas	SA	29[c]
Salicaceae	*Populus fremontii* Wats.	Bk	Arizona	FV	51[b]
Urticaceae	*Parietaria judaica* L.	Lf	Israel	LL	51[c]
Zygophyllaceae	*Fagonia cretica* L.	Lf	India	WM	51

[a] Abbreviations: bk = bark, fl = flower, lf = leaf, pl = whole plant, rt = root, sb = stem bark, st = stem.
[b] Original plant material supplied by College of Pharmacy, University of Arizona, Tucson.
[c] Original plant material supplied by Dr. Robert E. Perdue, Jr., U.S.D.A. Beltsville, Maryland.

TABLE XVIII
Cytotoxic Lignans

NSC No.	Supplier	Compound name	Molecular formula	Tumor system	Vehicle	Dose range tested (mg/kg)	Response (mg/kg)		Evaluation		
							MTD	MED	TWI(%)	ILS(%)	ED_{50}
24818	44	Podophyllotoxin	$O_8C_{22}H_{22}$	SA	CMC	0.175–15	~0.50	—	29		
				CA	CMC	0.13–1.1	~1.1	—	24		
				LL	CMC	1–4	~2	2	64		
				LE		0.14–2.70	~1.62	—		20	
				FV	CMC	0.135–1.1	0.55	—	17		
				D1	CMC	1.85–3.70	3.70	—	0		
				MM	CMC	1–10	~2.7	—	33		
				P1	CMC	1.85–3.70	~3.70	—	15		
				H1	Saline	0.0012–5	~0.0048	—	1		
				LZ	MC	5–180	23	—		9	
				PS	CMC	1–16	~10	~2		71	
				8P	CMC	0.9–4	~2.2		20		
				WM	CMC	0.9–13	~6	6	73		
				KB	Dioxane						<0.01
123,428	14	Burseran	$C_{22}H_{26}O_6$	WM	CMC	11–67	67	—	12		0.026
				KB	DMF						
403,148	44	Deoxypodophyllotoxin	$O_7C_{22}H_{22}$	SA	CMC	4–75	4	—	0		
				LL	CMC	5.15	~5	—	10		
				LE	Saline	6.25–400	200	~100[a]		27	
				PS	CMC	1.5–80	~10	5		48[b]	
				WM	Saline	2.5–160	20	—	41		
				KB	—						0.0012

[a] Single injection procedure; inactive in chronic test.
[b] Results not reproducible.

marginal activity in LE and low or moderate activity in PS. Since these compounds are more widely distributed than was once believed and since they are fairly easily isolated and identified, a list of the plants owing their activity largely to either of these compounds may be useful (Table XIX).

TABLE XIX
Plants Whose Cytotoxic Activity is Due to Lignans

Family	Genus and species	Plant part[a]	Origin of collection	Lignan[b]	Supplier
Burseraceae	*Bursera microphylla* Gray	St (fresh)	Arizona	DP; B	14
Burseraceae	*Bursera morelensis* Ramirez	St, lf	Mexico[c]	DP[d]	14
Pinaceae	*Callitris columellaris* F. Muell.	Lf	Australia[e]	DP[f]	29
Pinaceae	*Juniperus communis* L. var. *depressa* Pursh	St, lf, fr	Michigan[c]	DP[g]	29
Pinaceae	*Juniperus virginiana* L.	Lf, tw	Maryland[c]	PT[h]	29
Pinaceae	*Libocedrus decurrens* Torr.	St, lf	California[c]	DP[i]	29
Pinaceae	*Thuja occidentalis* S.E. Arbor Vitae leaves	Lf	—[j]	DP[k]	55

[a] Abbreviations: fr = fruit, lf = leaf, st = stem, tw = twig.
[b] Abbreviations: DP = deoxypodophyllotoxin, PT = podophyllotoxin, B = burseran.
[c] Original plant material supplied by Dr. Robert E. Perdue, Jr., U.S.D.A., Beltsville, Maryland.
[d] Private communication from Dr. J. R. Cole.
[e] Original plant material supplied by C.S.I.R.O., Australia.
[f] Unpublished results of Drs. S. M. Kupchan and Y. Aynehchi.
[g] Unpublished results of Drs. S. M. Kupchan and R. J. Hemingway.
[h] Kupchan *et al.* (1965b).
[i] Kupchan *et al.* (1967b).
[j] Original plant extract supplied by Meer Corp., New York.
[k] Unpublished results of Dr. M. E. Wall.

D. Plants Whose Cytotoxic Activity Is Due to Cucurbitacins

A few plants that show cytotoxicity (in KB) have been proved to owe their activity to the presence of the highly active cucurbitacins (see Section III,E and Table XI). Until recently, only plants belonging to the family Cucurbitaceae had been found to contain cucurbitacins, but lately the occurrence of these compounds in a few other plant families has been noted (Moss, 1966; Table XX). Although *in vivo* activity in this class of compounds has not been sufficient to justify further development into useful drugs, it may be of interest to present the list of plants in which they have been found in the CCNSC program to occur as the chief active components.

TABLE XX
PLANTS WHOSE CYTOTOXIC ACTIVITY IS DUE TO CUCURBITACINS

Family	Genus and species	Plant part[a]	Origin of collection	Compound	Supplier
Begoniaceae	*Begonia tuberhybrida*	Tu	Belgium	Cucurbitacin B; cucurbitacin D; dihydrocucurbitacin B	18[b]
Cucurbitaceae	*Citrullus colocynthis* S.E. Colocynth N.F. X	Pulp	—[c]	Cucurbitacin E[d]	55
Cucurbitaceae	*Marah oreganus* Howell	St, lf, fr	California	Cucurbitacin B; isocucurbitacin B; cucurbitacin E; dihydro-cucurbitacin B	29[e]

[a] Abbreviations: fr = fruit, lf = leaf, st = stem, tu = tuber.
[b] Doskotch (private communication); Doskotch *et al.* (1969).
[c] Original plant extract supplied by Meer Corp., New York.
[d] Dr. M. E. Wall, unpublished results.
[e] Kupchan *et al.* (1967c).

V. Conclusions

Recent developments in the field of antineoplastic principles in plants can be summarized in terms of specific compounds that have been isolated, certain generalizations that can be made, and fringe benefits in phytochemistry of secondary importance but possibly of some value to other workers in the field.

From this review, it is apparent that one of the main hopes originally held for this work is being realized, namely, that higher plants are yielding chemical compounds of a wide variety of types—alkaloids, sesquiterpene lactones, saponins, digitaloid glycosides, quinones, and proteins among others—active against many different experimental tumor systems. Furthermore, most of these compounds would have been inaccessible until their isolation from natural sources since not only would there have been no particular reason for attempted synthesis but also many of them could be synthesized only with great difficulty. As these compounds are subjected to extensive pharmacological testing designed to select out those that have clinical promise, most of them are eliminated as is to be expected. However, a sufficient proportion of them passes the criteria and reaches the level of clinical trial as to justify the large effort involved in the whole process.

Compounds previously known in the CCNSC program but tested according to earlier screening practices are being "rediscovered" by new isolation techniques and are being afforded a new examination. Analogously, related "synthetics" in the program are being reexamined in different tumor systems. In this way, natural products are contributing toward better utilization of the large store of synthetics on hand. Data have been, and are being, accumulated on which conclusions regarding structure-function relationships can be based. Chemists have always felt impelled to speculate in this area because of the attractive possibility of being able to plan the synthesis of new compounds with more assurance that the latter will be useful. While it must be admitted that, in the present work, such speculations have so far not been particularly rewarding, perhaps due in part to the small number of compounds yet available for study, at least certain broad classes of compounds are emerging as being worthy of further investigation. Certain other classes can be relegated at present to positions of lower priority. Within a given class of compounds the structural features necessary for activity in one or another tumor system are usually far from clear, but in individual cases it may be possible to see some relationships. These relationships are further complicated by the factor of the large number of experimental tumors on which data have accumulated. It is with the knowledge that the CCNSC screen is under constant modification to achieve better predictability of clinical effectiveness, and in the hope that other investigators may find the material here provided useful in developing more effective screens of their own, that data on so many different tumor systems are presented.

While a botanical discussion on the relationship of plants showing antitumor activity and their classification is outside the scope of this review, much thought has naturally gone into attempts to find such relationships with a view toward greater selectivity in plant collection. It may be stated briefly that antitumor activity in general has been found in 154 families of higher plants out of 270 families collected, and that probably the strongest reason for lack of activity in certain families is the small number of species studied. When one attempts to refine the search for correlation at a lower level of classification such as genus, one finds again that with all the additional variables to take into account, such as plant part, season of the year, geographical location, and tumor system used, the numbers of samples tested are too small for valid statistical consideration.

Among the several hundred different plant species that have been, or are still, under chemical fractionation, many plants have appeared that owe their antitumor activity to constituents—tannins, phytosterols, certain lignans, and cucurbitacins—which to date have not made useful drugs. Many other plants have appeared from which novel antitumor agents are being isolated. These agents provide a basis from which attempts can be made to develop practical drugs either directly or indirectly through chemical modification of the agents. Given several hundred thousand known species of higher plants, the fact that active agents may concentrate in certain plant parts, and the knowledge that plants are not distinct and reproducible materials but are complex living organisms whose metabolic processes can vary greatly with different environmental conditions, the possibilities for the isolation of a wide variety of novel antitumor agents are practically endless. More work should yield a better understanding of plant species-activity relationships and plant species-constituent relationships, thus making collection more efficient. The development of more predictive antitumor test systems should come with time. Since there is merit in the concept of chemotherapy of cancer, principles from plants should play an increasingly important role in this field as more become available.

REFERENCES

American Chemical Society (1966). *Abstr. Papers*, 152*nd Meeting*, *New York*, *Sept.* p. 27.

Balitskii, K. P., Vorontzova, A. L., and Karpukhina, A. M. (1966). "Medicinal Plants in the Therapy of Malignant Tumors." Zdorovia, Kiev. (In Russian.)

Bianchi, E., Caldwell, M. E., and Cole, J. R. (1968). *J. Pharm. Sci.* **57**, 696.

Boit, H.-G. (1961). "Ergebnisse der Alkaloid-Chemie bis 1960." Akademie Verlag, Berlin.

Buchalter, L., and Cole, J. R., (1967). *J. Pharm. Sci.* **56**, 1033.

Clark-Lewis, J. W., and Dainis, I. (1968). *Australian J. Chem.* **21**, 425.

Cole, J. R., and Buchalter, L. (1965). *J. Pharm. Sci.* **54**, 1376.

Cole, J. R., and Hammer, R. H. (1965). *J. Pharm. Sci.* **54**, 235.

Cole, J. R., Bianchi, E., and Trumbull, E. R. (1969). *J. Pharm. Sci.* **58**, 175.

Curcumelli-Rodostamo, M., and Kulka, M. (1967). *In* "The Alkaloids" (R. H. F. Manske, ed.), Vol. 9, pp. 133–174. Academic Press, New York.

Dalton, L. K., Demerac, S., Elmes, B. C., Loder, J. W., Swan, J. M., and Teitei, T. (1967). *Australian J. Chem.* **20**, 2715.

Dean, F. M. (1963). "Naturally Occurring Oxygen Ring Compounds." Butterworth, London and Washington, D.C.

de Mayo, P. (1959a). "Mono- and Sesquiterpenoids." Wiley (Interscience), New York.

de Mayo, P. (1959b). "The Higher Terpenoids." Wiley (Interscience), New York.

Doskotch, R. W., Malik, M. Y., and Beal, J. L. (1969). *Lloydia* **32**. In press.

Ebbell, B. (1937). "The Papyrus Ebers. The Greatest Egyptian Medical Document." Oxford Univ. Press, London and New York.

Farnsworth, N. F. (1966). *J. Pharm. Sci.* **55**, 225.

Fieser, L. F., and Fieser, M. (1959). "Steroids." Reinhold, New York.

Gellhorn, A., and Hirschberg, E., eds. (1955). Investigation of Diverse Systems for Cancer Chemotherapy Screening. *Cancer Res. Suppl.* **3**.

Gilbert, B. (1965). *In* "The Alkaloids" (R. H. F. Manske, ed.), Vol. 8, pp. 335–513. Academic Press, New York.

Goldin, A., Serpick, A. A., and Mantel, N. (1966). *Cancer Chemotherapy Rept.* **50**, 173.

Govindachari, T. R. (1967). *In* "The Alkaloids" (R. H. F. Manske, ed.), Vol. 9, pp. 517–528. Academic Press, New York.

Hartwell, J. L. (1967). *Lloydia* **30**, 379.

Hartwell, J. L. (1968). *Lloydia* **31**, 71.

Hartwell, J. L., and Schrecker, A. W. (1958). *Fortschr. Chem. Org. Naturstoffe* **15**, 83.

Herz, W., Santhanam, P. S., Subramaniam, P. S., and Schmid, J. J. (1967). *Tetrahedron Letters* No. 32, 3111.

Joachim, H. (1890). "Papyros Ebers." Reimer, Berlin.

Kapadia, G. J., and Zalucky, T. B. (1968). *Lloydia* **31**, 424.

Karrer, W. (1958). "Konstitution und Vorkommen der organischen Pflanzenstoffe." Birkhäuser, Basel.

Kupchan, S. M., Doskotch, R. W., Bollinger, P., McPhail, A. T., Sim, G. A., and Sáenz Renauld, J. A. (1965a). *J. Am. Chem. Soc.* **87**, 5805.

Kupchan, S. M., Hemingway, J. C., and Knox, J. R. (1965b). *J. Pharm. Sci.* **54**, 659.

Kupchan, S. M., Davies, A. P., Barboutis, S. J., Schnoes, H. K., and Burlingame, A. L. (1967a). *J. Am. Chem. Soc.* **89**, 5718.

Kupchan, S. M., Hemingway, R. J., and Hemingway, J. C. (1967b). *J. Pharm. Sci.* **56**, 408.

Kupchan, S. M., Gray, A. H., and Grove, M. D. (1967c). *J. Med. Chem.* **10**, 337.

Kupchan, S. M., Yang, T.-H., Vasilikiotis, G. S., Barnes, M. H., and King, M. L. (1967d). *J. Am. Chem. Soc.* **89**, 3075.

Kupchan, S. M., Hemingway, R. J., Knox, J. R., Barboutis, S. J., Werner, D., and Barboutis, M. A. (1967e). *J. Pharm. Sci.* **56**, 603.

Kupchan, S. M., Hemingway, R. J., Coggan, P., McPhail, A. T., and Sim, G. A. (1968a). Abstr.

Kupchan, S. M., Yang, T.-H., King, M. L., and Borchardt, R. T. (1968b). *J. Org. Chem.* **33**, 1052.

Lavie, D., Glotter, E., and Shvo, Y. (1965). *J. Chem. Soc.* p. 7517.

Leonard, N. J. (1960). *In* "The Alkaloids" (R. H. F. Manske, ed.), Vol. 6, pp. 35–121. Academic Press, New York.

Moss, G. P. (1966). *Planta Med.*, Suppl., 86.

Neuss, N., Johnson, I. S., Armstrong, J. G., and Jansen, C. J. (1964). *Advan. Chemotherapy* **1**, 133.

Neuss, N., Gorman, M., and Johnson, I. S. (1967). *In* "Methods in Cancer Research" (H. Busch, ed.), Vol. 3, pp. 633–702. Academic Press, New York.

Oettgen, H. F., Old, L. J., Boyse, E. A., Campbell, H. A., Philips, F. S., Clarkson, B. D., Tallal, L., Leeper, R. D., Schwartz, M. K., and Kim, J. H. (1967). *Cancer Res.* **27**, Pt. I, 2619.

Ourisson, G., Crabbé, P., and Rodig, O. (1964). "Tetracyclic Triterpenes." Holden-Day, San Francisco, California.

Rao, K. V., Wilson, R. A., and Cummings, B. M. Presented at the American Chemical Society meeting, New York, Sept. 13, 1966; also personal communication, 1967.

Romo, J., and Romo de Vivar, A. (1967). *Fortschr. Chem. Org. Naturstoffe* **25**, 90.

Šorm, F. and Dolejš, L. (1966). "Guaianolides and Germacranolides." Holden-Day, San Francisco, California.

Trumbull, E. R., and Cole, J. R. (1969). *J. Pharm. Sci.* **58**, 176.

Ulubelen, A., Caldwell, M. E., and Cole, J. R. (1965). *J. Pharm. Sci.* **54**, 1214.

Ulubelen, A., McCaughey, W. F., and Cole, J. R. (1967). *J. Pharm. Sci.* **56**, 914.

Venditti, J. M., and Abbott, B. J. (1967). *Lloydia* **30**, 332.

Wall, M. E., Wani, M. C., and Abernethy, G. S., Jr. (1968). *Proc. 5th Intern. Symp. Nat. Prod. (IUPAC), London* p. 417. (Abstr.)

Wall, M. E., Palmer, K. H., Wani, M. C., Cook, C. E., Sim, G. A., and McPhail, A. T. (1966a). *Proc. 4th Intern. Symp. Chem. Nat. Prod. (IUPAC), Stockholm* p. 103. (Abstr.)

Wall, M. E., Wani, M. C., Cook, C. E., Palmer, K. H., McPhail, A. T., and Sim, G. A. (1966b). *J. Am. Chem. Soc.* **88**, 3888.

Zee-Cheng K.-Y. and Cheng, C. C. (1969). *J. Med. Chem.* **12**, 157.

The Evaluation of Present Antileprosy Compounds

STANLEY G. BROWNE

Leprosy Study Centre,
57a Wimpole Street,
London, England

I. Introduction

Progress in the chemotherapy of human leprosy infections has hitherto been seriously hampered by two facts: first, notwithstanding numerous unconfirmed claims, the presumably causative organism, *Mycobacterium leprae*, could not be definitely and reproducibly cultivated on or in any laboratory medium; second, it was not possible by injecting this organism to reproduce in any laboratory animal a generalized and progressive bacilliferous granulomatous disease resembling human leprosy.

A. Recent History of Chemotherapy in Leprosy

Until recently, therefore, both the selection of drugs for trial in leprosy and the use of drugs in treating the established disease have been made empirically. Chaulmoogra oil entered reputable therapeutics from Burmese folklore, having been also used in China and India for centuries; other remedies had even less to commend them. Notwithstanding their dubious antecedents, chaulmoogra and hydnocarpus oils, together with their chemical derivatives, their esters (iodized or noniodized), and the basic salts formed from their weak acids, were subjected to clinical testing if not to objectively controlled investigation. Many workers followed Rogers, Muir, Cochrane, and others in affirming the definite if slight efficacy of these preparations in leprosy, particularly in those kinds of leprosy characterized by a vigorous host response to scanty organisms. No evidence of direct bactericidal action was forthcoming, or indeed sought. [See Jardin (1961) for an excellent and very full summary.]

Rational and experimental therapeutics in the late thirties demonstrated that diaminodiphenyl sulfone was bactericidal not only systemically against streptococci in mice and locally in streptococcal mastitis in cows, but also against *Mycobacterium tuberculosis* (both human and avian strains) *in vitro*, and modified the course of the disease in rabbits experimentally infected with avian tuberculosis. Early work with the drug suspended in oil and injected intramuscularly for human leprosy was abandoned by reason of its toxicity in the doses then advocated—now seen in retrospect to have been much too high: the thresholds of both the therapeutic and the toxic levels are considerably lower than those of the sulfonamides, which were mistakenly used as bases for dosage comparison. [Bushby (1964) provides a valuable review.]

In order to reduce dose-related signs of toxicity, the sulfone molecule was modified, and the compounds thus obtained were given in doses comparable with those of the sulfonamides then in vogue.

Several monosubstituted sulfones (e.g., Sulfon-Cilag) were synthesized in the decade 1940–1949 (Smith *et al.*, 1949) and shown to be effective in certain mycobacterial infections; some of these were active in human leprosy (Browne,

1955), but little knowledge accumulated concerning their mode of action or fate in the body. Various disubstituted derivatives (e.g., Promin, Diasone, Promacetin, and Promizole) were shown to have activity in clinical leprosy (Doob, 1961; *Intern. J. Leprosy*, 1967). It is suspected on analogy that the sulfones in general are bacteriostatic by competitive inhibition of some essential growth factor, e.g., *p*-aminobenzoic acid. Whether given orally, intravenously, or intramuscularly, most of these complex compounds appeared to exert their therapeutic effect roughly in proportion to the amount of mother sulfone (dapsone) made available in the circulating blood. Dapsone itself may exert its mycobactericidal effect either per se, or as a monosubstituted metabolite, a glucosonic acid monoconjugate (Bushby and Woiwod, 1956; Bushby, 1967). Some drugs active in certain experimental mycobacterial infections are clinically efficacious in leprosy: as a rule, compounds that are very active in experimental animal tuberculosis are also active in human leprosy, but those that are most active in naturally occurring human tuberculosis show slight activity in human leprosy (Guinto *et al.*, 1964).

B. Practical Considerations

Apart altogether from the restricted sphere of efficacy of antimycobacterial drugs in the treatment of the varied symptom-complex designated by the clinical term "leprosy," many practical considerations must be respected. Of the estimated 15 million leprosy patients in the world, fewer than 3 million are at present receiving treatment, and of these probably nine tenths are being treated as outpatients by paramedical workers. The untreated patients, like the majority of treated patients, live for the most part in economically poor and medically backward countries. Hence, to be of widespread use, an antileprosy drug should above all be cheap, and safe when given by partly trained medical assistants in mass treatment campaigns, in which visits to clinics to collect drugs may be possible at weekly intervals or less frequently. It should be active in all kinds of leprosy, and be reasonably free from serious side effects when taken for several years in circumstances where both medical supervision and laboratory cover may be virtually nonexistent. It should show minimal tendency to provoke drug resistance. There are practical advantages and disadvantages in both oral and parenteral routes. Divided daily doses are generally impracticable.

In centers where facilities exist for inpatient care (for patients sensitive to drugs or harboring drug-resistant strains, for those undergoing lepromatous exacerbations, etc.), individual treatment is possible, and a wider range of antileprosy drugs may be utilized. Moreover, at such centers medical supervision is assured and perhaps laboratory facilities are available, including microscopy of skin smears and biopsy specimens.

II. Experimental Evaluation of Drugs

A. Mouse Foot Pad as an Investigative Model

The absence until recently of any experimental basis for the demonstration and evaluation of the mycobactericidal properties of a drug supposedly active against *M. leprae* goes far to explain the confusions and contradictions in the literature. The hesitations and imprecisions that delayed for a decade the widespread oral use of the parent sulfone, dapsone, in nontoxic therapeutic doses could, in retrospect, have been resolved if, first, the then existing knowledge had been appreciated and applied, and second, if an experimental model had existed (Sato and Nishimura, 1967).

Thanks to the work of Shepard (1960) in demonstrating multiplication of *M. leprae* in the mouse foot pad, and the extension of his work by Shepard and Chang (1962) and Rees (1964) to the screening of drugs, it is now possible to demonstrate unequivocably if a drug shows partial or complete activity against *M. leprae* within the limits of the experimental model (and a possibly less-than-optimum microenvironment), and to determine the concentrations of drug that must be given in the diet or parenterally to achieve these results. Mouse foot-pad infection with *M. leprae* (Shepard, 1960; Rees, 1964) is characterized by a localized bacilliferous granuloma in which an inoculum of 10^4 *M. leprae* increases 100-fold in some 6–8 months, reaching a plateau. The bacilli have a generation time of 10–20 days, possibly longer. Similar infections are reported in the mouse ear, the ear and foot pad of the golden hamster, and the foot pad of the rat.

The essential details of the screening of drugs for their mycobactericidal or mycobacteriostatic activity consist of comparing the yield of bacilli in the foot pads of untreated mice and of those receiving known amounts of the trial drug in the diet or parenterally. The *M. leprae* to be injected are obtained from human skin or nasal washings, preferably from patients with pure lepromatous leprosy, untreated, and containing a high proportion of viable (i.e., morphologically normal, solid staining and uniformly staining) bacilli. The trial drug may be given before bacterial multiplication has begun (after a lag phase of several weeks), or after the first logarithmic phase of bacillary multiplication, that is, to ascertain if the drug is bactericidal as well as bacteriostatic. The model has been elegantly modified—by giving the drug for a predetermined period only, during the first 2 months of infection—to show that bacillary multiplication is thereafter resumed following a period in which, under the influence of the drug, bacilli do not multiply.

Using the experimental model of the mouse foot-pad technique, Shepard and Chang (1962, 1964) tested 11 drugs known to have antimycobacterial activity. All the drugs have been shown to be active *in vitro* against *M.*

tuberculosis except ditophal (Etisul, I.C.I.), the explanation of the failure in this latter case probably being that release of the active ethyl mercaptan from this compound results from metabolic cleavage *in vivo*. The drugs causing complete suppression of the growth of *M. leprae* in mice—with the single exception of dapsone—have minimal inhibitory concentrations against *M. tuberculosis in vitro* of 1 μg/ml, or less. Four drugs were most effective against *Mycobacterium lepraemurium*, viz., isoniazid, B 663, thiacetazone, and thiambutosine; of these, isoniazid and B 663 were active against *M. leprae* in the mouse foot pad. Five drugs caused complete suppression of multiplication of *M. leprae* in mice—dapsone, B 663, and the three first-line drugs used in human tuberculosis (viz., isoniazid, aminosalicylic acid, and streptomycin). Dapsone was not outstandingly active against either *M. tuberculosis* or *M. lepraemurium*, but was incontestably superior to the other drugs in its action against *M. leprae.*

Partial suppression of *M. leprae* was achieved by cycloserine and thiacetazone (amithiozone). Under the conditions of the investigation, thiambutosine, ethambutol, ditophal, and pyrazinamide were inactive. However, thiambutosine was found to be active against *M. leprae* by Rees (1967). It may be that some strains of *M. leprae* are sensitive to thiambutosine. Rees (1967) found that some identified metabolites of thiambutosine were active against *M. leprae*.

Rees (1967) independently came to the same conclusions as Shepard and Chang (1962, 1964) in respect of the activity of these drugs against *M. leprae.* He found full activity with sulfadimethoxine, sulformethoxine, and three diphenylthiourea compounds (including two metabolites of thiambutosine). Gaugas (1967), using the same technique, has confirmed the main findings of the workers already cited.

Shepard (1964) had shown by the same technique that capreomycin possesses activity against *M. leprae,* and more recently Rees (1968b) has found that rifampicin is active.

Further work utilizing this technique has demonstrated conclusively that not only are all strains of *M. leprae* (derived from many countries) so far tested sensitive to dapsone, but that they are sensitive to minute concentrations of the drug in the diet, as low as 0.001 to 0.00001%: this is equivalent to a daily intake of between 0.5 and 5 mg of dapsone, or 0.02 to 0.2 mg/kg body weight (Shepard *et al.*, 1966). These workers suggest that, on the experimental evidence submitted, the tissue levels of dapsone produced in the human subject taking 100 mg dapsone daily by the mouth are about a thousand times as high as those found effective in the mouse. *Mycobacterium leprae* is thus unusually sensitive to dapsone, the minimal inhibitory concentration being so low as not to be ascertainable by the Bratton and Marshall (1939) technique, or its modifications (Simpson, 1949; Glazko, 1950). The delicate fluorescent method of Glazko (Ellard and Gammon, 1968) is of value in demonstrating the presence and concentration of minute amounts of sulfone in the serum. Evidence, still unconfirmed, and denied by some, was offered by Chatterjee and Podder (1957) that ^{35}S-labeled dapsone was concentrated in lepromatous skin. Shepard (1967c) has recently developed a kinetic method for the experimental investigation of the activity of drugs against *M. leprae*. This method promises precise results.

The mouse foot pad as a model for screening drugs for their mycobactericidal activity in human leprosy will undoubtedly be increasingly utilized in the future, and precise identification of active constituents or chemical groupings or metabolites may provide information that is not only invaluable in therapeutic investigations but also of intrinsic pathological importance (Shepard, 1967a). This investigative model is also proving of value in the demonstration of the identity of *M. leprae* and the viability or nonviability of organisms obtained from patients, of drug-resistant strains (and the existence of partial resistance, and stepwise increase in resistance), of enhancement of systemic resistance to leprosy challenge by BCG vaccination, etc.

B. Systemic Leprosy Infection in the Mouse

A substantial advance in experimental animal infection with *M. leprae*, which will provide further opportunities for screening and precise evaluation of drugs for their activity in leprosy, has now been reported by Rees (1966) and Rees *et al.* (1967). Mice previously thymectomized and given whole body irradiation (at a dose of 900 r) to depress their immunological capacity, were found, after the intravenous injection of inocula of viable *M. leprae*, to develop generalized bacilliferous granulomatous lesions, particularly in the colder parts of the body, i.e., the paws, the face, the tail. Furthermore, the multiplication of *M. leprae* in the foot pads proceeded above the 10^6 ceiling postulated for normal mice.

A further advance in the utilization of the experimental mouse is announced by Gaugas and Rees (1968) and Gaugas (1968), who found that antilymphocytic globulin significantly enhanced the susceptibility of mice to infection with *M. leprae*. This work would suggest that cell-mediated immunity is an important factor in the host defense against the obligate intracellular mycobacterial parasites.

III. Controlled Clinical Trials

A. General Principles

Notwithstanding the considerable advances recently registered in the use of the mouse foot pad technique for the screening of drugs suspected of having an action against *M. leprae*, the final and only arbiter is still the patient actually suffering from active multibacillary leprosy, and the only way of demonstrating conclusively the clinical efficacy of any drug is some form of controlled clinical trial (World Health Organization, 1968a). The methodology of such trials in respect of an acute or subacute infection in which the pathology is relatively simple, the end point definite, and the clinical changes both directly dependent on the infection and in some way amenable to measurement may not be wholly reproducible in chemotherapeutic trials in leprosy.

Doull *et al.* (1960a,b, 1961, 1965, 1967) and his co-workers (Guinto *et al.*, 1964) have over many years conducted clinical trials in leprosy, mainly in connection with the Leonard Wood Memorial establishments in the Philippines, and enlisting the cooperation of other centers. These trials have not only made precise contributions to knowledge concerning the efficacy of reputed antileprosy drugs and their dosages, but have also provided a proving ground for the progressive development of the theoretical bases of drug trials in leprosy.

Jopling (1965) refers to the basic principles to be observed in carrying out a pilot therapeutic trial in leprosy, and Browne (1967a) refers to unemphasized factors. Useful indications may be derived from the intensive study of the results of therapy in a small series of lepromatous patients, even as few as ten.

More recently, excellent work along these lines has been both done and summarized by Waters *et al.* (1967). Emphasizing the importance of strict predetermined protocols, they refer to the work of Noordeen (1965), who estimated that only about a quarter of the drug trials reported in the decade 1954–1964 included adequate controls. On the other hand, a false impression of precision may be engendered by the inclusion of controls that are by no means adequate when judged by significant criteria: apparently similar clinical states may represent diverse tissue responses at different stages. The lepromin reaction and histological examination of material from typical lesions may each provide valuable confirmatory evidence of the classification of the individual leprosy patient at a given moment, but the slighter degrees of positivity of the lepromin reaction may vary in the same patient from time to time, and the histological picture may vary from lesion to lesion, from site to site in the same lesion, and even at different depths from the skin surface in the same lesion.

B. The Lepromin Reaction

The lepromin reaction is of value in two ways in connection with chemotherapeutic trials. First, it serves as a precise and measurable indication of the actual or potential immunological response of the individual to challenge with *M. leprae*. Subjects with some degree of tissue resistance—even slight—are unsuitable for inclusion in trials of possibly bactericidal drugs: they are apt to improve more rapidly, both bacteriologically and clinically, than their counterparts suffering from pure lepromatous leprosy, in whom the lepromin reaction is completely negative. [The early (Fernandez) reaction roughly parallels the late (Mitsuda) reaction, which attains its maximum reading about the third week or later.]

In the second place, the lepromin reaction, used experimentally, is of use in differentiating *M. leprae* from other acid-fast organisms. If a preparation made from these latter organisms is injected intradermally into patients with lepromatous leprosy (in whom the lepromin reaction should, of course, be completely negative), a variably positive response develops, indicating that the inoculated extract was obtained from organisms other than *M. leprae* (Shepard and Guinto, 1963).

C. The Bacterial Index

The Bacterial Index is a useful indication of the concentration of *M. leprae* in material obtained either by skin smears or by histological examination of skin. It takes account only of recognizable bacillary forms and disregards acid-fast dust and debris. It is expressed in different notations, which, however, show general correspondence: Cochrane (1952) has 6 degrees of positivity; Dharmendra (1950) 4; other workers 5; Ridley (1967a) 6. Uniformity of smearing technique is of paramount importance in assuring the approximate comparability of results between successive examinations in the same patient, between different patients, and between different centers.

On Ridley's scale (1967a), the Bacterial Index is the average of the index obtained from 6–8 stained smears, expressed as 6 degrees of positivity on a logarithmic scale (see Table I).

TABLE I

Bacterial Index According to Ridley's Scale[a]

Positivity	No. bacilli/microscopic field[b]
1+	1/100
2+	1/10
3+	1
4+	10
5+	100
6+	1000

[a] From Ridley (1967a).

[b] Refers to a field examined under the oil immersion (1/12 inch) objective.

The approximate corresponding figures in Dharmendra's notation (1950) are shown in Table II.

TABLE II
CORRESPONDING FIGURES IN DHARMENDRA'S NOTATION[a]

Dharmendra	Ridley
Very scanty, or 1/4+	1+
Scanty, or 1/2+	2+
1+	3+
2+	4+
3+	5+
4+	6+

[a] From Dharmendra (1950).

D. The Morphological Index

The imprecision, variability, and even the irrelevance (in the context of actual mycobactericidal activity) of many of the clinical findings in chemotherapeutic trials in leprosy are now to be considered in the light of recent work on the viability of *M. leprae* as seen in the skin smears and histological sections. Rees *et al.* (1960) provided evidence, long suspected on other grounds, that individual *M. leprae* that do not stain uniformly and deeply are almost certainly nonviable. Many workers (e.g., Davey, 1960; Waters and Rees, 1962; Browne, 1966a; and others) anticipating or applying these findings, have shown that the most sensitive—in fact, the only true—indication of the mycobactericidal activity of a drug is a progressive diminution in the proportion of viable *M. leprae* as seen in routine smears taken from selected skin (and nasal mucosa) sites by a standard technique at regular intervals. In patients with untreated lepromatous leprosy, the percentage of such viable forms may vary from 0 to 100, but is generally between 25 and 60. The figure depends *inter alia* on the phase of bacterial activity, the innate rate of death of bacilli, the rate of removal of effete forms, the criteria adopted for viability, etc. (It is, in passing, worthy of remark that in lepromatous leprosy—a form supposedly characterized by minimal or absent host resistance—morphologically degenerate bacilli are almost invariably present. This may be an expression of death of the individual bacilli after completion of their normal life span rather than an indication of some positive deleterious effect of unknown mechanism on the bacilli).

The arithmetical average of the percentages of normal bacilli found at the several sites smeared (termed the Morphological Index or M.I.), declines with effective therapy, attaining zero generally in from 6 to 9 months. Bactericidal activity can be demonstrated by this relatively sensitive test in 3 or 4 months (Waters *et al.*, 1967).

A notation with a similar object, the Granularity Index, was suggested by Ridley (1964; 1967b). It represents the proportion of granular (and hence nonviable) *M. leprae* in material obtained by the slit-smear method.

E. Other Indications of Bacterial Activity and Load

1. *The Histological Picture*

Additional information is obtainable from histological examination of a typical portion of whole thickness skin removed from a leprosy patient. Ridley (1958) has usefully summarized his utilization of serial biopsy examinations in therapeutic trials in leprosy. By special staining methods (e.g., TRIFF: Wheeler *et al.*, 1965) the presence, morphology, concentration, and disposition of *M. leprae* can be determined; and by standard staining techniques (preferably after fixation in Zenker's or Ridley's fixative, to avoid tissue distortion), the quality of the host reaction to the mycobacterial infection can be evaluated. By this means, Ridley and Jopling (1966) have elaborated a system of classification according to the immunological response, which is of value in codifying the patient's reaction to leprosy infection and in providing a yardstick for progress. Languillon (1964) also emphasizes the importance of immunological considerations in classifying cases of leprosy.

2. *The Biopsy Index*

Another numerical indication of bacterial density and the dimensions of the bacilliferous granuloma is afforded by the Biopsy Index (Ridley and Hilson, 1967).

3. *The Logarithmic Index*

A refinement of this index, called the Logarithmic Index of Bacilli (LIB) in biopsies (Ridley, 1967a) serves to indicate mathematically and more precisely bacterial density and the size of the granuloma in lepromatous leprosy, and should thus provide a delicate indication of the bacterial state of the patient and any changes occurring in that state during a drug trial, i.e., both the bactericidal activity of the drug and any concomitant clearing of bacillary debris: the latter effect may, of course, be unconnected directly with the former.

In general, reduction in the Bacterial Index appears to be completely or almost completely unrelated to and uninfluenced by mycobactericidal activity, but depends on the slow clearance by transporting macrophages of bacillary debris. The Bacterial Index falls regularly, attaining zero after the lapse of 3 to 6 years in the majority of patients with lepromatous leprosy; isolated viable bacilli may reappear in the routine examinations, depending on the hazards of smearing; solid-staining, but lighter-stained bacilli (probably nonviable) may also be seen from time to time. Very slow clearance of acid-fast debris is not unusual.

A most important field of investigation concerns the facilitation of removal of this mycobacterial debris—possibly by dissolution digestion, opsonization, stimulation of phagocytosis, etc.

F. Selection of Patients for Clinical Trials

Despite certain practical objections, clear indications are now available concerning the basic acceptable standards for selection of patients (suffering from pure and severe lepromatous leprosy, untreated, with high Bacterial Index and a high Morphological Index) and for assessment of clinical progress. Notwithstanding the enormous difficulties presented by a disease in which the host-parasite relation shows such a wide range, it is possible (by matched pairs and random allocation of patients to trial groups, and by independent and unbiased assessment of progress) to approach the standards achieved in less demanding clinical investigations. A trial may be scientifically controlled and present valid answers to the questions posed even if it is not double blind and based on strictly matched pairs.

The slight and slow changes in clinical appearances that may result from therapy may reflect not only the mycobactericidal action of the drug, but also (and mainly) the host reaction to the therapy or to the results of therapy; they may also depend upon the presence of bacterial debris in the lesions and the tissue response to the presence of acid-fast material. In other words, the direct action of a mycobactericidal drug may be overshadowed by hypersensitivity effects or by fibrosis (e.g., intraneural), and may produce no obvious and direct clinical amelioration. Other factors, such as the bulk of the bacilliferous granuloma, the precise phase of bacillary activity at the time the trial takes place, the complexity of the tissue response in leprosy, and the inherent variability of the disease must all be reckoned with. Ethical considerations loom large when dealing with a serious, chronic disease with emotional and social overtones. The use of the placebo in untreated patients for lengthy periods is impossible, and the double-blind procedure has its limitations. Hitherto, in many trials, an additive effect of the unknown drug has been sought initially when the drug was given as a complementary to standard dapsone therapy. But since combinations of drugs so far investigated do not accelerate either clinical improvement or elimination of mycobacterial debris (just as they do not accelerate the rate of fall of the Morphological Index, as shown above), it may be that drugs formerly discarded as valueless on the basis of the lack of additive effect should now be retested. Many clinicians report a distinct impression that change to another active antileprosy drug during a stationary phase in treatment may often appear to initiate again both clinical improvement and mycobacterial clearance.

An excellent summary of laboratory investigations in human and murine leprosy, with numerous references, is provided by Sato and Nishimura (1967).

IV. Modern Standard Therapy

A. Dapsone

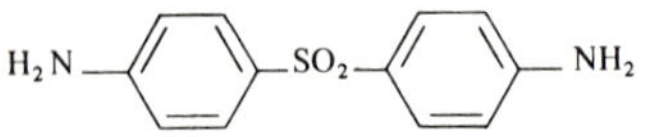

H_2N — SO_2 — NH_2

(I)

It is generally agreed that dapsone (I) (diaphenylsulfone, 4,4′-diaminodiphenylsulfone, DDS) is the drug of greatest usefulness for individual treatment of leprosy and in mass antileprosy campaigns. Its chemistry and pharmacology have been well investigated and documented (Doull, 1963; Bushby, 1964; Brown, 1967; *Intern. J. Leprosy*, 1965, 1967); its use in dermatitis herpetiformis and mycetoma (in well-tolerated doses of 200–300 mg daily, which incidentally are not reported to precipitate toxic polyneuritis) is established. It is toxic in high doses, giving rise to acute (Mathur and Karani, 1967) or chronic (Browne, 1965d) poisoning.

In leprosy, mono- and disubstituted derivatives possess little, if any, advantage over the parent sulfone, and apart from solapsone (Sulphetrone) (in a 50% aqueous solution, sterilized, with 0.5% phenol added as a preservative, given intramuscularly) are now rarely prescribed. They are in effect wasteful and costly ways of bringing dapsone itself (and possibly some unidentified metabolites) into contact with the bacilli in leprosy lesions, their activity having been shown to derive mainly from dapsone. Suspensions of dapsone in oil (arachis, coconut, olive, chaulmoogra, etc.), usually 20–25% w/v, or gelled with aluminum monostearate, have been given (mainly for administrative convenience) in mass-treatment campaigns, at weekly, fortnightly, or monthly intervals. Slow release of the product from intramuscular deposit, and even irregular release, with resulting transient high serum sulfone levels, appear to be equally efficacious clinically.

Differences exist in the recommended doses of orally administered dapsone. While the upper limits of dosage can be readily recognized by the toxic effects produced (especially irritating maculopapular rashes, "fifth week dapsone dermatitis," erythema multiforme, exfoliative dermatitis, toxic epidermal necrolysis, drug fever, etc.), the lowest effective doses are less easily determined in such a chronic infection in which the end point of therapy is uncertain. The official recommendation (World Health Organization, 1966) is that the maximum total weekly dose for an adult of 60 kg should be 600 mg, and that this dose may be given on one day, or divided into daily or twice-weekly doses.

1. *Low-Dose Dapsone Therapy*

Recent work suggests that much smaller doses may be equally effective, clinically and bacteriologically. Investigations along these lines were begun in an attempt to reduce the incidence of acute exacerbation (particularly in lepromatous leprosy) which may follow either high initial doses of dapsone or increments that are too large or made too rapidly. While this proposition is difficult to establish unequivocably in such a variable disease as leprosy—though reports are generally suggestive that this is so—the investigations to date provide evidence that the clinical and bacteriological progress of patients placed on lower dose regimes is comparable with that of similar patients given the previously advocated dose.

Browne (1965e) studied for 3 to 4 years a series of 13 Nigerian patients with severe untreated lepromatous leprosy, giving them 50 or 100 mg of dapsone in one weekly dose, and every month controlling the Morphological and Bacterial Indexes as determined from 6 skin and 2 nasal mucosal sites. Reporting good progress on all counts over a period of 4 years, he considered that complications had been less frequent and less severe than in a comparable series on higher doses. Subsequently, much larger series furnished similar results.

Ramu and Ramanujam (1965), basing their opinion on 135 Indian patients observed over a period of 18 months, considered that a dose of 200 mg weekly gave good clinical and bacteriological results in lepromatous leprosy, with a definitely lower incidence of lepra reaction.

Leiker and Carling (1966), in a limited trial comparing patients receiving dapsone in doses of 200, 400, and 800 mg weekly, and controlled by regular lesional biopsies as well as by routine skin-smear examinations, reported that the lower doses were at least as effective as the higher. Among the facts indicating that a lower dose of dapsone might be effective was the observation that the bacteriological improvement of patients attending irregularly to receive the standard dosage appeared to be comparable with that of patients whose attendance was regular. Moreover, the incidence of complications was lower in clinics that had a lower dosage scheme than those with higher.

Pettit and Rees (1967), giving 50 mg of dapsone twice weekly to 6 patients with untreated lepromatous leprosy, considered that the fall in the Morphological Index, over a period of $4\frac{1}{2}$ months, was sufficiently indicative of the equivalent efficacy of these low doses as compared with higher doses. The Bacterial Index could not be expected to show any significant fall in such a short period, and did not.

The tentative conclusion that oral administration of dapsone, in doses of 100 mg weekly or even lower, results in a rapid fall in the percentage of morphologically normal *M. leprae*, must be assessed in the light of the probably decreased accompanying incidence of acute exacerbation, permitting the continuation of leprosy treatment. The administrative advantages and the cost must be nicely balanced against the possibility that the lower dosage may favor the emergence of resistant strains.

The administrative advantages are not very substantial: the difference in cost between 600 and 100 mg of dapsone weekly is negligible, but the application by field workers of a regime equally suited to patients suffering from any of the clinical varieties of leprosy and unlikely to provoke acute exacerbation or sudden polyneuritis is a distinct gain. As for the risk of dapsone resistance, as long as the therapeutic dose is well above the minimal inhibitory doses as judged by the mouse foot-pad technique (Shepard *et al.*, 1966) and as long as the smaller doses are given regularly and not intermittently, this risk theoretically would appear to be quite small. One patient (Browne, 1969) receiving 50 mg of dapsone twice weekly, developed—after 52 months of supervised regular treatment (and 17 months after the last record of acid-fast material in the multiple smears)—new skin lesions replete with organisms proved by the mouse foot-pad inoculation technique to be resistant to dapsone. (The patient responded well to B 663, the Morphological Index in the lesions falling from 80 to 5% in 5 months.)

Whatever the lowest optimum dose of dapsone that eventually proves to be clinically efficacious and bacteriologically satisfactory (as shown by the progressive disappearance of morphologically normal forms of *M. leprae*), the dual problem remains—the clearance of nonviable organisms, and minimizing the effects of the continued presence of antigenic material in the tissues: this problem is apparently unresolved by dapsone or any other bacteriostatic drug.

At a dose of 100 mg daily by mouth, dapsone produces a blood concentration of 15 mg per 100 ml. Lowe (1952) found that a dose of dapsone of 30 mg daily produced a satisfactory, though not maximal response, with a blood level of 0.15 to 0.25 mg per 100 ml. Sulfone may be detected in the serum 3–4 weeks after a single oral dose of 100 mg (Browne, unpublished observations).

2. *Dapsone in Very Low Doses*

Evidence is now accumulating, from India (Karat, 1967) and Malaysia (Waters, 1968), that dapsone in doses of the order of 1–5 mg weekly for an adult is followed by clinical and bacteriological improvement (in particular, as shown by the rate of fall of the Morphological Index) comparable with that obtained with much higher doses. Progress is maintained for some months. It is not yet known if such low doses may favor the emergence of dapsone-resistant strains of *M. leprae* or clinical recrudescence. While the dose may appear to be homeopathically minute, it is still well above the theoretical level for bacteriostasis as suggested by extrapolation of the mouse foot-pad findings (Shepard *et al.*, 1966). These authors suggest, as the result of their investigations of the minimal inhibitory concentrations of dapsone in the mouse, that *M. leprae* is much more sensitive than other microorganisms to dapsone, and that standard doses of the drug in human leprosy produce a blood (or tissue) concentration approximately 1000-fold greater than that shown to be effective in the mouse. Even when the differences in the microenvironment are considered (e.g., the bulk of the bacilliferous granuloma, the size of the bacterial population and its rate of growth, and the possibility of mutants arising that are resistant to the concentration of drug that suppresses multiplication of normal *M. leprae*), the safety margin between the two levels seems unnecessarily large: on the basis of this reasoning, doses of dapsone much lower than 100 mg daily could be given to humans with equal therapeutic effect and without incurring a risk of facilitating the emergence of resistant strains.

The range of dapsone dosage in the mouse has been investigated down to concentrations of 0.00001% of dapsone in the diet—far below the lowest concentration (0.001%) that gives detectable blood sulfone levels (0.2–0.3 mg/ml)—without encountering the end point.

3. *Repository Preparations*

$$C_6H_5-\underset{SO_3Na}{CH}-CH_2-\underset{SO_3Na}{CH}-HN-C_6H_4-SO_2-C_6H_4-NH-\underset{SO_3Na}{CH}-CH_2-\underset{SO_3Na}{CH}-C_6H_5$$

Solapsone
(II)

$$H_3COC-HN-C_6H_4-SO_2-C_6H_4-NH-COCH_3$$

Dadds
(III)

a. Suspensions in Oil. Dapsone has been available for many years in oily suspension (20 or 25% w/v, commonly). The repository preparations have been thought to possess certain practical advantages, especially when infrequent treatment (weekly or fortnightly) only is possible. The therapeutic effect is comparable with that of orally administered dapsone, and depends on the slow release of the unchanged substance. There is, however, evidence that indicates that longer-spaced oral dapsone (at, e.g., fortnightly intervals) is equally efficacious as parenteral dapsone.

Other preparations have been investigated in an attempt to light on a formulation that would have a longer effective action: suspensions gelled with, e.g., aluminum monostearate, show no decided superiority.

b. Avlosulfon Soluble. Avlosulfon Soluble is supplied as a 41% w/w aqueous solution of disodium (*p*-1-sulfoethylaminophenyl) sulfone, which contains the equivalent of 200 mg of dapsone per ml, i.e., it releases approximately half its weight in the body as dapsone. Sterile, and given by intramuscular injection, it seems to act by virtue of the rapid release of dapsone (and possibly metabolites) into the circulation, giving high and unsustained blood levels. Davey (1956) reported good results from twice weekly injections of up to 2 ml of the solution, giving total sulfone blood levels of 0.003 mg/ml, and of extractable dapsone of less than 0.002 mg/ml.

c. Solapsone (Sulphetrone). Solapsone (Sulphetrone) (II) is tetrasodium di[*p*-(3-phenyl-1,3-disulfopropylamino)phenylsulfone. Given orally in doses up to 5 gm daily, commercial (impure) solapsone is largely broken down into a mixture of dapsone, monosubstituted sulfones, and known as well as unidentified metabolites. It is said to be less likely than dapsone to precipitate polyneuritis or acute exacerbation.

When given by intramuscular injection as a 50% solution twice weekly, it probably acts mainly by the unaltered disubstituted molecule. Solapsone in aqueous solution provides a convenient means for giving small and graduated amounts of sulfone for the purpose of desensitizing patients showing signs of sensitivity to dapsone (Browne, 1963) and the 0.5 gm tablets may be used for prophylaxis in children.

4. *Other Sulfones*

a. DADDS. Sulfones show activity against experimental malarial infection in animals and naturally occurring malarial infection in man. Initial observations of the apparent suppression of clinical malaria in leprosy patients taking dapsone (Leiker, 1956) suggested that the sulfones might be of value in the treatment of chloroquine-resistant malaria. Several repository sulfones active against *Plasmodium berghei* infections in mice, *P. cynomologi* in monkeys, and *P. falciparum* in man (Laing *et al.*, 1966) have been examined for their possible activity against experimental infection with *M. leprae* (Thompson, 1967).

4,4-Diacetyldiaminodiphenyl sulfone (CI-536; DADDS (III) is the most promising of the long-acting sulfones in respect of activity in leprosy. It is formulated in a benzyl benzoate and castor oil suspension containing 150 mg of drug in 1 ml.

Shepard (1967b) found that a dose of DADDS of 6 mg/kg gave almost complete suppression of *M. leprae* multiplication in the mouse foot pad for 2 months. Since a repository sulfone, releasing therapeutically effective amounts of dapsone into the circulation over prolonged periods, would be of practical use in countries where medical facilities and communications are limited, it could be employed both curatively and (if considered desirable) prophylactically in areas of high leprosy prevalence.

DADDS is probably metabolized into dapsone, or the monoacetyl derivative is slowly released in the tissue by deacetylating enzymes, and the observed activity of the drug against *M. leprae* is due to circulating dapsone, though the exact mechanism of the antibacterial action is obscure. The usual contraindications to dapsone therapy are to be observed in giving DADDS, and the usual toxic side effects are to be encountered—dapsone dermatitis, severe anemia, sulfone-precipitated psychosis, etc.—but in the dose recommended (225 mg every 75 days) toxic side effects should be minimal. Clinical trials are at present proceeding at several centers (Shepard, 1967b).

Since the therapeutic action of DADDS depends presumably on released dapsone, the indications and limitations of the compound are those applicable to dapsone itself, with the caveat that should patients develop persistent sulfone-induced or sulfone-precipitated exacerbation, the injected sulfone cannot be removed or its effects neutralized.

b. Complex sulfones. Compounds chemically related to the sulfones ranging from the relatively simple to the very complex condensation products formed with derivatives of chaulmoogra oil, certain antibiotics, or other antimycobacterial drugs have been synthesized from time to time and investigated for their activity in human leprosy. In some cases, it was hoped that the release of two active drugs after breakdown of the ingested compound would somehow accelerate bacterial clearance by a process of mutual potentiation; in others, the bringing of a chemically related molecule or of a further series of metabolites to bear on *M. leprae* was proposed. So far, none of the compounds investigated has shown any but the most marginal superiority over dapsone, and some, e.g., diaminodiphenylsulfoxide (Browne and Davey, 1961), have been abandoned because of nephrotoxicity or other undesirable side-effects.

B. Long-Acting Sulfonamides

In the early 1940's, short-acting sulfonamides (e.g., sulfathiazole and its cinnamylidenic derivative) were found to be moderately active in leprosy, but further work on this group was not pursued in view of the increasing availability

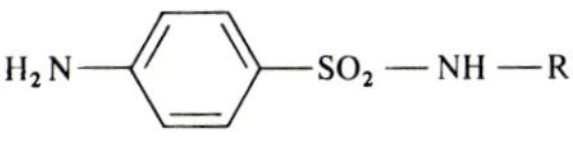

H_2N—⟨benzene ring⟩—SO_2 — NH — R

General formula

R =

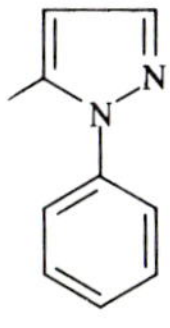

Sulfaphenazole (IV) — N-phenylpyrazolyl

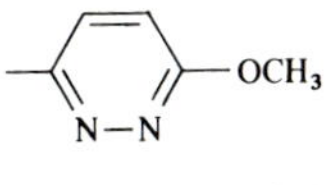

Sulfamethoxypyridazine (V) — OCH_3, N—N

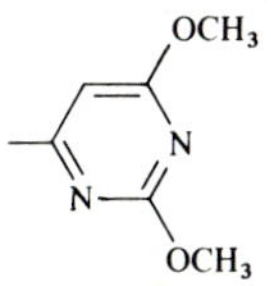

Sulfadimethoxine (VI) — OCH_3, N, N, OCH_3

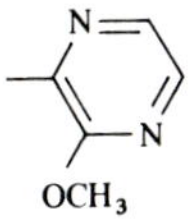

Sulfamethoxypyrazine (VII) — N, N, OCH_3

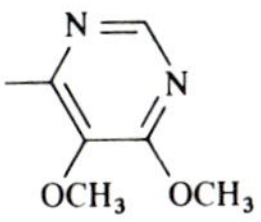

Sulformethoxine (VIII) — N, N, OCH_3 OCH_3

of certain active sulfone derivatives and, latterly, of the proved value of dapsone itself in correct (low) dosage. Some of the long-acting sulfonamides (e.g., sulfaphenazole) (IV) were shown to have but slight activity in lepromatous leprosy (Browne, 1961), possibly because the molecule was bound to plasma proteins (Newbould and Kilpatrick, 1960), although Schneider *et al.* (1960) were sufficiently impressed by the clinical evidence to recommend their widespread use in all forms of leprosy. Languillon (1966, 1968) gave sulfamethoxypyridazine (Kynex) (V) orally every 2 weeks, 20 ml of a 23% solution which produced a sustained blood level of 0.025 mg/ml. 2.5 mg%. He afterwards obtained excellent results with sulfadimethoxine (Madribon) (VI) orally administered at a dose of 0.75 gm every 2 days; and with sulfamethoxypyrazine (Sulfalène) (VII) and its acetyl derivative—both given orally—the latter at a dose of 2.5 gm once weekly. Sulformethoxine (sulforthomidine, Fanasil) (VIII) in the hands of several workers has given comparably good results in all forms of leprosy at a weekly oral dose of 1.5 gm. Languillon and Clary (1964) and Currie (1966) working in Africa, as well as several groups in South America, report excellent results with this compound, and a freedom from toxic side effects at the doses advocated.

Thus, several long-acting sulfonamides (e.g., sulfamethoxypyrazine, sulfadimethoxine, sulforthomidine, sulfamethoxypyridazine, acetylsulfamethoxypyrazine, sulfamethoxypyrimidine, sulfamethodiazine) have been shown to be active in leprosy by workers in French-speaking Africa, Argentine, Mexico, Japan, Nigeria, and Malawi. They act in both the multibacillary and the paucibacillary forms of leprosy, producing clinical and bacteriological amelioration, and their action in general is comparable with that of the sulfones. The resolution of tuberculoid lesions is, according to some workers, more rapid with the sulfonamides than with the sulfones. At the doses advised, the drugs are well tolerated, adverse reactions are uncommon, and no fatalities are recorded (Languillon, 1966). Their cost, and their known tendency to provoke serious skin sensitivities (including exfoliative dermatitis and the Stevens-Johnson syndrome), when taken in doses not far above the therapeutic, make for caution in advocating their use in mass treatment campaigns.

C. Thiacetazone

The use of thiacetazone (*p*-acetamidobenzaldehydethiosemicarbazone, amithiozone) (IX) in leprosy was suggested by its activity in experimental mouse and guinea-pig tuberculosis and in human tuberculosis. Lowe (1952)

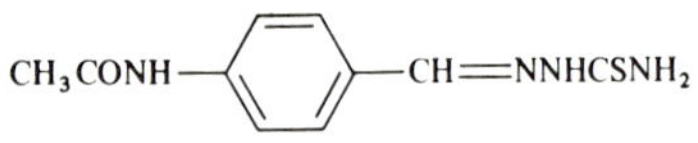

$$CH_3CONH—C_6H_4—CH{=}NNHCSNH_2$$

(IX)

reported that the drug was at least as effective as dapsone in human leprosy, but that its beneficial results were not maintained during the second year of treatment, possibly owing to the appearance of drug-resistant strains. Its toxicity (skin, kidney, liver, hemopoeietic system) did not apparently constitute a serious drawback in the early trials.

Although thiacetazone was at one time widely used in the treatment of leprosy and has recently fallen into disfavor, it still finds enthusiastic advocates, particularly in the Indian subcontinent and in South America (Alonso, 1959; Browne, 1967c). The indications for the prescription of thiacetazone in leprosy are worthy of reexamination, now that it is possible to demonstrate true resistance by the mouse foot-pad technique.

D. Thiambutosine

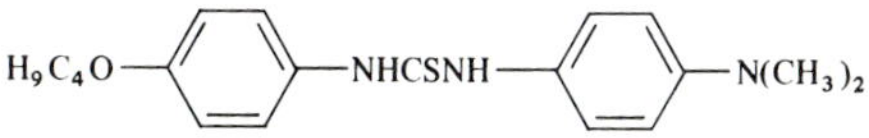

$$H_9C_4O{-}C_6H_4{-}NHCSNH{-}C_6H_4{-}N(CH_3)_2$$

(X)

Thiambutosine (X), a diphenylthiourea with the formula 1-(*p*-butoxyphenyl)-3-(*p*-dimethylaminophenyl)-2-thiourea, was investigated in leprosy because of its high activity in experimental guinea-pig tuberculosis and in murine tuberculosis. In these conditions, its action is similar to that of thiacetazone (Mitchinson and Lloyd, 1964). Although its use in human tuberculosis was disappointing, Davey and Currie (1956) reported favorably on its action in leprosy, and this success was confirmed by several workers, including Doull *et al.* (1961). It is commonly considered to be the best second-line all-purpose drug in leprosy (*Intern. J. Leprosy*, 1963). It has fewer side effects than dapsone, and shows less tendency to induce peripheral neuropathy or provoke psychosis; but it tends to lose its effect during the second year of treatment, possibly because of the appearance of drug-resistant strains of *M. leprae.* Rees (1967) has confirmed, by the mouse foot-pad inoculation test, the validity of this clinical suspicion. While the compound itself may (Rees, 1967) or may not (Shepard and Chang, 1964) be mycobactericidal in the mouse foot pad, certain metabolites of thiambutosine show definite activity (Rees, 1967).

The drug is poorly absorbed, and, given orally, rapidly excreted; hence it is not suitable for mass treatment in which a relatively costly drug has to be given orally in divided daily doses.

1. *Injectable Thiambutosine*

An injectable preparation, given weekly or fortnightly in a 20% w/v suspension, in doses of 5–10 ml, gives results comparable with those of the oral compound, and provides a more economical way of utilizing the drug (Browne, 1965c).

2. *Other Diphenylthioureas*

Thiocarlide, isoxyl,*N*,*N'*-di-(*p*-isopentyloxyphenyl)-thiourea (XI) is a tuberculostatic agent that has received favorable reports in small clinical trials in human tuberculosis. Buu-Hoi *et al.* (1961) used several related thiourea

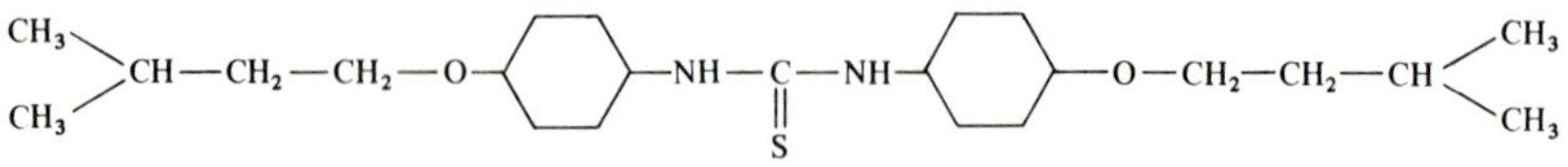

$$(CH_3)_2CH-CH_2-CH_2-O-C_6H_4-NH-C(=S)-NH-C_6H_4-O-CH_2-CH_2-CH(CH_3)_2$$

(XI)

derivatives in leprosy (Dialide or Etoxid) with some success, and Griffiths (1965), confirming Buu-Hoi's work, reported that thiocarlide gave good results in multibacillary leprosy, was well tolerated, and had no toxic effects. He used dosages of 100 mg daily, increasing by weekly increments of 100 mg daily to a maximum of 400 mg daily.

E. B 663

B 663 (or G 30,320) (XII) is 3-(*p*-chloroanilino-10-*p*-chlorophenyl)-2,10-dihydro-2 isopropyliminophenazine. It is one of a long series of phenazine com-

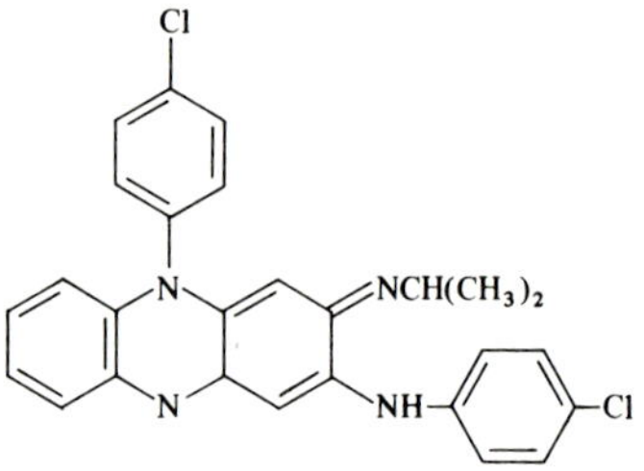

Cl; N; $NCH(CH_3)_2$; N; NH; Cl

(XII)

pounds, anilino*apo*safranines, rimino compounds, glyoxalinophenazines, *apo*safranones, etc., synthesized and described by Barry and his co-workers in a succession of valuable papers (Barry and Conalty, 1965).

Anilino*apo*safranine (B 283), the forerunner of these compounds, had been shown to inhibit the growth of *M. tuberculosis* in extremely low concentrations *in vitro*, causing complete inhibition of visible growth in Proskauer and Beck's synthetic medium at concentrations of 0.2 μg/ml or less, and to have activity in established experimental *M. tuberculosis* infections of the mouse and guinea pig. B 283 was used by Allday and Barnes (1952) in treating with success a small series of patients suffering from leprosy.

B 663 occurs as relatively coarse orange-red crystals, virtually insoluble in water, but freely soluble in fats. The stability of both the crystals and of solutions is excellent. Since the drug is poorly absorbed from the intestine (90% appearing unchanged in the feces) in man and the guinea pig, a micronized form (particle size not exceeding 5 μ) has been prepared. This is well absorbed from the intestinal tract, especially when given along with fat (e.g., 5 ml olive oil by mouth).

Weight for weight, B 663 is the most potent causal prophylactic known in experimental mouse tuberculosis, *in vitro* concentrations causing complete inhibition of growth of *M. tuberculosis* H 37 Rv being of the order of 1.3–3.3 μg/ml. In murine tuberculosis, B 663 is extraordinarily active, a single intraperitoneal dose of 1 mg on day 11 of an infection increasing the median survival time from 19 to 79 days, while in established infections in mice, hamsters, and rabbits, good curative effects have been demonstrated. In guinea pigs, monkeys, and man, the results of treatment of established infection with *M. tuberculosis* have been disappointing.

The high tissue levels of B 663 after oral administration are due to concentration of the drug in the cells of the reticuloendothelial system. When the cells are loaded with B 663 in crystalline form, they still take up carbon particles and tubercle bacilli. The low plasma concentrations bear no relation to therapeutic activity.

In established murine leprosy, B 663 is the most active drug yet investigated, increasing by a high factor the median survival time and causing an actual reduction in the extent of the established infection, the only drug to do so.

These facts suggested that B 663 should be tested clinically in volunteer leprosy patients. The initial good results claimed for this treatment have been experimentally attested by Shepard and Chang (1964), who have shown, using the elegant mouse foot-pad technique, that a dietary concentration of 0.01% B 663 causes complete suppression of the growth of *M. leprae.*

Of considerable interest is the report indicating that B 663 is an effective treatment for ulcers caused by mycobacteria resembling *Mycobacterium ulcerans* (Lunn and Rees, 1964) and that the growth of these and closely related organisms in the mouse foot pad is completely suppressed by dietary concentrations of 0.006% of B 663 (Rees, 1967).

Browne and Hogerzeil (1962a,b) treated unselected patients suffering from pure lepromatous (14) or borderline (2) leprosy, with B 663 in a dosage of approximately 5 mg/kg. The drug was given alone, or together with dapsone or ditophal, and with a small amount (5 ml) of vegetable oil to facilitate absorption. The tentative conclusion drawn after 6 months' trial, confirmed after 12 months, was that B 663 alone had definite bacteriological and clinical activity in leprosy. No symptoms of toxicity were noted except slight transient nausea and giddiness in 2 patients who were receiving relatively high doses for their weight. All patients developed a ruddiness of the skin, followed by hyperpigmentation, particularly of the areas of lepromatous infiltration.

After 12 months of treatment (Browne and Hogerzeil, 1962c) morphologically normal forms of *M. leprae* reappeared in the skin and nasal mucosa of these patients, suggesting that some kind of drug resistance was developing. Further experience indicated that this was a transient phenomenon and not true drug resistance. Reduced susceptibility, however, has been reported in monkeys infected with *M. tuberculosis*, but after repeated subculture the apparently resistant bacilli regained their susceptibility to the drug (Barry and Conalty, 1965).

Browne (1965b) in an appraisal after 3 years of the pilot trial with B 663, considered that the clinical improvement in 28 patients was more consistent and more rapid than in any similar group in his experience. The rate of fall in the Morphological Index and in the Bacterial Index was also rapid.

Pettit *et al.* (1967), from a study of 6 patients who received B 663 at a dose of 300 mg daily, concluded that reduction in the Morphological Index (an invaluable and sensitive indication of mycobactericidal activity) after 5 months' therapy was comparable with that seen with dapsone.

A novel observation was that while taking the drug patients seemed to be less liable to episodes of acute exacerbation (Browne, 1965a): only 2 patients out of 26 suffering from lepromatous leprosy developed signs of exacerbation (erythema nodosum leprosum, etc.), and in both instances the attack was slight and transient. This observation led Browne (1965a, 1966b) to postulate a possible anti-inflammatory action of B 663, which was confirmed by Williams *et al.* (1965) and others. At low doses (100 mg daily) B 663 did not, in the experience of Pettit (1967), suffice to control severe degrees of exacerbation, although Browne (1966b, 1967d) in a further series of patients, and Atkinson *et al.* (1967), Hastings and Trautman (1968), and Imkamp (1968) confirmed the earlier suggestion of anti-inflammatory action, given adequate dosage. The drug was found useful in patients with severe established or long-standing exacerbation, uncontrollable except with corticosteroids. All such patients could not only be weaned from dependence by adequate dosage of B 663, but their leprosy condition improved.

Treatment with B 663 of leprosy patients harboring dapsone-resistant *M. leprae*: Pettit and Rees (1966) treated with B 663, at a dosage of 300 mg daily for 6 days a week, the first 3 patients with proved dapsone-resistant leprosy. All 3 patients responded well—clinically, bacteriologically and histologically—to the drug, and the good results were maintained for over 2 years. A chemotherapeutic agent of different chemical constitution is thus shown to be effective in cases of dapsone resistance in leprosy. Hastings and Trautman (1968), and Browne (1968) also consider that dapsone resistance constitutes an important indication for the administration of B 663.

F. Drugs No Longer in Use or Insufficiently Investigated

1. *Methimazole* (Tapazole)

On rather slender theoretical assumptions, reinforced by some apparently impressive clinical results, O'Byrne (1960) suggested that certain antithyroid compounds (e.g., methimazole) deserved an extensive trial in leprosy. His findings have not been confirmed (Browne and Hogerzeil, 1962d).

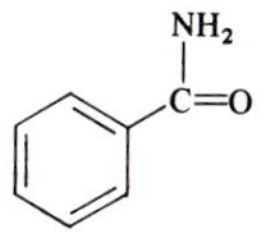

(XIII)

2. *Nicotinamide*

Nicotinamide (XIII), said to be very effective in murine leprosy, was not found by Doull *et al.* (1958) to have any additive effect in lepromatous leprosy when given together with standard doses of dapsone.

3. *Vadrine and Neovadrine*

Vadrine (XIV) and Neovadrine, aminosalicylic acid derivatives, are reportedly active in leprosy (Brechet and Cochrane, 1961; Jopling and Ridley,

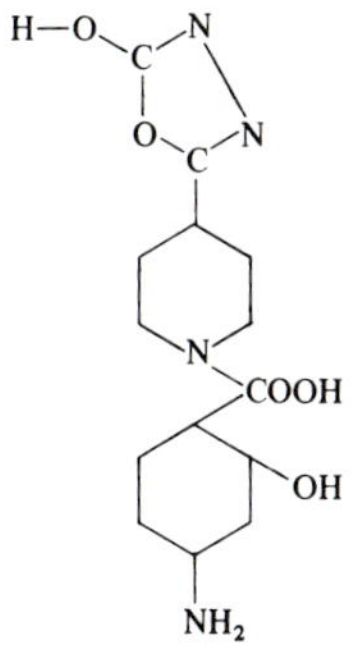

(XIV)

1961; Allan, 1961), but have not commended themselves for individual or mass treatment. They probably have an action in leprosy independent of dapsone, with which they were generally given in trials.

4. *Pyrazinamide* (XV)

Pyrazinamide (XV) is a diazine carboxamide related to nicotinic acid (XVI). It differs from nicotinamide in that a carbon atom in the para position is replaced by nitrogen. The suggestion is made by Smith (1964) that suitable modifications of the molecule of the hydrazide class of tuberculostatic compounds may confer on them antileprosy properties. Thus, the corresponding

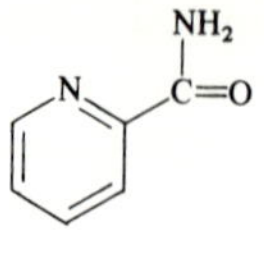

(XV)

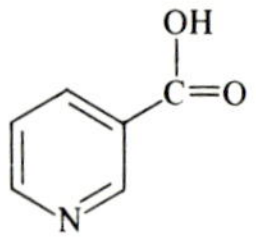

(XVI)

oxydiazolone or ozadiazolthione derivative may be antileprotic and may potentiate the action of dapsone. 4-Pyridylozadiazolone shows antileprotic properties distinct from those of isoniazid.

McDermott *et al.* (1954) reported that a combination of pyrazinamide and isoniazid was effective in experimental mouse tuberculosis, and Chang (1954) suggested that, since pyrazinamide was active in experimental murine leprosy, it should be tried in human leprosy. Doull *et al.* (1960a), giving pyrazinamide and isoniazid to 26 lepromatous patients for 24 weeks, concluded that the results did not justify further trials.

5. *Ethambutol*

Ethambutol (Wilson, 1967) is the dextrorotatory isomer of 2,2′-ethylenedimino-di-1-butanol dihydrochloride. It is an antimycobacterial agent, active (orally) in human tuberculosis, and is used especially in drug-resistant chronic disease. Shepard and Chang (1964) found it to be inactive against *M. leprae* in the mouse foot pad. The results of pilot clinical trials in leprosy are awaited.

6. *Ditophal*

Several groups of workers (e.g., Davies and Driver, 1957) have shown that certain ethyl mercaptan compounds are active in experimental murine tuberculosis. Ditophal (diethyldithiolisophthalate, Etisul or ETIP (XVII) is active after percutaneous absorption (Bushby, 1964). Davies and Driver (1958)

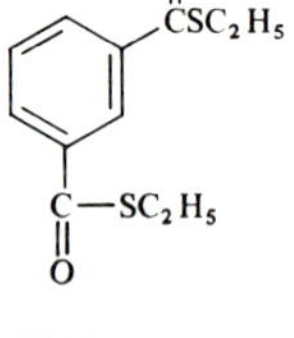

(XVII)

suggested in explanation that ethyl mercaptan, released in the tissues, interfered with a biological methylating or thiomethylating system.

Davey and Hogerzeil (1959) reported enthusiastically on its value in leprosy, but warned that drug resistance might develop rapidly. Subsequent workers have been less laudatory; Guinto *et al.* (1964) and others have found that the addition of ditophal to standard dapsone therapy does not accelerate bacterial clearance or shorten the total length of treatment required. Despite partly successful attempts to mask its objectionable odor, ditophal encounters considerable patient resistance and is unlikely to have a permanent place in therapy. Shepard and Chang (1964) found ditophal to be inactive against *M. leprae* in the mouse foot pad, but as Bushby (1964) has pointed out, this drug (like macrocyclon) may still influence the infection although it may not have demonstrable and direct mycobactericidal properties.

7. *Macrocyclon*

Macrocyclon is a polyethylene glycol of a *p-tert*-octylphenolformaldehyde cyclic tetramer. Its chemical antecedents and the history of its chemotherapeutic uses are summarized by Bushby (1964) and Waters (1963). Experimentally, it appears to potentiate the action of streptomycin, and is itself active against mouse and guinea-pig tuberculosis. In murine tuberculosis, but not in advanced human tuberculosis, macrocyclon may possess some property modifying the surface lipids of intracellular mycobacteria, a property that indicates that it might modify a mycobacterial infection against which it has no direct action. Its antituberculous action can be demonstrated in tissue culture of mouse macrophages infected with human *M. tuberculosis* (D'Arcy-Hart, 1968). Apparently the macrocyclon is stored in macrophages (Lovelock and Rees, 1955), probably in association with the lysosomes. It is possible that this association causes changes in the permeability of the lysosome membranes that tend to inhibit the growth of mycobacteria (D'Arcy-Hart, 1968). In the carefully controlled trial reported by Waters (1963), the addition of macrocyclon to standard dapsone therapy in patients with lepromatous leprosy failed to increase the rate of improvement—clinical, histological, or bacteriological. The failure to show any additive or synergistic effect by a drug presumably acting in a physical rather than in a protoplasmic mycobactericidal fashion should not shut the door to future investigations along similar or related lines.

G. Combinations of Drugs

After experience in the chemotherapy of tuberculosis, few physicians would pin their faith to one drug for individual or mass treatment. In leprosy, however, given the rarity of proved dapsone resistance, the lack of success of combined drug regimens in reducing either the period of contagiousness or the total period of treatment necessary for arrest of the disease process, and the general failure of such regimes to reduce the risk of peripheral neuritis or of acute lepromatous exacerbation or of relapse, it is not surprising that the use of one drug at a time is general. The question of cost is also relevant in developing countries, as is the observation that the toxic side effects of antileprosy drugs may be additive or potentiated, with no corresponding advantages. Studies of combined drug regimens have been reported by Guinto *et al.* (1964) and Doull *et al.* (1960a,b, 1961, 1965, 1967) in a series of excellent papers emanating from the Leonard Wood Memorial Laboratories in the Philippines, the general conclusions being that combinations of drugs in leprosy fail to show any but the slightest marginal differences.

Combinations of drugs have not given better results than the individual drugs given alone: diasone and dihydrostreptomycin, dihydrostreptomycin with either aminosalicylic acid or isoniazid, dapsone with either nicotinamide or ditophal (Guinto *et al.*, 1964). Other workers (e.g., Schulz *et al.*, 1966) have arrived at similar conclusions.

Situations in which a trial drug is added to a drug of known efficacy in leprosy provide the ethical justification for the introduction of the drug of suspected but undemonstrated activity; the results, however, are seldom or never clear-cut, and a definite clinical answer necessarily awaits the trial of the drug alone in suitable patients.

H. Antibiotics in Leprosy

Despite its taxonomic affinity with *M. tuberculosis*, *M. leprae* has not shown itself outstandingly susceptible to the antibiotics that appear among the first-line or the second-line drugs used in the treatment of human tuberculosis If dapsone were not as effective as it is, or if leprosy were commoner in the economically richer, medically advanced countries, investigations into the place of antibiotics in the treatment and control of leprosy would undoubtedly have been prosecuted with greater vigor and persistence. As it is, and despite the proved activity of certain antibiotics in the treatment of multibacillary leprosy, their cost and the mode of administration necessary (parenterally, and at frequent intervals) restrict their practicable usefulness to selected and hospitalized patients presenting special indications for such treatment.

1. *Streptomycin*

Streptomycin has been shown to be active in leprosy, both clinically (Doull *et al.*, 1965), and in the mouse foot pad (Shepard and Chang, 1964). Given with dapsone, dihydrostreptomycin has no additive action. Recent reports from Karat *et al.* (1964) indicate its dramatic value when given with isoniazid in patients showing multiple ulcerations of the lesions of acute lepromatous exacerbation; and Price and Fitzherbert (1966) suggest that the rare histoid nodules of lepromatous leprosy, which are notably indolent and unresponsive to standard therapy, regress and subside under combined streptomycin and isoniazid therapy.

2. *Penicillin Hydroxyprocaine*

Trappmann (1961) found penicillin useful in lepromatous and especially in borderline leprosy, with results comparable to those of dapsone.

3. *Viomycin*

Basset *et al.* (1964) found rapid improvement in patients with lepromatous leprosy, in doses of 1 gm intramuscularly 3 times a week. The Bacterial Index was said to have fallen by 50% in a year. Toxic reactions were less than with kanamycin.

4. *Streptonicozid* (*Streptohydrazid*)

This compound is a condensation product of streptomycin salts and isoniazid. Dreisbach and Cochrane (1958) reported favorably on the clinical response to treatment, and in particular, rapid healing of nodulations and ulcerations of the upper respiratory tract. Guinto *et al.* (1964) found that the drug exerted an action comparable to that of other effective drugs given singly or in combination.

5. *Kanamycin*

Kanamycin is an antibiotic elaborated by *Streptomyces kanamyceticus*. Japanese workers (Yanagisawa and Asami, 1958) and Chang (1959) have reported on its inhibitory action in murine leprosy. Languillon (1963) tried it in a small series of 4 patients with untreated lepromatous leprosy, finding rapid improvement (especially clinical) over a period of 12 months.

6. *Oxytetracycline*

This drug was given by intramuscular injection to 6 patients suffering from various kinds of leprosy (Mariano, 1963). Opromolla *et al.* (1965) report favorably on oxytetracycline (Terramycin), given by intramuscular injection to 22 patients, at a dose of 100 mg every 12 hours for 12 months.

7. *Cycloserine*

Cycloserine, produced by *Streptomyces orchidaceus* or *S. garyhalus*, or synthetically, has been shown by Doull *et al.* (1960b) and others to have an effect in leprosy comparable to that of dapsone. Some workers (e.g., Neto and Revelles, 1958) consider that the drug acts directly on *M. leprae* and in ways different from that of the sulfones. Hence, according to them, a combined therapy might be indicated. In the mouse foot pad, Shepard and Chang (1962) found partial suppression of *M. leprae* multiplication. Alonso (1963) reported that cycloserine gave results comparable with those of dapsone and thiacetazone. When given together with the latter drug, it did not enhance its action.

Chambon and Pestel (1960), treating patients with lepromatous leprosy with D-cycloserine, found that it precipitated controllable reactions, with ultimate benefit to half the patients. Opromolla and Quagliato (1960) reported favorably on cycloserine given with isoniazid, but mentioned the apparent precipitation of reaction some 5 days after treatment was begun.

8. *Capreomycin*

Capreomycin, an antimycobacterial agent isolated from *Streptomyces capreolus*, is a cyclic polypeptide. It shows some cross-resistance with kanamycin and neomycin, but not with streptomycin or cycloserine or other antimycobacterial agents (Wilson, 1967). It is active against *M. tuberculosis*, but resistance is said to develop somewhat rapidly. Shepard (1964) and Rees (1967) have shown that it is active against *M. leprae*, using the mouse foot-pad technique. Despite its ototoxic and nephrotoxic properties, clinical trials are recommended in patients with leprosy, provided due precautions are observed.

9. *Rifamycin SV* (XVIII)

Rifamycin SV (XVIII) is a monobasic acid derived from rifamycin B, which is a member of a group of antimicrobial substances (rifamycins) isolated by Sensi *et al.* (1961) from a strain of *Streptomyces mediterranei*. Obtained by the reduction of rifamycin S with ascorbic acid, it is the least toxic of all the rifamycins so far isolated and investigated. No cross-resistance with other antibiotics has been demonstrated.

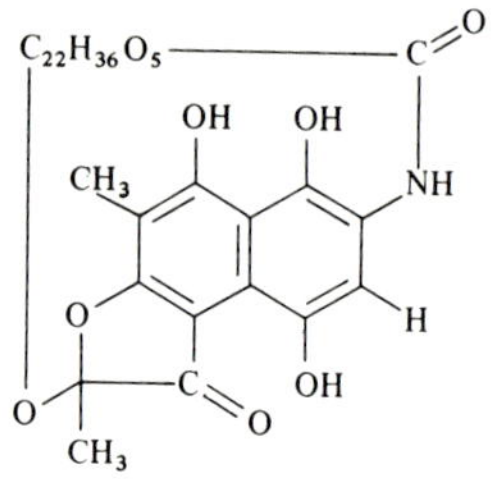

(XVIII)

Its use in leprosy was first suggested rather by its *in vitro* activity against *M. tuberculosis* than by its efficacy in established clinical tuberculosis in man. The minimal inhibitory concentration of rifamycin SV for *M. tuberculosis* (human and bovine varieties) has been shown to be from 0.02–1.0 μg per ml. A similar range obtains for gram-positive bacteria, while for gram-negative bacteria the upper and lower limits of the range would be approximately 100 times as great. Against *M. tuberculosis in vitro*, rifamycin SV shows greater activity than both streptomycin and aminosalicylic acid, and similar activity to isoniazid.

In the treatment of patients with tuberculosis, rifamycin SV is usually given by intramuscular injection in doses of 500–1000 mg daily in divided doses. When administered orally, the drug attains therapeutically active concentrations only after excretion in the biliary tract, whereas after intramuscular injection, the plasma concentration rapidly attains a peak.

In leprosy, the small clinical trials conducted at several centers have been sufficiently encouraging to warrant more extended investigations not only of rifamycin SV itself but also of numerous related compounds. The mode of action of the rifamycins on mycobacteria in general requires elucidation, as do also the effects of the drugs both on the viability of *M. leprae* and on the clearance of nonviable bacilli from the tissues.

The doses given in reported trials were based empirically on accepted dose scales for patients suffering from tuberculosis. Furthermore, although skin concentrations of the drug in animals are low compared with plasma concentrations, persisting high levels of the drug may be observed in superficially situated granulomata. On these grounds, therefore, it might be expected that rifamycin SV would show greater activity in leprosy than the blood concentration of the drug suggests (no investigations with a tagged rifamycin have yet been reported). The proportion of morphologically normal forms of *M. leprae* is said to fall, suggesting that rifamycin SV is bactericidal. The clearance of acid-fast debris was not uniformly expedited in all patients: in 7, the bacterial load decreased, while in 2 it remained unchanged, and in 2 it actually increased.

Farris and Baccaredda-Boy (1963) briefly reported a series of 15 patients with lepromatous leprosy who were treated for 8 months with rifamycin SV, 500–1000 mg daily, intramuscularly every 12 hours for periods of 15–45 days, alternating with rest periods of 10–15 days. The clinical and bacteriological results were encouraging, but some patients developed erythema nodosum leprosum with pyrexia.

As the result of 2–3 months' treatment with twice-weekly subcutaneous injections of rifamycin SV, Merklen and Cottenot (1964) reported rapid regression of widespread tuberculoid skin lesions in 1 patient, and improvement in 2 patients with long-standing lepromatous leprosy. The authors warn that local reaction to the injection might render prolonged treatment difficult.

Further work is proceeding on derivatives of rifamycin that may prove to be of therapeutic interest in leprosy. For example, rifampicin has been shown by Rees (1968b) to be inhibitory against *M. leprae* in the mouse foot-pad test as follows: at concentrations of 0.01, 0.005, and 0.0025% in the diet, which are respectively equivalent to 20, 10, and 5 mg/kg body weight.

10. *Systemic Fungicides*

These substances have received scant attention in leprosy. No improvement was reported in 2 patients treated with Griseofulvin (Pfaltzgraff and Cochrane, 1963).

I. Vaccines in Leprosy

1. *Marianum Antigen*

Marianum antigen has been given by Ondoua *et al.* (1964) as an adjuvant to dapsone therapy, or alone (Bagalanis *et al.*, 1966), with satisfactory results, but Tolentino (1957) failed to find any bacteriological improvement attributable to the antigen.

2. *BCG Vaccination*

No evidence was found by Doull *et al.* (1958) that BCG vaccination conferred any benefit on patients with lepromatous leprosy who were being given standard treatment with dapsone.

J. γ-Globulin

Trautman and Callaway (1965) gave γ-globulin to 5 patients with severe lepromatous leprosy, with good results in 2. They suggest that γ-globulin may be of value in intractable cases of leprosy.

K. Lysozyme

Pupo (1963), and Silva and Andrade (1963) report encouraging results with lysozyme (with or without calciferol) in treating leprosy, ascribing the results mainly to its desensitizing properties in reactive states. Further work is indicated along these lines, especially to ascertain if the clearance of effete mycobacteria can be facilitated or expedited by these or related means. Opromolla *et al.* (1965) considered, on the basis of treating 11 patients suffering from lepromatous leprosy, that the drug was remarkably effective. Of the patients, 8 were treated for about a year, the remaining 3 for 5 months (2 patients) and 9 months, respectively. No serious toxic effects were attributed to the drug, though 1 patient complained of pruritus, another had an urticarial rash, and 2 others had jaundice and gastric troubles which subsided within 2 weeks of discontinuance of the treatment.

V. Relapse in Leprosy

If World Health Organization (1966) recommendations for length of treatment are observed, e.g., regular treatment for at least 4 years in patients with lepromatous or borderline leprosy, or for at least 2 years after all signs of clinical and bacteriological evidence of activity have disappeared, relapse is uncommon (Browne, 1965f). Adequately treated lepromatous or tuberculoid leprosy tends to remain quiescent, though some authorities advocate, for the former, treatment for life at half the therapeutic dose. Patients having one of the intermediate (borderline, or dimorphous) types of leprosy, which may respond very satisfactorily to therapy (with rapid clearance of the clinical lesions, and very rapid fall in both the Morphological Index and the Bacterial Index) show a distinct tendency to relapse when treatment is discontinued too soon; the relapse rate may be as high in some series as 30%.

Relapse in leprosy is in reality a reactivation of the disease from foci of viable bacilli in deep tissues (liver, nerves, bone marrow, etc.), and is not a reinfection (about which nothing definite is at present known). Relapse is not to be compared with slow response to therapy (with persistence of viable bacillary forms, or more commonly of degenerate forms), or with the transient reappearance of morphologically normal forms. Bacteriological relapse in patients with lepromatous leprosy usually precedes by some months signs of renewed clinical activity. The bacilli are susceptible to the drug used initially with success. Rarely, relapse is due to the appearance of drug-resistant strains of *M. leprae*, and hence requires a drug of different chemical design (Pettit and Rees, 1964).

VI. Drug Resistance

Mycobacterium leprae had long been suspected, on clinical grounds that are scientifically inadequate, of developing resistance to many drugs used in the treatment of leprosy, e.g., dapsone, thiambutosine, thiacetazone, ditophal. In most cases, the unsupported suspicion may be capable of one of several possible explanations, such as failure to take the drug or to absorb the drug, slow response to treatment, persistence or transient reappearance of pockets of morphologically normal bacilli, etc. On the other hand, true resistance to dapsone, regarded on clinical grounds as being extremely rare, has now been demonstrated by Pettit and Rees (1964) and others by the use of the mouse foot-pad inoculation technique. Drug resistance, fortunately, is not as common in leprosy as it is in tuberculosis and other infections. The determining factors in the development of demonstrable drug resistance have not been precisely identified, but in practice intermittency and very low doses of drug may be important. Furthermore, cross-resistance to drugs of related chemical composition has been demonstrated by the mouse foot-pad inoculation technique; cross-resistance to drugs of dissimilar chemical structure awaits investigation. The detection of spontaneously arising resistant mutants, while unlikely in an experimental system providing a plateau of 10^6 bacilli, is not impossible in one in which a count of 10^8 or even 10^9 is attainable (Rees, 1967).

Rees (1967) has also provided evidence for the existence of thiambutosine-resistant strains of *M. leprae*, and has shown that such strains show cross-resistance to thiacetazone, as has been reported against *M. tuberculosis* (Konopka *et al.*, 1955). Resistance may be developed in a stepwise process (Morrison, 1968), and partial resistance may occur (Pearson *et al.*, 1968). A strain of *M. leprae* may be inhibited by a concentration of drug that is not bactericidal (Shepard, 1967a). There is a wide range of dapsone resistance apparent in strains derived from patients showing presumptive evidence of resistance. The most precise clinical data so far available indicate that a total of 22.4 gm dapsone, given at a dose of 50 mg twice weekly over 52 months, preceded the development of proven dapsone resistance (which responded to B 663) (Browne, 1969). Up to the present Rees (1968a) has demonstrated resistance in 18 strains of *M. leprae* against dapsone, and 5 against thiambutosine.

VII. Drugs Used in Acute Exacerbation of Lepromatous Leprosy

To keep this section within a reasonable compass, reference will be highly selective and purposely limited to some recent reports of methodology, experimental investigations, and clinical trials, ignoring most of the drugs reputedly effective in controlling acute exacerbation, e.g., the antimonials, chloroquine, etc.

A. Therapeutic Trials

The principles to be observed in the conduct of therapeutic trials in these conditions are well set out by Waters *et al.* (1967). In a clinical syndrome manifesting such diversity, variability, and spontaneous remissions (short-lived or definitive), the utmost care should be exercised before attributing improvement to any treatment given.

B. Relevant Clinical Considerations

While all types of leprosy (except the indeterminate) may undergo acute inflammation, it is in lepromatous leprosy that some kind of acute exacerbation (*Intern. J. Leprosy*, 1963) (indifferently called reaction, erythema nodosum leprosum, lepra fever, lepra reaction, etc.), is most serious. It occurs at any stage of the disease (but most frequently in the established, rather than in the early, condition); in the untreated, as well as in those being treated with standard drugs; in a varying proportion of patients, rising to three quarters; it may be transient, recurrent, or persistent, merging imperceptibly into "chronic lepra reaction"; it may necessitate prolonged interruption of antileprosy therapy, and be accompanied by acute polyneuritis, iridocyclitis, and other serious signs of a hypersensitive state. Standard medical treatment consists of analgesics, antimonials, antimalarials, and corticosteroids—in that order, the latter being used only when the former have failed.

C. Immune Suppressive Drugs

Since it has been suggested that immunosuppressive drugs should be given to control acute lepromatous exacerbation, the work of Shepard and Redus (1967) is relevant. These workers gave the antineoplastic drugs, amethopterin, 6-mercaptopurine, and cyclophosphamide to mice experimentally infected with *M. marinum* (*balnei*). The principal effect was an increase in the proportion of viable bacilli. Mice infected with *M. tuberculosis* died sooner after being given these drugs. In *M. leprae* infections, no promotion of bacterial growth was noted; the dose of cyclophosphamide had to be reduced because of drug-associated mortality.

Having given cyclophosphamide by inadvertence to 8 leprosy patients, Davison *et al.* (1964) suggested that the drug might be used to inhibit acute leprosy reactions, but Schulz and Falkson (1965) later found no improvement in 9 patients already suffering from erythema nodosum leprosum.

Schulz and Falkson (1965) gave Natulan (RO 4-6467), a cytostatic agent, to 6 patients without benefit: leukopenia was induced in 4. The same authors (Schulz and Falkson, 1967) report no beneficial effect from Ancyte and Vercyte, cytostatic agents.

D. Thalidomide (XIX)

A chance observation by Sheskin (1965a) that within 48 hours thalidomide (α-phthalimidoglutarimide) (XIX) given as a sedative controlled the severe

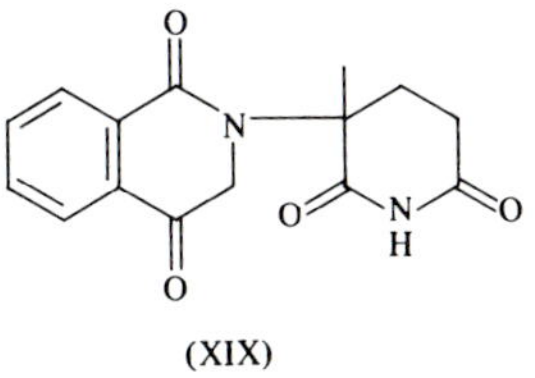

(XIX)

manifestations of acute lepromatous exacerbation led to the investigation of the drug as an immunosuppressive in a series of such patients. Sheskin and Convit (1966) then carried out a double-blind trial of thalidomide, giving 173 treatments; the results were very good. Sheskin (1965b), after observing 6 patients, gave up to 400 mg of the drug daily for 7 months to 13 patients, with good results, but noted toxic effects. Cazort and Ye Kun Song (1966) were similarly impressed with the results in 24 patients given 300 mg daily, though relapse occurred after withdrawal. Opromolla *et al.* (1966) confirm the efficacy of the drug, and recommend its widespread use. De las Aguas and Contreras Dueñas (1966) report rapid disappearance of the signs of reaction when thalidomide is given at a dose of 100 mg daily.

Despite the toxic manifestations in skin, gastrointestinal tract, and nervous system following its use, and despite the recurrence of signs of exacerbation after withdrawal and the danger of teratogenic effects, thalidomide or related compounds (Sheskin and Sagher, 1968) may have a place in the treatment of severe and persistent exacerbation in lepromatous leprosy. The drug has no action on the underlying disease; in fact, its use may actually suppress some beneficial inflammatory response (Convit *et al.*, 1967; Sheskin *et al.*, 1968). Mellin and Katzenstein (1962) have summarized the teratogenic and toxic properties of thalidomide.

E. Corticosteroids and Antileprosy Chemotherapy

Because prolonged corticosteroid administration in a chronic disease like leprosy entails a high risk of serious side effects, corticosteroids are not advised except in certain well-defined situations, such as acute lepromatous exacerbation that has failed to respond to standard measures. It may be necessary to give minimal maintenance doses of corticosteroids in patients with persistent and uncontrollable exacerbation and to resume antileprosy medication under corticosteroid cover.

Shepard and McRae (1965) have provided evidence that, in the experimental mouse, daily cortisone injections (0.1 mg cortisone acetate), after an initial slow increase of the growth of *M. leprae* in the foot pad, actually appeared to stimulate bacterial multiplication. An anti-inflammatory corticosteroid-like agent that was also mycobactericidal would be invaluable in suppressing the signs of acute exacerbation while not favoring bacterial multiplication in nerves and skin.

F. B 663

Browne (1965a, 1966b) suggested that B 663 (XII) might have such an anti-inflammatory action, suppressing the development of signs of acute exacerbation in lepromatous leprosy. Further evidence seems to support this claim (Williams *et al.*, 1965; Hastings and Trautman, 1968; Imkamp, 1968); moreover, when given in appropriate doses, B 663 is effective in controlling the signs of severe established exacerbation, enabling corticosteroid-dependent patients to be weaned from steroids while at the same time being exposed to a mycobactericidal drug.

VIII. Prophylaxis

Although perhaps the prophylaxis of leprosy is in the strict sense excluded from consideration in this paper, the subject is so important and so apposite to any practical discussion of the chemotherapy of leprosy that it must be referred to, however briefly.

A. BCG Vaccination

Since the suggestion was first put forward by Fernandez (1939) that BCG vaccination might afford some protection against leprosy, numerous investigations have been reported, but the results were equivocal methodologically and unconvincing statistically. More recently, Brown and Stone (1966) and Brown *et al.* (1968), observing apparently unassailable protocols, have produced evidence suggesting that BCG vaccination will protect children exposed to intrafamilial leprosy challenge against the development of overt leprosy lesions in approximately 80% over a period of 2 years, and up to 87% over $3\frac{1}{2}$ years. The protective effect is presumably due to common- or group-antigenic activity. If these results are confirmed and are applicable to other countries (including those where the lepromatous/tuberculoid ratio is higher than in Uganda), and if the protection afforded is maintained and potent against the appearance of lepromatous leprosy, a most valuable means of control will be made available. BCG vaccine, given routinely to all infants, may prove the best and the cheapest method of leprosy control.

Results of similar trials in other countries, conducted under similarly adequate statistical control, are up to the present not so convincing. In Karimui (Papua and New Guinea), in an isolated population exposed to leprosy but not to tuberculosis, BCG vaccination appears to protect about 56% of children exposed to leprosy challenge (Russell *et al.*, 1964, 1968; Scott *et al.*, 1966). In Burma, where the prevalence of leprosy is high, and where the lepromatous/tuberculoid ratio is also high, the World Health Organization team reports (1968b) that preliminary findings do not suggest that BCG vaccination affords protection to exposed children.

Experimental support for the clinical evidence of a certain measure of protection afforded by BCG vaccination in children exposed intrafamilially to leprosy comes from Shepard (1965a,b). When given to mice within 2 months before challenge with *M. leprae*, or within the same interval after challenge, BCG appears to give some protection. The intracutaneous route of administration is better than the subcutaneous or the intraperitoneal. Revaccination during the incubation period gives increased protection. The protection afforded decreases progressively after some months. While all these findings may not be directly applicable to man challenged by *M. leprae*, they do furnish an experimental basis for the assumption that some protection may be given by BCG vaccination, but suggest that subcategories of recipients classified according to degree and duration of exposure to *M. leprae* from the index case, the viability of *M. leprae* shed from the putative index case, the interval between cessation of exposure and vaccination, the innate responsiveness to injected lepromin, and the presence and degree of any change noted after BCG vaccination, should be subject to critical analysis.

B. Dapsone

Dharmendra *et al.* (1965, 1967) and Wardekar (1967) have shown that small graduated doses of dapsone, given to intrafamilial child contacts of known leprosy patients in weekly (or twice-weekly) doses for some years, will apparently confer protection against leprosy to about 75% of the children. While the proposition may not be in dispute—although it does need confirmation by repetition elsewhere—practical objections relate to such questions as the cost, the length of control necessary, the manpower required, the risks of adverse drug reactions, etc.

IX. The Way Ahead

The state of leprosy control and treatment in the world as a whole, while less bleak than in the presulfone era, remains highly unsatisfactory. The application of existing knowledge of mycobactericidal drugs in mass treatment campaigns could conceivably break the cycle of transmission of viable intracellular host-dependent *M. leprae* from the disseminator to the susceptible recipient. Such an application, however, is generally proving too costly in precisely those countries where leprosy is a problem of medical and economic importance.

Hence, the real need for further research (Browne, 1967b) lies along the following lines: (*a*) A long-acting chemical prophylactic; (*b*) a rapidly-acting mycobactericidal drug; (*c*) an agent that will accelerate the removal of acid-fast mycobacterial debris from the tissues; and (*d*) a drug that will minimize or abolish the results of tissue sensitization to undetermined mycobacterial antigens.

These drugs should be inexpensive; they should be effective orally and at long intervals; they should be suitable for mass treatment at the hands of medical auxiliaries. An impossible demand? I hope not.

REFERENCES

Allan, J. A. (1961). *Leprosy Rev.* **32**, 191.

Allday, E. J., and Barnes, J. (1952). *Irish J. Med. Sci.* **322**, 421.

Alonso, A. M. (1959). *Intern. J. Leprosy* **27**, 321.

Alonso, A. M. (1963). *Vol. Serv. Nacl. Lepra (Rio de Janeiro)* **22**, 15.

Atkinson, A. J., Sheagren, J. N., Barba Rubio, J., and Knight, V. (1967). *Intern. J. Leprosy* **35**, 119.

Bagalanis, A., Oh, E., and Whang, E. (1966). *Leprosy Rev.* **37**, 51.

Barry, V. C., and Conalty, M. L. (1965). *Leprosy Rev.* **36**, 3.

Basset, A., Sicard, D., Faye, I., and Basset, M. (1964). *Bull. Soc. Méd. Afrique Noire Langue Franç.* **9**, 418.

Bratton, H. C., and Marshall, E. K. A. (1939). *J. Biol. Chem.* **128**, 537.

Brechet, R., and Cochrane, R. G. (1961). *Leprosy Rev.* **32**, 180.

Brown, G. M. (1967). *Intern. J. Leprosy* **35**, 580.

Brown, J. A. K., and Stone, M. M. (1966). *Brit. Med. J.* **i**, 7.

Brown, J. A. K., Stone, M. M., and Sutherland, I. (1968). *Brit. Med. J.* **i**, 24.

Browne, S. G. (1955). *Intern. J. Leprosy* **23**, 284.

Browne, S. G. (1961). *Intern. J. Leprosy* **29**, 502.

Browne, S. G. (1963). *Brit. Med. J.* **ii**, 664.

Browne, S. G. (1965a). *Leprosy Rev.* **36**, 9.

Browne, S. G. (1965b). *Leprosy Rev.* **36**, 13.

Browne, S. G. (1965c). *Leprosy Rev.* **36**, 21.

Browne, S. G. (1965d). *Leprosy Rev.* **36**, 53.

Browne, S. G. (1965e). *Leprosy in India* **37**, 299.

Browne, S. G. (1965f). *Intern. J. Leprosy* **33**, 273.

Browne, S. G. (1966a). *Leprosy Rev.* **37**, 23.

Browne, S. G. (1966b). *Leprosy Rev.* **37**, 141.

Browne, S. G. (1967a). *Leprosy Rev.* **38**, 7.

Browne, S. G. (1967b). *Trans. Roy. Soc. Trop. Med. Hyg.* **61**, 265.

Browne, S. G. (1967c). *Practitioner* **199**, 525.

Browne, S. G. (1967d). *Intern. J. Leprosy* **35**, 395.

Browne, S. G. (1968). *Intern. J. Leprosy* **36**, (4), Pt. 2, Abstr. No. 202.

Browne, S. G. (1969). *Intern. J. Leprosy* **37**, (in press).

Browne, S. G., and Davey, T. F. (1961). *Leprosy Rev.* **32**, 194.

Browne, S. G., and Hogerzeil, L. M. (1962a). *Leprosy Rev.* **33**, 6.

Browne, S. G., and Hogerzeil, L. M. (1962b). *Leprosy Rev.* **33**, 182.

Browne, S. G., and Hogerzeil, L. M. (1962c). *Leprosy Rev.* **33**, 185.

Browne, S. G., and Hogerzeil, L. M. (1962d). *Leprosy Rev.* **33**, 190.

Bushby, S. R. M. (1964). *In* "Leprosy in Theory and Practice" (R. G. Cochrane and T. F. Davey, eds.), p. 344. Wright, Bristol, England.

Bushby, S. R. M. (1967). *Intern. J. Leprosy* **35**, 572.

Bushby, S. R. M., and Woiwod, A. J. (1956). *Biochem. J.* **63**, 406.

Buu-Hoi, N. P., Bang, T. V., Kim Mong-Don, T. T., and Xuong, N. D. (1961). *Chemotherapia* **2**, 122.

Cazort, R. J., and Ye Kun Song (1966). *Current Therap. Res.* **8**, 6.

Chambon, L., and Pestel, M. (1960). *Intern. J. Leprosy* **28**, 239.

Chang, Y. T. (1954). *Intern. J. Leprosy* **22**, 331.

Chang, Y. T. (1959). *Am. Rev. Tuberc. Pulmonary Diseases* **79**, 673.

Chatterjee, K. R., and Podder, R. K. (1957). *Proc. Soc. Exptl. Biol. Med.* **94**, 122.

Cochrane, R. G. (1952). *Leprosy Rev.* **23**, 135.

Convit, J., Soto, J. M., and Sheskin, J. (1967). *Intern. J. Leprosy* **35**, 446.

Currie, G. (1966). *Leprosy Rev.* **37**, 205.

D'Arcy-Hart, P. (1968). *Science* **162**, 686.

Davey, T. F. (1956). *Leprosy Rev.* **27**, 6.

Davey, T. F. (1960). *Trans. Roy. Soc. Trop. Med. Hyg.* **54**, 199.
Davey, T. F., and Currie, G. (1956). *Leprosy Rev.* **27**, 94.
Davey, T. F., and Hogerzeil, L. M. (1959). *Leprosy Rev.* **30**, 61.
Davies, G. E., and Driver, G. W. (1957). *Brit. J. Pharmacol.* **12**, 434.
Davies, G. E., and Driver, G. W. (1958). *Nature* **182**, 664.
Davison, A. R., Schulz, E. J., Falkson, G., and Egnal, M. L. (1964). *Lancet* **ii**, 1138.
de las Aguas, T., and Contreras Dueñas (1966). *Rev. Leprol. (Fontilles)* **6**, 449.
Dharmendra, (1950). *Leprosy in India* **22**, 46.
Dharmendra, Mohammed, Ali P., Noordeen, S. K., and Ramanujam, K. (1965). *Leprosy in India* **37**, 447.
Dharmendra, Noordeen, S. K., and Ramanujam, K. (1967). *Leprosy in India* **39**, 100.
Doob, L. (1961). *Med. Chem.* **5**, 350.
Doull, J. A. (1963). *Intern. J. Leprosy* **31**, 143.
Doull, J. A., Rodriguez, J. N., Davison, A. R., Tolentino, J. G., and Fernandez, J. V. (1958). *Intern. J. Leprosy* **26**, 219.
Doull, J. A., Rodriguez, J. N., Tolentino, J. G., and Fernandez, J. V. (1960a). *Intern. J. Leprosy* **28**, 12.
Doull, J. A., Rodriguez, J. N., Tolentino, J. G., and Fernandez, J. V. (1960b). *Intern. J. Leprosy* **28**, 18.
Doull, J. A., Rodriguez, J. N., Tolentino, J. G., Fernandez, J. V., Guinto, R. S., Rivera, J. N., and Mabalay, M. C. (1961). *Intern. J. Leprosy* **29**, 291.
Doull, J. A., Tolentino, J. G., Rodriguez, J. N., Guinto, R. S., Rivera, J. N., Fernandez, J. V., and Mabalay, M. C. (1965). *Intern. J. Leprosy* **33**, 2, 186.
Doull, J. A., Tolentino, J. G., Guinto, R. S., Rodriguez, J. N., Leano, L. M., Fernandez, J. V., Rivera, J. N., and Fajardo, T. T., Jr. (1967). *Intern. J. Leprosy* **35**, 128.
Dreisbach, J., and Cochrane, R. G. (1958). *Leprosy Rev.* **29**, 136.
Ellard, G. A., and Gammon, P. T. (1968). *Intern. J. Leprosy* **36**, (4) Pt. 2, Abstr. No. 197.
Farris, G., and Baccaredda-Boy, A. (1963). *Intern. J. Leprosy* **31**, 560.
Fernandez, J. M. M. (1939). *Rev. Argentina Dermatosif.* **23**, 425.
Gaugas, J. M. (1967). *Leprosy Rev.* **38**, 225.
Gaugas, J. M. (1968). *Intern. J. Leprosy* **36** (4), Pt. 2, Abstr. No. 35.
Gaugas, J. M., and Rees, R. J. W. (1968). *Nature* **219**, 408.
Glazko, A. J. (1950). *Intern. J. Leprosy* **18**, 247.
Glazko, A. J. (1968). Unpublished observations. Quoted in Ellard and Gammon (1968).
Griffiths, P. G. (1965). *Leprosy Rev.* **36**, 23.
Guinto, R. S., Tolentino, J. G., and Doull, J. A. (1964). *Intern. J. Leprosy* **32**, 168.
Hastings, R. C., and Trautman, J. R. (1968). *Leprosy Rev.* **39**, 3.
Imkamp, F. M. J. H. (1968). *Leprosy Rev.* **39**, 119.
Intern. J. Leprosy (1963). Panel on Lepra Reaction **31**, 480.
Intern. J. Leprosy (1965). Research Problems in Leprosy **33**, 397.
Intern. J. Leprosy (1967). Symposium on Sulfones **35**, 563.
Jardin, C. (1961). "Agents Thérapeutiques et Remèdes Traditionnels Contre la Lèpre." Imprimerie Robert, Marseille.
Jopling, W. H. (1965). *Leprosy Rev.* **36**, 69.
Jopling, W. H., and Ridley, D. S. (1961). *Leprosy Rev.* **32**, 188.
Karat, A. B. A. (1967). *Intern. J. Leprosy* **35**, 623.
Karat, A. B. A., Job, C. K., and Karat, S. (1967). *Leprosy Rev.* **38**, 25.
Konopka, E. C., Gisi, T., Eisman, P. C., and Mayer, R. L. (1955). *Proc. Soc. Exptl. Biol. Med.* **89**, 388.
Laing, A. G. B., Pringle, G., and Lane, F. C. T. (1966). *Am. J. Trop. Med. Hyg.* **15**, 838.

Langullon, J. (1963). *Bull. Soc. Méd. Afrique Noire Langue Franç.* **7**, 409.
Languillon, J. (1964). *Bull. Soc. Pathol. Exotique* **57**, 424.
Languillon, J. (1966). *Méd. Trop.* **26**, 131.
Languillon, J. (1968). *Bull. Assoc. Léprol. Langue Franç.* **1**, 89.
Languillon, J., and Clary, J. (1964). *Bull. Soc. Pathol. Exotique* **57**, 431.
Leiker, D. L. (1956). *Leprosy Rev.* **27**, 66.
Leiker, D. L., and Carling, D. (1966). *Leprosy Rev.* **37**, 27.
Lovelock, J. E., and Rees, R. J. W. (1955). *Nature* **175**, 161.
Lowe, J. (1952). *Leprosy Rev.* **23**, 4.
Lunn, H. F., and Rees, R. J. W. (1964). *Lancet* **i**, 247.
McDermott, W., Ormond, K., Muschenheim, C., Deuschle, K., McCure, R. M., Jr., and Tompsett, R. (1954). *Am. Rev. Tuberc.* **69**, 319.
Mariano, J. (1963). *Rev. Brasil. Leprol.* **31**, 45.
Mathur, S. N. M., and Karani, H. (1967). *Leprosy in India* **34**, 8.
Mellin, G. W., and Katzenstein, N. (1962). *New Engl. J. Med.* **267**, 1238.
Merklen, F. P., and Cottenot, F. (1964). *Presse Méd.* **72**, 48.
Mitchinson, D. A., and Lloyd, J. (1964). *Tubercle* **45**, 360.
Morrison, N. E. (1968). *Intern. J. Leprosy* **36** (4), Pt. 2, Abstr. No. 199.
Neto, E. de A., and Revelles, J. P. (1958). *Rev. Brasil. Leprol.* **26**, 63.
Newbould, B. B., and Kilpatrick, R. (1960). *Lancet* **i**, 887.
Noordeen, S. K. (1965). *Leprosy in India* **37**, 10.
O'Byrne, A. (1960). *Intern. J. Leprosy* **28**, 401.
Ondoua, P., Prost, M. T., and de la Trinité, M. (1964). *Leprosy Rev.* **35**, 297.
Opromolla, D. V. A., and Quagliato, R. (1960). *Rev. Brasil. Leprol.* **28**, 185.
Opromolla, D. V. A., Mendes, J. P., and De Souza Lima, L. (1965). *Rev. Brasil. Leprol.* **33**, 3.
Opromolla, D. V. A., Lima, L. S., and Marques, M. B. (1966). *Hospital (Rio de Janeiro)* **69**, 827.
Pearson, J. M. H., Pettit, J. H. S., and Rees, R. J. W. (1968). *Intern. J. Leprosy* **36**, 171.
Pettit, J. H. S. (1967). *Intern. J. Leprosy* **35**, 11.
Pettit, J. H. S., and Rees, R. J. W. (1964). *Lancet* **ii**, 673.
Pettit, J. H. S., and Rees, R. J. W. (1966). *Intern. J. Leprosy* **34**, 391.
Pettit, J. H. S., and Rees, R. J. W. (1967). *Intern. J. Leprosy* **35**, 140.
Pettit, J. H. S., Rees, R. J. W., and Ridley, D. S. (1967). *Intern. J. Leprosy* **35**, 25.
Pfaltzgraff, R. E., and Cochrane, R. G. (1963). *Leprosy Rev.* **34**, 5.
Price, E. W., and Fitzherbert, M. (1966). *Intern. J. Leprosy* **34**, 367.
Pupo, J. A. (1963). *Rev. Brasil. Leprol.* **31**, 59.
Ramu, G., and Ramanujam, K. (1965). *Leprosy in India* **37**, 293.
Rees, R. J. W. (1964). *J. Exptl. Pathol.* **45**, 207.
Rees, R. J. W. (1966). *Nature* **211**, 657.
Rees, R. J. W. (1967). *Trans. Roy. Soc. Trop. Med. Hyg.* **61**, 69.
Rees, R. J. W. (1968a). *Intern. J. Leprosy* **36** (4), Pt. 2, Abstr. No. 194.
Rees, R. J. W. (1968b). Personal communication.
Rees, R. J. W., Valentine, R. C., and Wong, P. C. (1960). *J. Gen. Microbiol.* **22**, 443.
Rees, R. J. W., Waters, M. F. R., Weddell, A. G. McD., and Palmer, E. (1967). *Nature* **215**, 599.
Ridley, D. S. (1958). *Leprosy Rev.* **29**, 45.
Ridley, D. S. (1964). *In* "Leprosy in Theory and Practice" (R. G. Cochrane and T. F. Davey, eds.), p. 620. Wright, Bristol, England.
Ridley, D. S. (1967a). *Intern. J. Leprosy* **35**, 187.
Ridley, D. S. (1967b). *Trans. Roy. Soc. Trop. Med. Hyg.* **61**, 84.

Ridley, D. S., and Hilson, G. R. F. (1967). *Intern. J. Leprosy* **35**, 184.
Ridley, D. S., and Jopling, W. H. (1966). *Intern. J. Leprosy* **34**, 255.
Russell, D. A., Scott, G. C., and Wigley, S. C. (1964). *Intern. J. Leprosy* **32**, 235.
Russell, D. A., Scott, G. C., and Wigley, S. C. (1968). *Intern. J. Leprosy* **36** (4), Pt. 2, Abstr. No. 122.
Sato, S., and Nishimura, S. (1967). "Mykobacterien und mykobakterielle Krankheiten," Vol. 9. Fischer, Jena.
Schneider, J., Languillon, J., Clary, J., and Picart, P. (1960). *Méd. Trop.* **20**, 543.
Schulz, E. J., and Falkson, G. (1965). *Lancet* **i**, 912.
Schulz, E. J., and Falkson, G. (1967). *Leprosy Rev.* **38**, 221.
Schulz, E. J., Egnal, M. L., and Doevendans, G. (1966). *Leprosy Rev.* **37**, 47.
Scott, G. C., Wigley, S. C., and Russell, D. A. (1966). *Intern. J. Leprosy* **34**, 139.
Sensi, P., Ballotta, R., Greco, A. M., and Gallo, G. G. (1961). *Farmaco (Pavia), Ed. Sci.* **16**, 165.
Shepard, C. C. (1960). *J. Exptl. Med.* **112**, 445.
Shepard, C. C. (1964). *Science* **146**, 403.
Shepard, C. C. (1965a). *Am. J. Epidemiol.* **81**, 150.
Shepard, C. C. (1965b). *J. Immunol.* **96**, 279.
Shepard, C. C. (1967a). *Intern. J. Leprosy* **35**, 616.
Shepard, C. C. (1967b). *Proc. Soc. Exptl. Biol. Med.* **124**, 430.
Shepard, C. C. (1967c). *Intern. J. Leprosy* **35**, 429.
Shepard, C. C., and Chang, Y. T. (1962). *Proc. Soc. Exptl. Biol. Med.* **109**, 636.
Shepard, C. C., and Chang, Y. T. (1964). *Intern. J. Leprosy* **32**, 260.
Shepard, C. C., and Guinto, R. S. (1963). *J. Exptl. Med.* **118**, 195.
Shepard, C. C., and McRae, D. H. (1965). *J. Bacteriol.* **89**, 365.
Shepard, C. C., and Redus, M. A. (1967). *Intern. J. Leprosy* **35**, 348.
Shepard, C. C., McRae, D. H., and Habas, J. A. (1966). *Proc. Soc. Exptl. Biol. Med.* **122**, 893.
Sheskin, J. (1965a). *Clin. Pharmacol. Therap.* **6**, 303.
Sheskin, J. (1965b). *Leprosy Rev.* **36**, 183.
Sheskin, J., and Convit, J. (1966). *Hautarzt* **17**, 548.
Sheskin, J., and Sagher, F. (1968). *Leprosy Rev.* **39**, 203.
Sheskin, J., Sagher, F., Dorfman, M., and von Schrader-Beielstein, H. W. (1968). *Israel J. Med. Sci.* **4**, 901.
Silva, N. C., and Andrade, R. S. C. (1963). *Intern. J. Leprosy* **31**, 555.
Simpson, I. A. (1949). *Intern. J. Leprosy* **17**, 208.
Smith, A. E. W. (1964). *Leprosy Rev.* **35**, 55.
Smith, M. I., Jackson, E. L., and Bauer, H. (1949). *N.Y. Acad. Sci.* **52**, 704.
Thompson, P. E. (1967). *Intern. J. Leprosy* **35**, 605.
Tolentino, J. G. (1957). *Intern. J. Leprosy* **25**, 351.
Trappmann, R. (1961). *Intern. J. Leprosy* **29**, 46.
Trautman, J. R., and Callaway, J. C. (1965). *Intern. J. Leprosy* **33**, 206.
Wardekar, R. V. (1967). *Leprosy in India* **39**, 155.
Waters, M. F. R. (1963). *Leprosy Rev.* **34**, 173.
Waters, M. F. R. (1968). Personal communication.
Waters, M. F. R., and Rees, R. J. W. (1962). *Intern. J. Leprosy* **30**, 266.
Waters, M. F. R., Rees, R. J. W., and Sutherland, I. (1967). *Intern. J. Leprosy* **35**, 311.
Wheeler, E. A., Hamilton, E. G., and Harman, D. J. (1965). *Leprosy Rev.* **36**, 37.
Williams, T. W., Mott, P. D., Wertlake, P. T., Barba Rubio, J., Adler, R. C., Hill, G. J., Perez Suarez, G., and Knight, V. (1965). *Intern. J. Leprosy* **33**, 767.

Wilson, T. M. (1967). *Practitioner* **199**, 817.

World Health Organization (1966). Expert Committee on Leprosy, Third Report World Health Organ. Tech. Rept. Ser. **319**.

World Health Organization (1968a). *World Health Organ. Tech. Rept. Ser.* **403**.

World Health Organization (1968b). *Intern. J. Leprosy* **36** (4), Pt. 2, Abstr. No. 123.

Yanagisawa, K., and Asami, N. (1958). *La Lepro* **27**, 107.

Chemotherapy of Chlamydial Infections

ERNEST JAWETZ

Departments of Microbiology, Medicine, and Pediatrics,
University of California Medical Center,
San Francisco, California

I. Introduction—Biological Characteristics of Chlamydiae—Types of Clinical Disease

The agents of psittacosis, lymphogranuloma venereum [LGV], and trachoma are a large group of nonmotile, gram-negative, obligate intracellular parasites possessing a similar morphology and a common group antigen. These agents multiply in the cytoplasm of their host cells by a distinctive developmental cycle. The group includes some important human and animal pathogens. In the interest of brevity the generic term "chlamydiae" will be used here to denote agents of the psittacosis-LGV-trachoma group (Moulder, 1966; Page, 1966).

Because of their obligate intracellular parasitism, these agents were once considered viruses. However, the chlamydiae differ from true viruses in the following important characteristics (Moulder, 1964, 1966):

(1) They contain both RNA and DNA; viruses have only one nucleic acid in their extracellular form.

(2) They multiply by binary fission; viruses never do.

(3) They possess a cell wall of the bacterial type, with mucopeptide containing muramic acid; viruses never do.

(4) They possess ribosomes; viruses never do.

(5) They have a variety of metabolically active enzymes, e.g., they can liberate CO_2 from glucose. Some chlamydiae can use extracellular *p*-aminobenzoic acid to synthesize folates.

(6) Their growth can be inhibited by many antimicrobial drugs. Chlamydiae may be considered as gram-negative bacteria, which lack some important mechanisms for the production of energy and are thereby restricted to an obligate intracellular existence.

The above list of characteristics clearly defines chlamydiae as very closely related to bacteria. Possessing a bacterial cell wall, they can be expected to be subject to inhibitors of cell-wall synthesis, such as penicillin and cycloserine. Those chlamydiae that require extracellular *p*-aminobenzoic acid and must synthesize their own dihydropteroic and folic acids can be expected to be susceptible to the sulfonamides. Some bacterial type of protein synthesis is required for growth and development of chlamydiae, and thus they may be inhibited by tetracyclines, chloramphenicol, and erythromycin-like drugs. The relative efficacy of these different agents in experimental or natural infections will be described in subsequent sections.

All chlamydiae share a general sequence of events in their reproduction. The infectious particle is small ("elementary body"), measuring about 0.3 μ in diameter with an electron-dense center. It enters susceptible host cells, perhaps by phagocytosis. A vacuole, derived from host cell membranes, forms around the small particle, and it is then reorganized into a larger one ("initial body"), which measures 0.5–1.0 μ in diameter and has no electron-dense center. Within the membrane-bound vacuole the large particle grows in size and divides repeatedly by binary fission, until the entire vacuole becomes filled with small particles, and forms an "inclusion" in the host cell cytoplasm. Some chlamydiae (e.g., trachoma-inclusion conjunctivitis (TRIC), LGV) form inclusions which contain a glycogen-like matrix in which particles are embedded. This matrix stains brown with dilute Lugol's iodine. All mature chlamydial inclusions stain dark purple by Giemsa's method because of the densely packed mature particles. Finally, the newly formed small particles may be liberated from the ruptured host cell cytoplasm to infect new cells. The entire developmental cycle takes 24 to 48 hours.

An outstanding characteristic of chlamydial infections is the balance that is often reached between host and parasite, resulting in prolonged, often lifetime infections. Subclinical infections with chlamydiae are the rule, and overt disease is the exception in the natural hosts of these agents. Spread from one species to another (e.g., bird to man) or disturbance of natural host resistance (e.g., shipment of birds; bacterial conjunctivitis in man) may precipitate overt disease. While chlamydial infection is commonly associated with the development of antibodies, these globulins often have little protective effect against exacerbation of disease or reinfection. Immunization of animals or man has been singularly unsuccessful in protecting against infection. At best immunization, or prior infection, has induced partial resistance which could result in milder disease after challenge or reinfection (Meyer and Eddie, 1962). Very intensive, early, prolonged treatment with antimicrobial drugs can suppress antibody formation and occasionally can result in the elimination of the infectious chlamydiae. More commonly, however, the administration of antimicrobial drugs suppresses active replication of chlamydiae and thereby aids in clinical recovery, but fails to eliminate the infectious agent. Ultimately, eradication of infection is a function of host responses. It is in this general framework that chemotherapy of chlamydial infections must be considered.

II. Action of Antimicrobial Drugs on Chlamydiae in Experimental Models

Until recently, chlamydiae had been considered viruses because of their obligate intracellular habitat, and reviews on viral chemotherapy mentioned the effects of sulfonamides and antibiotics on the "large viruses" of the psittacosis-LGV-trachoma group (Cutting *et al.*, 1947; Eaton, 1950; Hurst and Hull, 1956). In view of the facts presented above, this notion must be discarded. Antibacterial drugs act on chlamydiae because chlamydiae in essence are bacteria (Moulder, 1964), and it can be postulated that the mechanism of drug action on chlamydiae is probably comparable to that on bacteria.

Many different experimental infections have been employed in attempts to quantify and compare the activity of antimicrobial drugs on chlamydiae. The infected mouse, embryonated egg, and cell culture have been used most widely. Each of the models has its own peculiarities, and no model entirely mirrors treatment of infection in the natural host. The greatest weight must therefore be given to controlled therapeutic studies in natural hosts, e.g., man or bird. Regrettably, only few adequately controlled treatment trials are available, and most clinical reports rely on the anecdotal method. The greatest hazard in attributing therapeutic significance to a drug given to only a few patients is the failure to acknowledge that spontaneous, sometimes dramatic, recovery is part of the natural history of infectious diseases. This is a particular problem in chlamydial infections, because they exhibit a very wide spectrum of clinical severity. Disease patterns vary greatly with time and place, even within a single well-defined clinical entity.

Among experimental models, different variables and parameters must be considered. The mouse may be infected intracerebrally or intraperitoneally, may receive drug prophylactically or therapeutically, in a single dose or multiple doses. The earlier a drug is administered and the longer high levels are maintained, the greater is the likelihood of survival of the animal, or even eradication of the infectious agent. The later drug administration is started, the greater the probability of persistent infection in surviving animals.

The yolk sac of the embryonated egg permits growth of all chlamydiae (Cox, 1938). It provides a relatively uniform system for drug testing. However, it often permits the administration of only a single dose of drug, and therefore emphasizes relative drug lability. While embryonated eggs are virtually devoid of natural host defenses, intermittent periods of insusceptibility to infection may vitiate the usefulness of the system (Jawetz *et al.*, 1962a).

Cell culture approaches an ideal assay system for quantitative drug-susceptibility testing of chlamydiae, comparable to the testing of bacteria *in vitro*. Obviously, cell culture assay results are not directly applicable to drug action in the intact host. There are also differences in the susceptibility of different cell lines, and certain types of chlamydiae are altogether incapable of unlimited replication in cell culture (Jawetz, 1964). The end point for assay of drug action must be chosen arbitrarily, e.g., the formation of inclusions, the release of infective particles, the maturation of chlamydiae as evidenced by acridine-orange staining, or others. In spite of these variables, it is likely that the study of drug action in cell culture will reveal important relationships between drugs and chlamydiae, and that some of this information may be applicable to therapeutic problems.

In the following section, I shall briefly discuss each major class of drugs. Because of the diversity of the models employed in different studies, I shall emphasize general conclusions which appear valid rather than individual specific results.

A. Sulfonamides

It came as a shock to many virologists when some casual experiments (McCallum and Findlay, 1938) indicated that the "large virus" of LGV in mice was susceptible to sulfonamides. Later, other chlamydiae were shown to be inhibited by sulfonamides in various hosts, including man. Little would be gained by listing the many reports which describe in some detail the activity of one or another sulfonamide against different chlamydiae. Instead, just two points will be discussed: The first concerns the evidence that the chlamydiae which are inhibited by sulfonamides possess the enzymatic machinery to utilize extracellular *p*-aminobenzoic acid for the synthesis of folic acid, and thus are analogous to sulfonamide-susceptible bacteria (Moulder, 1962). The second point discusses the claim that chlamydiae can be subdivided into two distinct groups on the basis of sulfonamide-susceptibility, and that this character is sufficiently stable to serve as the basis of classification (Moulder, 1966; Page, 1968).

Sulfonamides inhibit the growth of bacteria by blocking the incorporation of *p*-aminobenzoic acid (PABA) into the folic acid molecule. Folic acid is a component of all living cells, participating in essential enzymatic reactions. Bacteria that make their own folic acid from PABA are sulfonamide-sensitive, whereas bacteria that require exogenous preformed folic acid, and animal cells, are sulfonamide-resistant. Morgan (1948) and others showed that the sulfonamide inhibition of some chlamydiae was reversed by PABA, as is the case with sulfonamide-sensitive bacteria. Moulder (1962) summarized the evidence that chlamydiae, which are sulfonamide-sensitive, possess the machinery for synthesis of folic acid and carry out folic acid metabolism entirely equivalent to that of bacteria.

All bacteria are inhibited by structural analogs of folic acid such as aminopterin because the formation of the coenzyme form of folic acid is prevented. Aminopterin also inhibits the early stages of psittacosis agent replication in cell culture, and this inhibition can be reversed by folinic acid (Pollard and Sharon, 1963). This further emphasizes the similarity between bacteria and chlamydiae.

In early studies on LGV (Shaffer *et al.*, 1944; Jones *et al.*, 1945), it had been observed that some LGV isolates were relatively resistant to sulfonamides and that sulfonamide-treated mice sometimes yielded drug-resistant strains of the agent. Hurst *et al.* (1950) pointed out that LGV strains varied markedly in the degree of sulfonamide sensitivity. Golub (1948) demonstrated rapid development of resistance to sulfonamides in psittacosis strains passed through eggs containing drug. A high degree of sulfonamide resistance emerged in mouse pneumonitis agent passed through the lungs of mice receiving the drug, and the variants subsequently remained resistant when passed in the absence of sulfonamides (Loosli *et al.*, 1954–1955). Most TRIC agent isolates tested thus far have been susceptible to sulfonamides, but Johnston *et al.* (1962) and Shiao *et al.* (1967) have reported observations on some relatively sulfonamide-resistant TRIC isolates. Tests in the treatment of infected monkey eyes, however, failed to confirm the relative *in ovo* sulfonamide resistance of certain isolates (Shiao *et al.*, 1967). It may be assumed that the various sulfonamide-resistant variants represent mutants which are resistant by virtue of requiring an exogenous supply of folic acid.

The examples listed above illustrate the relative ease with which sulfonamide-resistant mutants can be selected from sulfonamide-sensitive populations of chlamydiae. This raises serious doubts as to the validity of employing the sulfonamide marker as a means of classification. Yet such a classification of chlamydiae has been proposed (Page, 1968).

Gordon and Quan (1965) divided chlamydiae into two groups on the basis of inclusion morphology and glycogen deposition. Subgroup A (including LGV, mouse pneumonitis, TRIC agents, etc.) form compact inclusions which regularly contain glycogen. Subgroup B (including avian psittacosis strains, and various mammalian isolates) form diffuse inclusions which do not contain glycogen. Lin and Moulder (1966) noted that most subgroup A strains are inhibited by sulfadiazine 4 μM per embryo, whereas most group B strains (except psittacosis strain 6 BC) are resistant to that amount of drug. Only 13 strains were examined in comparative tests. Nevertheless, the description "growth in the yolk sac of the chicken embryo is inhibited by sodium sulfadiazine, 1 mg per embryo" now forms part of an official key to the speciation of chlamydiae (Page, 1968). The wisdom may be questioned of including a marker of such evident instability in a classification scheme. At least one other psittacosis agent strain (Gleason) is known to be sulfonamide-sensitive (Meiklejohn *et al.*, 1946), whereas one recent isolate from clinical LGV is sulfonamide-resistant (Schachter, 1967).

B. Penicillins and Cycloserine

Chlamydiae have a cell wall of the bacterial type (Perkins and Allison, 1963). Therefore, inhibitors of cell wall synthesis may be expected to inhibit chlamydial replication. Penicillin G was shown quite early to inhibit chlamydial growth in embryonated eggs (Early and Morgan, 1946; Meiklejohn *et al.*, 1946; Eaton *et al.*, 1948; Weiss, 1950) or in mice (Bedson, 1959; Wiseman *et al.*, 1946). However, relatively large quantities of penicillin were required for inhibition, e.g., 250 units prior to infection of eggs with a psittacosis strain, in keeping with the resemblance of chlamydiae to gram-negative, rather than gram-positive, bacteria. Smaller amounts of penicillin G (e.g., 50–200 units per egg) did not completely inhibit TRIC agent replication, and permitted T'ang *et al.* (1957) to isolate the first strains of trachoma agent. However, similar amounts of penicillin protected eggs from death with established TRIC strains.

All derivatives of 6-aminopenicillanic acid, possessing antibacterial activity, act by the same mechanism. It is not surprising, therefore, that other penicillins, e.g., ampicillin, are inhibitory for chlamydiae (Allison and Busby, 1962).

Penicillin-resistant variants of chlamydiae have been selected by prolonged passage of sensitive strains in eggs containing subinhibitory concentrations of penicillin (Moulder *et al.*, 1955; Gordon *et al.*, 1957, 1960a,b). Most of the variants bred true and thus appeared to be stable mutants. Some exhibited additional changes in biologic characteristics, e.g., loss of lethality, altered antigenic features or change in susceptibility to other drugs (Woodroofe and Moulder, 1960; Greenland, 1961). Chlamydiae do not produce penicillinase. The exact nature of their penicillin resistance is not understood but probably resides in structural changes of the cell wall architecture.

Cycloserine also inhibits bacterial cell wall formation, probably because it is a structural analog of D-alanine, and inhibits the incorporation of that amino acid into the mucopeptide. Cycloserine inhibits chlamydiae of subgroup A (Gordon and Quan, 1965; Lin and Moulder, 1966) much more efficiently than those of subgroup B. This suggests a fundamental difference in the cell wall structure of groups A and B. The inhibition of cycloserine, 5–10 μM per embryonated egg, of group A chlamydiae can be completely reversed by D-alanine 1 mole per 0.4 mole of cycloserine (Moulder *et al.*, 1963), whereas this does not apply to group B. This association of cycloserine inhibition with group A of chlamydiae is incomplete: At least one group A (mouse pneumonitis) strain is resistant to cycloserine and at least one group B (goat) strain is susceptible (Lin and Moulder, 1966).

There are great variations in the quantity of penicillin required for the inhibition of different strains of TRIC agents in eggs (Jawetz and Hanna, 1960; Jawetz *et al.*, 1962b; Shiao *et al.*, 1967). At a given concentration of penicillin (e.g., 3–5 μg per egg), there may be a thousandfold range in the amounts of TRIC agent of different strains inactivated.

In cell cultures as little as 0.1 μg/ml penicillin G sometimes interfered with the production of infective chlamydiae, but even a thousandfold larger concentration did not completely prevent the production of early developmental forms seen microscopically (Bernkopf *et al.*, 1962). The inhibition of cell wall formation of penicillin may lead to bizarre structural forms of chlamydiae observed by light microscopy (Weiss, 1950; Kravchenko *et al.*, 1961; Bernkopf *et al.*, 1962) and electron microscopy (Bernkopf *et al.*, 1962; Armstrong and Reed, 1967). Under the influence of penicillin, very large, vacuolated forms develop, perhaps as a result of continuing growth of initial bodies which fail to divide. Perhaps these forms are analogous to bacterial spheroplasts. In addition to inhibiting cell wall formation, penicillin also blocks the formation, or deposition, of glycogen in inclusions of chlamydiae belonging to subgroup A (Becker *et al.*, 1962; Bernkopf *et al.*, 1962; Gordon and Quan, 1962). Evidently, penicillin does not influence the toxic factor of chlamydiae in mice, in spite of protecting the animals against death from infection (Manire and Meyer, 1950).

C. Tetracyclines

Wong and Cox (1948), Gogolak and Weiss (1950), Allen *et al.* (1953), and others initially demonstrated the efficacy of tetracyclines in suppressing chlamydial infection in embryonated eggs and mice. One milligram of chlortetracycline per egg or per mouse was sufficient to permit survival of the host, but from surviving mice chlamydiae could be recovered. Because chlortetracycline was the first tetracycline to be proved effective, this most labile member of the group remained prominent in clinical treatment of chlamydial infections for several years. For instance, it is surprising that for a decade chlortetracycline was used in millions of persons infected with trachoma in spite of the availability of more stable tetracyclines. Perhaps the initial good results with chlortetracycline in embryonated eggs, infected with chlamydiae by the yolk sac route, were made possible by a substance in yolk which protected the drug from rapid breakdown at incubator temperature (Womack *et al.*, 1950).

Subsequently, other, more stable tetracyclines were shown to be effective drugs in laboratory models (Eaton, 1950; Loosli *et al.*, 1954–1955; Hurst, 1962; Bedson, 1959). During the last decade, tetracyclines have maintained their position as the most effective of all available drug groups in chlamydial infections. Most observations indicate that tetracyclines suppress chlamydial growth and replication but fail to eliminate the agent from an infected host. In bacteria, tetracyclines do not affect the synthesis of nucleic acids, but they block protein synthesis, perhaps by interfering with the transfer of amino acids from the activated transfer RNA (tRNA) to the growing peptide chain on the ribosome. It is assumed that the mechanism of tetracycline action is the same in chlamydiae, although Pollard and Tanami (1961) stated that tetracycline "interrupted the cytochemical sequence which reflected maturation of the virus," whereas penicillin and sulfonamides only delayed maturation.

By weight, tetracyclines appear to be more effective than penicillin. From 1 to 10 μg tetracycline HCl per egg prevent death from chlamydial infection in contrast to 5 to 50 μg penicillin G per egg required for the same effect (Jawetz *et al.*, 1962; Shiao *et al.*, 1967; Tarizzo and Nabli, 1967). Different strains of chlamydiae differ up to a thousandfold in their susceptibility to tetracyclines, as estimated by the amount of infectious agent inactivated by a given drug concentration (Jawetz *et al.*, 1962b; Shiao *et al.*, 1967). To some extent, tetracycline susceptibility is a strain characteristic, but the overlap between strains is too great to permit use of this characteristic for classification.

Rare tetracycline-resistant mutants can be selected from chlamydial populations (Gordon *et al.*, 1957, 1960a; Moulder *et al.*, 1965). Some of these mutants are stable, and there is a suggestion that the genetic trait of tetracycline-resistant mutants may be transmitted from heat-inactivated, resistant to viable, susceptible chlamydiae (Gordon *et al.*, 1960b). Some tetracycline-resistant mutants are also resistant to cycloserine, perhaps reflecting a genetically controlled change in surface structure (Moulder *et al.*, 1965).

Clinical and epidemiologic impressions have suggested from time to time that chlamydiae of increasing resistance to tetracyclines might gain prevalence. Shiao *et al.* (1967) performed detailed quantitative susceptibility tests on TRIC agents in order to find objective laboratory evidence regarding this possible emergence of resistance. They estimated the reduction in infective agent at various drug levels, as done earlier by Jawetz *et al.* (1962b). The results of these tests revealed a wide range of susceptibility of different clinical isolates, with some more resistant to tetracyclines than the mean of the group. Isolates obtained from a single locality (Taiwan) five years apart did not differ in their responses. The results of drug-susceptibility tests in embryonated eggs are somewhat variable and must be confirmed extensively before they can be accepted as meaningful. Tarizzo and Nabli (1967) have proposed another method for drug-susceptibility testing of chlamydiae which is said to be highly reproducible. At the present time, however, there is no reliable correlation between the results of any laboratory test and the clinical experience which may point to the possible emergence of tetracycline resistance in chlamydiae.

D. Chloramphenicol, Erythromycins

In 1946, chloramphenicol was shown to be effective in protecting mice and chick embryos against psittacosis agent (Smadel and Jackson, 1947). Quantitative comparisons, however, indicated that chloramphenicol was 3- to 10-fold less active by weight than tetracyclines (Wells and Finland, 1949; Eaton, 1950; Hurst, 1962; Johnston *et al.*, 1962; Jawetz, 1964; Bietti and Werner, 1967). This seems somewhat surprising because in most bacterial systems chloramphenicol is a more potent inhibitor of protein synthesis than tetracycline, and it also penetrates tissues and cells more readily. Perhaps some specific chlamydial characteristic of protein synthesis is reflected in the lower efficacy of chloramphenicol in laboratory models and in man.

The activity of erythromycins (erythomycin, oleandomycin, triacetyloleandomycin, carbomycin, tylosin, etc.) in laboratory models of chlamydial infection was similar to that of tetracyclines in some investigations (Endo, 1964; Tarizzo and Nabli, 1967) and much lower in others (Loosli *et al.*, 1954–1955; Hurst, 1962; Jawetz *et al.*, 1962b; Bietti and Werner, 1967). Pollard and Tanami (1961) believed that tylosin tartrate interrupted the cytochemical sequence of chlamydial maturation in cell cultures more effectively than other drugs. There is no support for this sentiment in other studies.

E. Aminoglycosides, Polymyxins, Bacitracin, Vancomycin, Nystatin

These drugs are of particular importance in experimental work with chlamydiae, because they permit chlamydial growth in concentrations which effectively inhibit certain bacteria or fungi (Early and Morgan, 1946; Gordon and Quan, 1962; Jenkin and Hung, 1967). The aminoglycosides (streptomycin, neomycin, kanamycin) are particularly useful in this regard because they inhibit many common contaminants, which might occur in specimens designed for the isolation of chlamydia.

Streptomycin (1–10 mg per egg, or 16 μg/ml in cell culture) does not impair replication of most strains of chlamydiae. Higher concentrations may have a slight inhibitory effect (Gordon and Quan, 1962). T'ang *et al.* (1957) employed streptomycin (5 mg per egg, or more) in the first successful isolation of trachoma agents. Kanamycin or neomycin 0.1% may be applied to eyes infected with TRIC agents prior to the removal of specimens for TRIC agent isolation. They can also be mixed with the specimen and inoculated into eggs (Sowa *et al.*, 1965). These drugs tend to suppress bacterial flora of the conjunctiva but do not suppress chlamydiae. The lack of antichlamydial action of the aminoglycosides may be attributed, in part, to their poor penetration into cells. It has been long known, and was recently reemphasized (Ekzemplyarov, 1965) that streptomycin does not enter cells readily; and that intracellular concentrations are only a small fraction of extracellular drug levels. By contrast, tetracyclines may owe part of their efficacy against chlamydiae to their good cell penetration which results in similar intra- and extracellular drug levels.

Vancomycin (1.5 mg/ml) permitted growth of chlamydiae in eggs and cell cultures and inhibited some gram-positive bacterial contaminants (Jenkin and Hung, 1967). Bacitracin (1000 units per egg) did not inhibit chlamydial growth, but in cell culture this drug may have a suppressive effect—perhaps due to surface action on host cells (Gordon and Quan, 1962). Similarly polymyxin B (100 μg per egg) does not inhibit chlamydial growth, but in cell culture this drug may be inhibitory.

Nystatin (3000 units per ml) has been used to reduce fungal contamination, without inhibiting chlamydial growth in eggs (Gordon and Quan, 1962).

In summary the drugs mentioned in this section are important because they may permit the isolation of chlamydiae from specimens contaminated with bacteria or fungi.

III. Psittacosis and Ornithosis: Natural Infection in Birds

Chlamydial infections are exceedingly common in virtually all avian species. Infection in psittacine birds (e.g., parrots, cockatoos, parakeets) is traditionally called psittacosis, whereas chlamydial infections in other birds is often called ornithosis. Infection of birds is frequently latent, with chlamydiae being present in some organs, especially the spleen and liver, and shed in feces. Natural transmission occurs commonly from latently infected adults, who shed chlamydiae in feces, to nestling birds. Latent avian infection may be transformed into active disease by stresses induced by crowding, shipment, deprivation of water or food, and other drastic changes in environmental conditions. Birds with active, progressive disease develop sepsis, lesions in many organs, wasting, and they may die. Sick birds excrete much larger quantities of infectious chlamydiae than latently infected animals and therefore are more commonly the cause of chlamydial infections in man. On the other hand, repeated and prolonged exposure of man to latently infected birds may also result in infection. Among the personnel of poultry farms involved in the dressing, packing, and shipping of ducks, geese, turkeys, and chickens, chlamydial infection (subclinical or clinical) is relatively frequent.

Chemotherapy of chlamydial infections in birds was stimulated largely by the economic problems of aviaries which sell psittacine birds. Such birds often present a health hazard to their human contacts. Therefore, restrictive legislation was employed in the past to limit importation of birds, and infected aviary stocks of birds were subject to seizure and destruction. As an alternative measure, treatment of birds could be used to rid them of suspected or proved infection.

After it had been established that tetracyclines were highly effective drugs in experimental models of chlamydial infection, some field trials for the treatment of infected birds were undertaken.

Meyer *et al.* (1958) summarized the results of extensive trials in aviaries which compared the efficacy of tetracyclines administered to psittacine birds by injection, or mixed in food or water. Intramuscular injection of 1 mg tetracycline in aqueous solution twice daily for 14 days was effective but cumbersome and expensive. Tetracycline in oily suspension injected intramuscularly on only two occasions was also effective but expensive and not without risk to the birds. Tetracyclines in feed in daily doses of approximately 2.5–5 mg given for 15 days not only suppressed signs of illness but also eradicated the chlamydiae from a high proportion of birds. Tetracycline in drinking water was somewhat less reliable because of irregular intake.

After some additional years of experience, Meyer (1962) developed the following recommendations: Psittacine birds weighing 200 to 1000 gm should receive for 30 days or more a medicated feed containing tetracycline 10 mg per gm of feed. Such treatment could eliminate chlamydiae from a majority of birds. Reinfection from contacts was possible, of course, but animals that had been cured of an infection were somewhat more resistant to disease from reinfection. Additional controlled studies added some further information (Arnstein, 1967). Cooked grain rations containing 0.5% to 1.0% chlortetracycline (the cheapest bulk drug) were fed to infected parrots daily for 45 days. Within the first two to five days, birds developed levels of 2–4 μg tetracycline per milliliter of plasma. At the end of the treatment period, most infected birds given drug-free rations yielded chlamydiae from blood and feces, whereas the drug-treated birds did not. At the end of a 6-month observation period, there was a 74.5% mortality in infected controls compared to a 12.0% mortality among originally infected but treated birds. Tetracycline treatment was much more effective in salvaging parrots and eliminating infection from aviaries than experimental administration of inactivated vaccines (Arnstein, 1967).

Drug prophylaxis of ornithosis in turkey poults was also effective. Turkey poults were experimentally inoculated at 3 weeks of age with psittacosis chlamydiae, while receiving feed containing various quantities of chlortetracycline (Davis and Delaplane, 1958). Poults on feed without tetracycline had a mortality rate of 81%. Those receiving 100 or 200 gm of chlortetracycline per ton of feed survived but exhibited signs of infection and developed lesions which yielded chlamydiae. Poults receiving 400 to 800 gm of chlortetracycline per ton of feed had no disease, no lesions, and yielded no chlamydiae. Thus prophylaxis on a commercial scale seems possible, although certainly not uniformly successful. If a great deal of commercially used poultry feed were to contain tetracycline, one wonders what influence this might have on the emergence of tetracycline-resistant mutants of chlamydiae. At the present, no epidemiologic information is available in that regard. During the above-mentioned trials, no tetracycline-resistant mutants were isolated from birds whose tissues still contained chlamydiae after tetracycline treatment.

IV. Psittacosis in Man

The term psittacosis, applied to human disease, signifies a chlamydial infection of man acquired through direct or indirect contact with birds. While many mammals are infected with chlamydiae, their role in transmission to man is not established. Human infection is most commonly acquired through the respiratory tract, by inhalation of dried bird feces, or infected aerosols. Subclinical infection is very common in exposed persons. If illness develops, there is usually an incubation period of 7–14 days, followed by a sudden onset of fever, malaise, anorexia, sore throat, and severe headache. The illness may resemble influenza and resolve without specific signs in a few days. On the other hand, it may progress to severe prostration, suggestive of sepsis with or without symptoms and signs pointing to pulmonary involvement. Clinical and radiologic signs may show widespread diffuse pneumonitis, which often resolves slowly. Fatality rates vary with different outbreaks; in elderly untreated patients, they may be as high as 20%.

The clinical suspicion of psittacosis is often supported by epidemiologic evidence of contact with birds, and by marked rise in complement-fixing antibody titer, or by laboratory isolation of the chlamydiae from blood or sputum.

With the recognition that antibacterial drugs were able to inhibit chlamydiae in laboratory models, virtually every drug has undergone occasional use in clinical psittacosis. However, no extensive series of cases has been published to illustrate any one drug regimen, and no controlled clinical trials have been carried out. Most records refer to single cases or to small outbreaks. The variability of the disease often does not permit an objective assessment of the value of the drugs used.

Isolated cases of psittacosis were treated with sulfonamides in the early 1940's (Bedson, 1959). In spite of the recent speciation proposal (Page, 1968), which removes any chlamydial isolate inhibited by sulfadiazine (1 mg per egg) from *Chlamydia psittaci*, there can be little doubt that some strains of psittacosis agent (6 BC and others) are sulfonamide-susceptible (Bedson, 1959). However, the majority of patients suffering from psittacosis are probably not helped by sulfonamide therapy. Individual cases are reported whose chlamydial pneumonitis progressed during the administration of sulfadiazine or sulfamerazine 3–4 gm daily (Flippen *et al.*, 1945; Perlman and Milzer, 1954).

When it was established that penicillin could suppress the growth of psittacosis agents in mice and eggs, certain patients were treated with penicillin from 1944 on. In an occasional case, a sudden improvement (return of temperature to normal, clearing of lungs) was associated with the administration of very small doses, e.g., 100,000 units daily of penicillin G (Flippin *et al.*, 1945). More commonly the response was a gradual one to daily doses of 300,000 to 600,000 units of penicillin daily. At times both penicillin and a tetracycline were administered simultaneously (Perlman and Milzer, 1954; Grist, 1964). It is difficult to decide in most published cases whether the clinical improvement occurred spontaneously as part of the natural course of disease or whether the drug treatment was responsible. If one calculates a human curative dose of penicillin from the dose effective in a laboratory model, it becomes apparent that at least 10 to 20 million units in a 7-day period must be administered. Most of the penicillin treatments between 1940 and 1955 employed far smaller doses which were probably inadequate. When a dose of 12 million units was given in 7 days to a patient in 1948, he apparently responded fairly promptly (Bedson, 1959). Treatment of a chronic human carrier with penicillin 8 million units given intramuscularly in 10 days, together with the inhalation of 50,000 units every 3 hours during the same period, had some questionable clinical effects but definitely failed to eradicate the infectious agent from the lung. Psittacosis chlamydiae were recovered from sputum 40 and 60 days and 2 years after this treatment (Meyer and Eddie, 1951).

In summary, penicillins could possibly be employed for the treatment of human psittacosis, provided very large doses were given. In the small doses employed in the past, penicillin is not a useful drug in human psittacosis, and recent cases of psittacosis have progressed during penicillin administration (Schaffner *et al.*, 1967).

The success of chlortetracycline in experimental infections with chlamydiae (Wong and Cox, 1948; Hurst *et al.*, 1950) was rapidly followed by the application of this drug to human psittacosis. The administration of 2–3 gm of tetracycline per day often resulted in striking improvement within 36 to 48 hours, and the response seemed sufficiently constant to attribute it to the drug (Green, 1950; Perlman and Milzer, 1954). The variability of the clinical course in human psitttacosis, however, must be considered in evaluating tetracycline effects. Thus Pollard *et al.* (1954) treated their own laboratory infections very promptly after onset of symptoms, using only 1 gm of tetracycline daily for 2–4 days. Response was rapid in all three individuals—but was it spontaneous improvement, or effective early treatment? A family outbreak in 1954 led to the entire spectrum of disease, from one rapidly fatal case to one very mild infection requiring no treatment and one asymptomatic infection. The fourth person in this family responded gradually while being treated with tetracycline, 2 gm per day (Prouty and Jordan, 1956). A similar spectrum on severity of disease was proposed by Goto *et al.* (1961). A series of middle-aged women who developed erythema nodosum during their psittacosis infection received tetracycline treatment and all recovered—but the response was equivocal (Sarner and Wilson, 1965). Three of 9 patients seen at Vanderbilt University failed to respond to tetracycline, whereas the remainder did (Schaffner *et al.*, 1967).

In spite of rather fragmentary evidence, there is a prevailing belief that tetracyclines are probably the drugs of choice in psittacosis infection. For persons exhibiting significant illness, full systemic doses (2 gm daily for adults) are recommended (Grist, 1964; Barrett and Greenberg, 1966; Schaffner *et al.*, 1967) in articles and in textbooks. Occasionally protracted drug administration of more than one course of 2 weeks' treatment is considered to reduce the chances for relapse and enhance the opportunity for eradication of the chlamydiae. There is no solid basis for this suggestion. In mild or localized psittacosis infections, tetracycline, 1 gm daily for several weeks, has been prescribed (Schachter *et al.*, 1968) but, again, the response was by no means dramatic and infectious chlamydiae were isolated weeks after inception of treatment.

A few reports mention the use of choramphenicol (1–2 gm daily for adults) in place of tetracycline, or even with tetracycline. Slow response, followed by relapse was seen in exceedingly ill patients with pneumonia (Schaffner *et al.*, 1967), but patients with milder psittacosis appeared to respond (Valasek, 1967).

When children acquire psittacosis infection, the majority have only a mild illness in spite of the ease with which chlamydiae can be isolated from the blood. Tetracycline in full systemic doses (20–40 mg/kg/day for 14 days) is recommended, but the evidence for benefit from such treatment is marginal (Berman *et al.*, 1955; Grantova and Milek, 1968).

From the evidence quoted, and many other clinical reports, one can conclude that tetracyclines are probably the drugs of choice in human psittacosis infection, but that the response is irregular. The great variability of the disease makes it difficult to clearly separate spontaneous improvement from a therapeutic response to the drug.

V. Lymphogranuloma Venereum (LGV)

Lymphogranuloma venereum (LGV) is a systemic infection usually acquired as a venereal disease. A small papule develops on genitalia 5–20 days after sexual exposure. This lesion is painless, often not noticed, and heals spontaneously. The infectious chlamydiae spread through lymphatics to reach the regional lymph nodes and the blood stream. Enlargement of regional nodes begins about 2 weeks after the appearance of the primary lesion and is determined by its location. If the primary lesion is on penis or vulva, the inguinal glands often become involved, suppurate, and drain pus through multiple sinuses. If the primary lesion is in the vagina or in the rectum, the perirectal and para-aortic glands become involved. There is often fever, and occasionally arthritis, meningoencephalitis, and a variety of rashes. Involvement of regional lymph nodes may subside spontaneously and rapidly or may persist for months or years. Chronic inflammation of lymphatics may induce fibrosis, proctitis, rectal strictures (especially in women or homosexual males) or elephantiasis of genitalia.

The disease picture can be notoriously variable, and the results of treatment are therefore difficult to evaluate. The most definite responses to treatment may be seen in persons who have suffered for months or years with active proctitis or inflammatory stricture, i.e., lumen narrowed by inflammation of wall, and are abruptly improved after antimicrobial drug treatment for just one or two weeks (Greenblatt, 1952).

During active early LGV, the skin test group antigen (Frei test) tends to become positive, and complement-fixing antibodies with group reactivity appear in the serum. Eradication of the infection may lead to disappearance of these antibodies. This disappearance of antibodies has been employed as a possible criterion for therapeutic success.

Early studies in laboratory models indicated the susceptibility of the chlamydiae of LGV to both sulfonamides and to penicillin (McCallum and Findlay, 1938; Meiklejohn *et al.*, 1946). Shaffer *et al.* (1944) and Hurst *et al.* (1950) stressed that there were marked differences in the degree of sulfonamide sensitivity of different strains of LGV. In early clinical use, sulfonamides were believed to be effective in altering the natural course of the disease. Some preference for sulfonamides was expressed because they would not tend to mask syphilitic infection coexisting with LGV (Bedson, 1959). In recent years, however, sulfonamides have lost favor because of the belief that many LGV infections were not affected by their administration in full dosage. Patients systemically ill with LGV usually also failed to respond to penicillin (Jawetz, 1948), although it is clear that treatment with large doses was not attempted.

After Wong and Cox (1948), Hurst *et al.* (1950) and others had established the effectiveness of chlortetracycline in laboratory models of LGV infection, the tetracyclines soon became the favorite drugs for treatment of clinical LGV. Wright *et al.* (1948) demonstrated the regression of buboes after 4–8 days of chlortetracycline [20 mg injected once daily (!)] in 8 patients, and the improvement in proctitis in 3 patients; 14 persons with rectal strictures showed no definite change. In retrospect, one may wonder whether the pain associated with the intramuscular injection of chlortetracycline may have acted as a deterrent to the subsequent promiscuity of these patients.

Greenblatt (1952) applied his large experience with LGV to an evaluation of drug treatment. Of 21 patients with LGV proctitis or stricture, 15 were definitely improved by oral tetracycline (1–2 gm daily for 7 to 60 days), and 3 of 6 patients were similarly improved by chloramphenicol. However, the complement-fixing antibody titer remained unchanged in virtually all these patients, suggesting persistence of the infection. The number of patients in any one group was too small to evaluate possible differences between chlortetracycline, oxytetracycline, or chloramphenicol, but the latter was given less credit for therapeutic efficacy.

Erskine (1958) reviewed 61 cases of LGV, many of whom were treated with oxytetracycline (2 gm daily for 10 days) and then given a second identical course of treatment after 1 week's interval. Of 21 patients with early LGV, 19 were considered "cured," with their antibody titers declining. Of 39 patients in later stages of LGV, at least 10 failed to respond to two courses of tetracycline treatment, but in a majority the degree of improvement was difficult to assess. Another British study (Goldberg and Banov, 1956) failed to detect a fall in antibody titer in late cases of LGV treated with tetracycline (15–25 gm) and then followed for 1–2 years. While there was questionable symptomatic improvement in a few patients, the constant antibody titer was taken to indicate failure of the drug to eradicate the chlamydiae.

A major attempt at a controlled study of LGV treatment to date was made by Greaves *et al.* (1957). These authors clearly recognized the extreme variability of the disease caused by LGV and the obvious need to compare patients who receive only symptomatic treatment with those who are treated with specific antimicrobial drugs. Forty-three patients were seen 1 to 37 days after onset of a bubo and were assigned in rotation to one of four treatments or to a control group. Patients received antibiotic (chloramphenicol, chlortetracycline, oxytetracycline) 1 gm initially followed by 0.5 gm 4 times daily for 14 days, or sulfadiazine 2 gm initially followed by 4 gm daily for 10 to 28 days, or comparable numbers of aspirin tablets. Fourteen patients were lost from the study. In the 26 patients who finished antimicrobial treatment, the total mean duration of the bubo was 31 days, as compared to 69 days in the controls. This shortened clinical course is of marginal statistical significance. The patients receiving sulfadiazine or oxytetracycline fared somewhat better than the other two drug groups, but the numbers are too small for statistical evaluation. The number of persons developing complications (bubonic relapse after healing, skin lesions, or sinus formation) was too small to permit valid comparisons; however, in each instance complications were more common among those treated symptomatically.

The serologic response to treatment was unequivocal. In all 26 patients who had received antimicrobial drugs, the antibody titer had decreased 4-fold or more 1 year after treatment, whereas only 7 of 17 patients treated symptomatically showed this decline. It was concluded that all antimicrobial drugs had a beneficial effect, that none was clearly superior (within the limitations of the study), and that sulfonamides might well be the drugs of choice because of availability and low cost.

An attempt was made to evaluate the treatment of LGV in Jamaica by using a complex scoring system (Sigel, 1962). Both clinical response and movement of antibody titer were considered. Tetracyclines and sulfonamides were quite successful, chloramphenicol and erythromycin-like drugs less so. In this series, as in all reported ones, several general observations were made. The earlier treatment was administered, the more striking the response. Whereas some patients responded well, all series mention individual failures. In view of the type of host-parasite relationship involved in LGV and the very chronic disease process, short-term results mean relatively little and long-term follow-up seems essential for comprehensive evaluation of treatment. Clearly, there is great need for a controlled clinical study of comprehensive nature to provide guide-lines for optimal therapy.

During the last few years, there has been an increasing number of LGV infections among American military personnel in Southeast Asia. Some of these patients have exhibited fairly severe systemic disease, reminiscent of the cases I observed in 1946 (Jawetz, 1948). There is a prevalent impression that tetracycline (4 gm daily) for several weeks is necessary to improve these patients and that sulfonamides are not regularly of benefit. There is, however, no detailed evidence available at the time of this writing to substantiate these impressions.

VI. Trachoma-Inclusion Conjunctivitis (TRIC)

This group of infections characteristically involves the eye and the genital tract. Tissue reactions involve hyperemia, exudate, follicular hypertrophy and scarring, with comparable changes occurring in conjunctiva, urethra, and cervix. In addition, neovascularization and scarring of the cornea may lead to pannus formation, opacity, and blindness. The chlamydiae causing trachoma and those causing inclusion conjunctivitis cannot be distinguished from each other in the laboratory with certainty at present. It is also becoming clear that either type of agent can induce a complete spectrum of disease from minimal and self-limited to fulminant and blinding. The classic forms of each disease picture are given below.

A. Trachoma

The onset is often insidious, with lacrimation, mucopurulent discharge, and conjunctival hyperemia. This is followed by follicular hypertrophy, epithelial keratitis, subepithelial infiltration, and extension of vessels into the cornea (pannus). Over a period of months or years, the pannus may progress across the cornea, there may be scarring of conjunctivae, lid deformity, secondary bacterial infection, and blindness. It is estimated that over 400 million people throughout the world are infected, of whom 20 million people have been blinded. The disease is most prevalent in Africa and Asia, particularly where water is scarce and hygienic conditions are poor. Transmission is most probably mechanical—from eye to eye by fingers and fomites.

B. Inclusion Conjunctivitis

Most commonly this occurs as an acute purulent conjunctivitis of the newborn, involving particularly the lower lids. The disease tends to be self-limited so that after several weeks of intense inflammation the process subsides, and the conjunctiva becomes normal in several months. Pannus and scarring do not usually develop in the child. The newborn acquires the infection from the mother's cervix during the passage through the birth canal. Inclusion conjunctivitis is fundamentally an infection of the adult human genital tract, and is spread primarily through sexual contact. The infection of the adult female is often asymptomatic, or produces cervicitis. In the adult male, infection is often asymptomatic or associated with urethritis. While the adult disease is typically a venereal disease, the adult eye may be infected and a clinical picture indistinguishable from trachoma may result (Jones and Collier, 1962).

Trachoma is a disease well-recognized since antiquity and involving vast numbers of people. The literature concerning its treatment includes several hundred major titles. Many of the more important contributions are listed in the monumental review of Bietti and Werner (1967), to which the reader is directed for specific references. Only a few selected issues will be discussed here, in an attempt to evaluate the available evidence. The literature is replete with enthusiastic claims, testimonials, authoritarian statements and recommendations, but there is great dearth of objective evidence or controlled studies. Among the many reasons for the difficulty in evaluating the treatment of TRIC-agent eye disease, a few may be listed:

(1) There is great variability in the severity of disease, influenced by locale, climate, availability of water, socioeconomic standing, race, age, etc.

(2) Clinical trachoma is often a composite of chlamydial infection and bacterial infection. The suppression of bacterial superinfection alone may result in marked improvement.

(3) TRIC agents may remain latent in the conjunctiva for months or years, then become reactivated to produce disease. Endogenous relapse and exogenous reinfection cannot be differentiated unequivocally. Absence of clinical signs following treatment does not mean eradication of the infectious agent.

(4) The criteria for clinical activity, regression, and healing vary greatly from one study to another; there is also a very large, probably unavoidable observer error in clinical evaluation.

C. Sulfonamides

From antiquity until the mid-1930's, treatment consisted of the application of metal salts and vegetable compounds to the eye, combined with surgical procedures. The use of sulfonamides topically and systemically from 1937 on was received with enormous enthusiasm. There was little doubt that these drugs were capable of modifying in a dramatic fashion the course of progressive eye disease attributed to trachoma and its bacterial complications, and that with prolonged treatment the cytoplasmic inclusions typical of active infection with TRIC agents tended to disappear. The prevalence of clinical trachoma in the southwestern part of the United States permitted Forster and McGibony (1944) to treat a very large number of patients with sulfanilamide given orally 60 mg per kg per day for 3 weeks. It was estimated that blood levels of sulfanilamide exceeded 3 mg% in all and 5 mg% in many of the patients. On the basis of clinical follow-up examinations performed from 1 to 6 months after the end of treatment, it was estimated that about 75% of "over 20,000 patients" were clinically cured by a single 3-week course. Those that still showed activity were given a second course of sulfanilamide, resulting in a 90% cure rate. No improvement was noted from the topical application of sulfanilamide.

After such initial successes virtually all other sulfonamides were tried at one time or other in chronic trachoma. Emphasis was placed on convenience of administration, safety, and speed and completeness of clinical response. With the more rapidly excreted sulfonamides, it was neceessary to give several doses daily, for several days each week, making mass treatment cumbersome. The advent of slowly excreted, long-acting sulfonamides (e.g., sulfadimethoxine, sulfamethoxypyridazine) permitted the administration of a single dose (100 mg/kg) once every week for 12 weeks, with marked clinical improvement of from one third to two thirds of active cases (Bietti and Werner, 1967). Endless varieties of treatment schedules were employed in different countries. Thus one group in northern India employed sulfadimethoxine (100 mg/kg once weekly for 3 months) and estimated a 50% cure rate in trachomatous children (Shukla *et al.*, 1966). Another group in India employed sulfadimethoxine (250 mg twice weekly every fourth week for 6 months) in 3- to 6-year-old children and found that "as a result of treatment the active trachoma was reduced from 68.4 to 36.4%, whereas in the control village 64.2% of children were active initially and 65.1% at the final examination" (Gupta, 1966). Investigators in Italy (Ghione *et al.*, 1967) expressed the belief that prolonged presence of low levels of well-diffusing drugs were a paramount requirement of effective sulfonamide treatment. Bietti *et al.* (1967) believed that some long-acting sulfonamides may be administered in low dose (e.g., 20 mg/kg) by mouth once every 10–15 days for 3 months, to yield cure rates of about 80%, when clinical examinations are carried out at the end of treatment. Reassessment was urged 3 and 6 months later because recurrences were seen in 10% to 15% of apparently "cured" individuals. The possibility of relapse, rather than reinfection had not been given much weight in most of these studies.

These glowing reports on successful treatment with sulfonamide must be contrasted with the experiences in controlled trials, where matched individuals received either drug or placebo and the evaluations were conducted by double-blind methods and evaluated statistically. Foster *et al.* (1966) conducted a controlled trial of treatment in American-Indian children and found that "cure rates" were 60% 6 months after treatment with either topical tetracycline, oral sulfonamides, or a placebo. Woolridge *et al.* (1967) found a cure rate of 16% in sulfonamide-treated, and of 22% in placebo-treated children on Taiwan, 6 months after the end of a course of trisulfapyrimidines, 3 gm daily for 4 weeks.

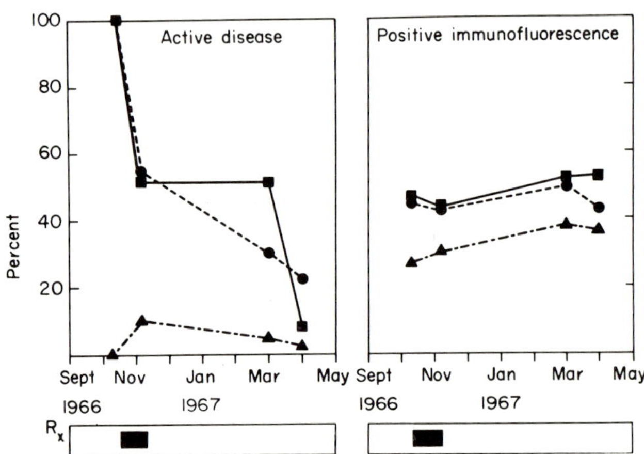

FIG. 1. Results of oral sulfisoxazole therapy (4 gm daily for 3 weeks) for trachoma. ■, placebo (33 schoolchildren); ●, sulfisoxazole (34 schoolchildren); ▲, not active October, 1966 (203 schoolchildren). Reproduced from Lancet **ii**, 961, 1967 by permission.

Our group (Dawson *et al.*, 1967) introduced another type of evaluation into controlled trials by estimating not only the clinical activity of disease but also the prevalence of the infectious agent in conjunctival scrapings examined by immunofluorescence. Groups of American-Indian children residing in a boarding school during and for 6 months after the treatment trials were treated in a double-blind fashion, either with an oral suspension of sulfisoxazole, 4 gm daily, for 3 weeks, or with placebo. Clinical and laboratory examinations were carried out before, during, and at intervals after the treatment trial. Figure 1 summarizes the results of clinical examinations and of immunofluorescence. There was a marked diminution in the number of children with clinical activity, but the incidence of positive immunofluorescence remained constant during the 7 months' observation. There was no difference between the drug and the placebo group by either form of examination. The marked improvement in environmental hygiene seemed to be the responsible beneficial influence, leading to reduction of clinical activity, but the immunofluorescence findings suggested that the persistence of the etiologic agent was not influenced by either drug or environment. Subsequent studies were carried out by our group in two boarding schools for American-Indian children, with similar results, employing trisulfapyrimidines given orally, 3.5 gm daily, for 21 consecutive days. Blood samples were obtained on day 12 and 16, respectively, of the treatment program, from all children, about 1–2 hours after the second daily dose. The average blood levels of sulfonamide (expressed as the equivalent of sulfanilamide both free and combined) in one school were 7.90 mg% (range 1.7–15.8 mg%) and in the other school 7.61 mg% (range 1.8–16.2 mg%). All 32 children on drug therapy had measurable sulfonamide levels, whereas only 1 of the 32 children on placebo had a sulfonamide level of 5.9 mg%. This child was eliminated from the analysis of results, because it was not clear whether she might have received drug instead of placebo, or whether the blood sample had been mislabeled accidentally. Figure 2 summarizes the findings in one of the schools.

It is again evident that the incidence of immunofluorescence is unchanged by either residence at the boarding school or the administration of sulfonamide drugs. In one school, the group receiving either drug or placebo were entirely comparable from the standpoint of clinical examinations with both groups, showing marked improvement in clinical appearance at all examinations during the 7-month observation period. In the other school, however, the group receiving sulfonamide had significantly less clinical activity for 2 months following the drug treatment than did the placebo group. At the end of the observation time, the difference between the groups was no longer significant.

It must be stated with great emphasis that these trials do not reflect the trachoma problem as it appears in the field in most hyperendemic countries. There, trachoma is almost universally complicated by bacterial infection, and these bacterial infections greatly aggravate both the signs of active disease and the progression toward blindness. By contrast, the controlled trials in American-Indian children were carried out in the virtually complete absence of bacterial infection. These children have "pure" chlamydial eye infection which rarely progresses to blindness. Thus the trials of chemotherapy evaluated only the "antichlamydial effect" in very small groups but cannot be considered

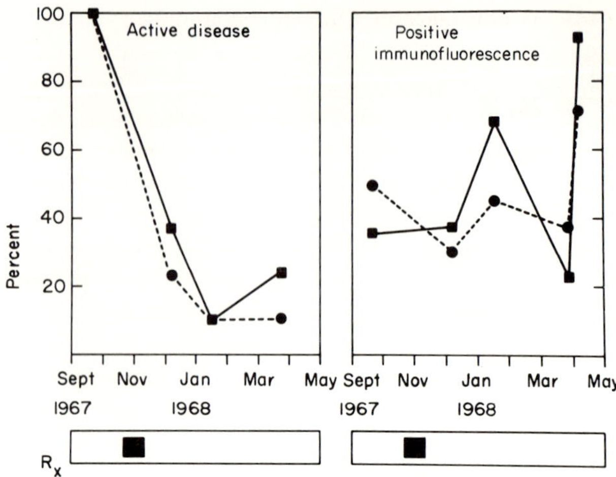

FIG. 2. Results of oral trisulfapyrimidines therapy (3.5 gm daily for 3 weeks) for trachoma. ■, placebo (14 schoolchildren); ●, trisulfapyrimidines (15 schoolchildren).

applicable to situations where bacterial superinfection forms an important and universal part of trachomatous eye disease. It is hoped that future controlled drug trials will be performed in areas of the world where trachoma is severe and commonly complicated by bacterial superinfection. It must also be remembered that the total treatment period in the controlled trials was only 3–4 weeks. Perhaps sulfonamide levels are required for a much longer period of time (e.g., 3–4 months) in order to permanently eliminate the infectious agent.

One of the most central problems in the treatment of chronic trachoma is the well-established host-parasite relationship. By contrast acute TRIC-agent infection is far more susceptible to treatment, and eradication of the chlamydiae should be possible. In the earliest volunteer inoculations performed with egg-grown TRIC agent, Collier *et al.* (1960) observed complete clinical recovery after 10 days' treatment with a sulfonamide. Khaw *et al.* (1963) observed the rapid and apparently permanent cure of experimentally infected volunteers treated with sulfonamides. Jawetz *et al.* (1967) studied acute TRIC-agent infection in volunteers and its response to treatment. Soon after the inception of sulfisoxazole administration (3 gm daily for 2 weeks) marked clinical improvement was accompanied by negative immunofluorescence. Several patients relapsed microbiologically, with immunofluorescence becoming positive again, although clinical relapse was rare. A second, identical course of sulfisoxazole was regularly followed by permanently negative immunofluorescence, i.e., apparent eradication of the acute infection (Fig. 3). We have not yet seen a relapse after such a second course of sulfonamide in an acutely infected volunteer.

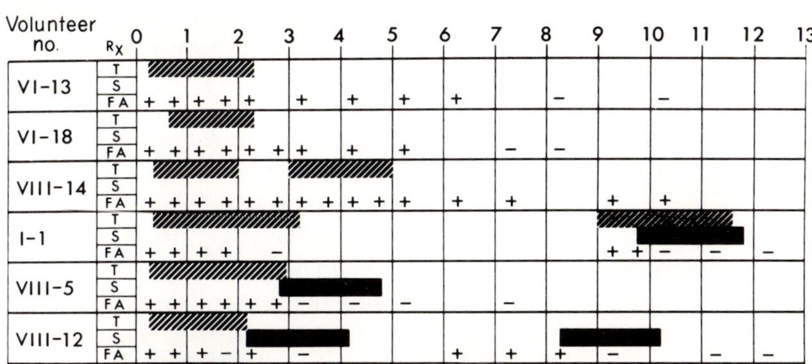

FIG. 3. Acute TRIC-agent infection in volunteers and their response to treatment. T, topical tetracycline HCl (1%) ointment, 3 times daily; S, sulfisoxazole, 1 gm by mouth, 3 times daily; FA, results of immunofluorescent stain of conjunctival scraping.

In this summation of sulfonamide effects, I have made no attempt to weigh the possible side effects of various types of drugs. There can be little doubt that the highly soluble preparations (e.g., trisulfapyrimidines, sulfisoxazole) tend to induce fewer renal complications and a lower incidence of serious hypersensitivity reactions, particularly in children, than long-acting preparations (e.g., sulfadimethoxine, sulfapyridazine). This review attempts only to evaluate the efficacy of drugs that are acceptable for general use. In any consideration of treatment, the physician must weigh the benefits of a given drug against its probable risk.

D. PENICILLINS

While penicillin has a marked effect on TRIC agents in laboratory models, the effect in the human eye is marginal, perhaps due to inadequate levels achieved locally. Gilkes *et al.* (1958) noted marked abnormalities in TRIC-agent inclusions in the eyes of patients soon after penicillin injections were begun. Later there was marked clinical improvement and inclusions disappeared altogether for days or weeks. Patients were not followed sufficiently well to establish microbiologic relapse. Acutely infected volunteers (Collier *et al.*, 1960) improved only slightly during the injection of penicillin (1 million units daily for 10 days) and relapsed clinically soon thereafter. The predominantly negative attitude toward penicillin in the therapy of TRIC-agent infections is reviewed by Bietti and Werner (1967).

E. Tetracyclines

The advent of chlortetracycline in the therapy of ocular infections was greeted with enthusiasm. Topical application of a 1% solution was proclaimed to be effective in inclusion conjunctivitis (Braley and Sanders, 1948). The impact of this finding was diminished by the claim that chlortetracycline was also effective in dendritic keratitis (caused by herpes simplex virus) and in epidemic keratoconjunctivitis (caused by adenovirus type 8) virus infections, which are certainly not susceptible to tetracycline action. However, enthusiastic acceptance of tetracyclines continued: "The treatment of trachoma . . . has reached a point where modern antibiotic treatment is so effective that a few days on local Terramycin or Aureomycin is all that is necessary. It is nothing short of a miracle when one considers that this worldwide scourge can be cured within two weeks" (Braley, 1952). The rosy glow subsided somewhat when Mitsui *et al.* (1951) treated 173 patients with chronic trachoma by the application of 1% tetracycline ointment 3 times daily for 8 weeks and did careful clinical follow-up examinations. Among severe cases, 53% were "clinically cured," among mild cases 83%. There was no laboratory follow-up. Based on these and many other reports, the World Health Organization attempted a mass treatment campaign among school children in Morocco (Reinhards *et al.*, 1959). Chlortetracycline ointment 1% was applied to the eyes of nearly 9000 schoolchildren with active trachoma two or three times daily for 60 days, and "cure" rates were claimed to approach 80%. Oxytetracycline, 1% in oil instilled into children's eyes twice daily for 5 days per month for 6 consecutive months resulted in a "cure" rate of 75% in India in 1962–1963 (Nema *et al.*, 1965). These accounts, and dozens more (Bietti and Wener, 1967), support the belief that tetracycline applied topically is an effective method to suppress the clinical signs of trachomatous eye disease in endemic populations, provided a sufficient dose (0.5% ointment) is given 4–6 times daily for a sufficient period of time (6 weeks) with adequate follow-up.

It is difficult to evaluate the basis for this apparent success. In part, it is likely that suppression of the bacterial superinfection is important. TRIC agents can also be suppressed in the eye by topical tetracycline, but even in acute disease chlamydiae are not easily eradicated (Jawetz *et al.*, 1967). Thus one might expect the most spectacular success of topical tetracycline treatment in areas of the world where there is extensive bacterial superinfection of trachoma. This might explain the failure of this treatment in Taiwan or in schools for American-Indians where bacterial infection is rare (Dawson *et al.*, 1967; Woolridge *et al.*, 1967). Yet another explanation might be the emergence of tetracycline resistance among the prevalent strains of TRIC agents, but there is little support for this belief (Shiao *et al.*, 1967).

Acute infection with TRIC agents is much more susceptible to tetracycline treatment (as was the case with sulfonamides) than chronic, established disease. An example might be the inclusion conjunctivitis of the newborn which rapidly improves with the topical administration of tetracycline ointment (Chiang *et al.*, 1968) and usually heals completely. By contrast, infection with similar agents, resulting in "inclusion conjunctivitis of the adult," becomes chronic and then is difficult to eradicate (Schachter *et al.*, 1967). In this context, it must be remembered, however, that infection and disease of the newborn tend to be self-limited even without antimicrobial therapy, and that even in the adult, infection with inclusion conjunctivitis agents is said to regress spontaneously. In volunteers acutely infected with TRIC agents, the topical administration of tetracycline ointment generally suppressed the signs of clinical activity within a few days. While the inflammatory lesions were suppressed, there was often progression of subepithelial infiltrates (perhaps a manifestation of hypersensitivity). Furthermore, the chlamydiae often persisted in the conjunctiva during tetracycline administration, as evidenced by positive immunofluorescence. Even two courses each consisting of the application of ophthalmic tetracycline ointment 0.5% 3 times daily for 14 days, did not promptly eliminate the chlamydiae (see Fig. 3). This provides striking illustration for the inhibitory activity of tetracyclines but their lack of chlamydiacidal activity.

Orally administered tetracyclines have had only limited trial. Children with active trachoma receiving 0.5 gm oxytetracycline by mouth twice daily for 6–8 weeks had a "cure" of about 50% when examined 2 months after the end of treatment. They received no topical drug (Bietti and Werner, 1967). In a later trial, 21 children with active trachoma (trachoma II) in Sardinia were given demethylchlortetracycline, 300 mg by mouth once every other day for 3 months. One month after the end of therapy, 76% were considered clinically cured, and 2 months later 85.5% were in that category. Less frequent, or shorter, administration of the same drug had less effect (Bietti and Lanzieri 1957).

If one considers that tetracyclines are the most active drugs against chlamydiae in laboratory models, and that their penetration and diffusion are good, systemic treatment with tetracyclines might be expected to be highly successful in TRIC infections. Unfortunately, there have been no controlled trials.

F. Chloramphenicol and Erythromycin

Chloramphenicol is looked upon with less favor by ophthalmologists who treat TRIC infections, and it has the reputation of being less effective both in laboratory models and in man (Bietti and Werner, 1967). Oral chloramphenicol, 3 gm daily for 3–8 days, then 1.5 gm daily for 2–4 more days, was given to trachomatous adults by Pijoan *et al.* (1950). Blood levels of 8–12 μg/ml were reached and the treatment "resulted in amelioration of the disease." No meaningful prolonged follow-up or extended treatment were reported.

The role of erythromycin in the treatment of TRIC infections is equally uncertain. Button (1955) treated Navajo Indian children with oral erythromycin, 4–6 mg/kg every 4–6 hours for 12 days. The clinical appearance of their trachoma is said to have improved significantly. However, there are marked differences in the absorption of erythromycin preparations, and it is not certain what systemic levels were achieved in this trial which, in any case, was uncontrolled. A comparative study of the action of erythromycin and chlortetracycline was carried out in Tunis (Nataf *et al.*, 1963). Groups of children with active trachoma were given ointment containing one or the other drug in comparable 1% concentration, twice daily for 5 days per week, for 6 weeks. Both groups improved, the clinical signs diminished, but chlamydiae could be isolated after the treatment from at least one patient who had improved clinically. There was no difference in the response of the groups treated with erythromycin or tetracycline ointment. The investigators felt that the antibiotics were suppressive, but were unlikely to eliminate the infectious agent. Cure would depend on factors of individual resistance in addition to the effect of drugs.

Our group has employed oral erythromycin estolate (1.5 gm daily for 10 days) in the treatment of acute TRIC infection in 11 volunteers. The clinical signs of active inflammation subsided very slowly, and chlamydiae persisted throughout the course of treatment in a majority of volunteers as evidenced by positive immunofluorescence and prompt clinical relapse after the end of treatment. These were uncontrolled observations only, and we could not be certain that each volunteer ingested his drug doses regularly and reliably. Nevertheless, these observations are not encouraging toward the usefulness of erythromycins in TRIC infections, in spite of favorable impressions from laboratory models (Pollard and Tanami, 1961).

In conclusion, it appears that acute TRIC infection of short duration can be cured effectively by systemic sulfonamides or topical tetracyclines administered for several weeks. Systemic tetracyclines are probably equally effective, but the evidence for other drugs is—thus far—unconvincing.

Chronic trachoma presents a complex problem in which environmental and personal hygiene greatly contribute to the outcome of any treatment. Systemic sulfonamides in full doses or topical tetracyclines can suppress clinical signs, if treatment is of sufficient duration. However, there is no convincing evidence at present that any presently accepted form of treatment will regularly eliminate TRIC agents from the chronically infected eye.

VII. Summary

Chlamydiae are obligate intracellular parasites, related to gram-negative bacteria but quite distinct from viruses. They produce a variety of human and animal infections, which are characterized by great chronicity and latency, some of which produce disease in millions of individuals. Chlamydiae are susceptible to a variety of antibacterial drugs in laboratory models. While acute infections in animals or man can sometimes be cured by the administration of certain drugs, treatment of chronic infection is difficult. Often drug administration results in the suppression of signs and symptoms of disease but fails to eradicate the infectious agent. Prolonged administration of relative large doses of drugs is advisable in treating chronic chlamydial infections. The present status of various drugs has been reviewed and their efficacy compared in laboratory models and in human infections. The need for more quantitative and controlled studies is emphasized.

ACKNOWLEDGMENTS

Supported, in part, by research grants from the National Institutes of Health (NB 00604 and 5 TO1 AI00299) and from the Burroughs Wellcome Fund.

I have not attempted to conduct a formal survey of the literature or to list the many hundreds of papers that bear some relationship to the topic of discussion. I have mentioned a few papers published as late as May 1968. Miss Lavelle Hanna and Dr. J. Schachter have reviewed the manuscript and made valuable suggestions. However, the selection of material is my responsibility and the opinions expressed are mine.

REFERENCES

Allen, E. G., Girardi, A. J., Sigel, M., and Klein, M. (1953). *J. Exptl. Med.* **97**, 783.

Allison, A. C., and Busby, D. (1962). *Brit. Med. J.*, **ii**, 834.

Armstrong, J. A., and Reed, S. E. (1967). *J. Gen. Microbiol.* **46**, 435.

Arnstein, P. (1967). *Am. J. Ophthalmol.* **63**, 1260.

Barrett, P. K. M., and Greenberg, M. J. (1966). *Brit. Med. J.* **ii**, 206.

Becker, Y., Mashiah, P., and Bernkopf, H. (1962). *Nature* **193**, 271.

Bedson, S. P. (1959). *J. Roy. Inst. Public Health Hyg.* **22**, 131.

Berman, S., Freudlich, E., Glaser, K., Abrahamov, A., Ephrati-Elizur, E., and Bernkopf, H. (1955). *Pediatrics* **15**, 752.

Bernkopf, H., Mashiah, P., and Becker, Y. (1962). *Ann. N.Y. Acad. Sci.* **98**, 62.

Bietti, G. B., and Lanzieri, M. (1957). *Rev. Intern. Trachome* **34**, 270.

Bietti, G. B., and Werner, G. H. (1967). "Trachoma: Prevention and Treatment." Thomas, Springfield, Illinois.

Bietti, G. B., Pannarale, C., and Milano, C. (1967). *Am. J. Ophthalmol.* **53**, 1569.

Braley, A. E. (1952). *Ann. N.Y. Acad. Sci.* **55**, 1056.

Braley, A. E., and Sanders, M. (1948). *J. Am. Med. Assoc.* **138**, 426.

Button, R. R. (1955). *Am. J. Ophthalmol.* **39**, 223.

Chiang, W. T., Alexander, E. R., Wei, P. Y., and Fresh, J. W. (1968). *Am. J. Obstet. Gynecol.* **100**, 422.

Collier, L. H., Duke-Elder, S., and Jones, B. R. (1960). *Brit. J. Opthalmol.* **44**, 65.

Cox, H. R. (1938). *Public Health Rept.* (*U.S.*) **53**, 2241.

Cutting, W. C., Dreisback, R. H., Halpern, R. M., Irwin, E. A., Jenkins, D. W., Proescher, F., and Tripi, H. B. (1947). *J. Immunol.* **57**, 379.

Davis, D. E., and Delaplane, J. P. (1958). *In* "Progress in Psittacosis Research and Control" (F. R. Beaudette, ed.). Rutgers Univ. Press, New Brunswick, New Jersey.

Dawson, C. R., Hanna, L., and Jawetz, E. (1967). *Lancet* **ii**, 961.

Early, R. L., and Morgan, H. R. (1946). *J. Immunol.* **53**, 151.

Eaton, M. D. (1950). *Ann. Rev. Microbiol.* **4**, 223.

Eaton, M. D., Dozois, T. F., Van Allan, A., Parish, V. L., and Schwahm, S. (1948). *J. Immunol.* **58**, 251.

Ekzemplyarov, O. N. (1965). *Antibiotiki* **10**, 425.

Endo, K. (1964). *Acta Soc. Ophthalmol. Japan* **68**, 1794.

Erskine, D. (1958). *Brit. J. Venereal Diseases* **34**, 163.

Flippen, H. F., Gaydosh, M. J., and Fittipoldi, W. V. (1945). *J. Am. Med. Assoc.* **128**, 280.

Forster, W. G., and McGibony, J. R. (1944). *Am. J. Ophthalmol.* **27**, 1107.

Foster, S. O., Powers, D. K., and Thygeson, P. (1966). *Am. J. Ophthalmol.* **61**, 451.

Ghione, M., Brivio, R., Sanfilippo, A., and Schioppacassi, G. (1967). *Am. J. Ophthalmol.* **63**, 1573.

Gilkes, M. J., Smith, C. H., and Sowa, J. (1958). *Brit. J. Ophthalmol.* **42**, 478.

Gogolak, F. M., and Weiss, E. (1950). *J. Infect. Diseases* **87**, 264.

Goldberg, J., and Banov, L., Jr. (1956). *Brit. J. Venereal Diseases* **33**, 37.

Golub, O. J. (1948). *J. Lab. Clin. Med.* **33**, 1241.

Gordon, F. B., and Quan, A. L. (1962). *Ann. N.Y. Acad. Sci.* **98**, 261.

Gordon, F. B., and Quan, A. L. (1965). *J. Infect. Diseases* **115**, 186.

Gordon, F. B., Andrew, V. W., and Wagner, J. C. (1957). *Virology* **4**, 156.

Gordon, F. B., Bloom, H. H., Mamay, H. K., and Trimmer, R. W. (1960a). *Virology* **11**, 474.

Gordon, F. B., Mamay, H. K., and Trimmer, R. W. (1960b). *Virology* **11**, 486.

Goto, T., Shoda, H., Nakamura, H., Naito, H., Matsushima, S., Murano, J., Shimano, K., and Matumoto, M. (1961). *Japan J. Exptl. Med.* **31**, 249.

Grantova, H., and Milek, E. (1968). *Muench. Med. Wochschr.* **110**, 1130.

Greaves, A. B., Hilleman, M. R., Taggart, S. R., Bankhead, A. B., and Feld, M. (1957). *Bull. World Health Organ.* **16**, 277.

Green, T. W. (1950). *J. Am. Med. Assoc.* **144**, 237.

Greenblatt, R. B. (1952). *Ann. N.Y. Acad. Sci.* **55**, 1082.

Greenland, R. M. (1961). *J. Infect. Diseases* **108**, 287.

Grist, N. R. (1964). *Brit. Med. J.* **ii**, 21.

Gupta, U. C. (1966). *Brit. J. Ophthalmol.* **50**, 262.

Hurst, E. W. (1962). *Ann. N.Y. Acad. Sci.* **98**, 275.

Hurst, E. W., and Hull, R. (1956). *Pharmacol. Rev.* **8**, 199.

Hurst, E. W., Peters, J. M., and Melvin, P. (1950). *Brit. J. Pharmacol.* **5**, 611.

Jawetz, E. (1948). *Stanford Med. Bull.* **6**, 289.

Jawetz, E. (1964). *Ann. Rev. Microbiol.* **18**, 301.

Jawetz, E., and Hanna, L. (1960). *Proc. Soc. Exptl. Biol. Med.* **105**, 320.

Jawetz, E., Chino, S., and Hanna, L. (1962a). *J. Immunol.* **89**, 80.

Jawetz, E., Hanna, L., Chino, S., and Zichosch, J. (1962b). *Proc. Soc. Exptl. Biol. Med.* **109**, 205.

Jawetz, E., Hanna, L., Dawson, C. R., Wood, R., and Briones, O. (1967). *Am. J. Ophthalmol.* **63**, 1413.

Jenkin, H. M., and Hung, S. C. (1967). *Appl. Microbiol.* **15**, 10.

Johnston, P. B., Grayston, J. T., and Chen, P. C. (1962). *Ann. N.Y. Acad. Sci.* **98**, 280.

Jones, B. R., and Collier, L. H. (1962). *Ann. N.Y. Acad. Sci.* **98**, 212.

Jones, H., Rake, G., and Stearns, B. (1945). *J. Infect. Diseases* **76**, 55.

Khaw, O. K., Lin, H. M., Wang, S. P., Woolridge, R. L., and Grayston, J. T. (1963). *Chinese Med. J. (Republic of China)* **10**, 97

Kravchenko, A. T., Gudima, O. S., and Milyutin, V. N. (1961). *Probl. Virol. (USSR) (English Transl.)* **6**, 321.

Lin, H. S., and Moulder, J. W. (1966). *J. Infect. Diseases* **116**, 372.

Loosli, C. G., Hamre, D., Grayston, J. T., and Alexander, E. R. (1954–1955). *Antibiot. Ann.* p. 490.

McCallum, F. O., and Findlay, G. M. (1938). *Lancet* **ii**, 136.

Manire, G. P., and Meyer, K. F. (1950). *J. Infect. Diseases* **86**, 233.

Meiklejohn, G., Wagner, J. C., and Beveridge, G. W. (1946). *J. Immunol.* **54**, 1.

Meyer, K. F. (1962). *Schweiz. Med. Wochschr.* **92**, 1632.

Meyer, K. F., and Eddie, B. (1951). *J. Infect. Diseases* **88**, 109.

Meyer, K. F., and Eddie, B. (1962). *Ann. N.Y. Acad. Sci.* **98**, 288.

Meyer, K. F., Eddie, B., Richardson, J. H., Shipkowitz, N. L., and Muir, R. J. (1958). *In* "Progress in Psittacosis Research and Control" (F. R. Beaudette, ed.), pp. 163–196. Rutgers Univ. Press, New Brunswick, New Jersey.

Mitsui, Y., Tanaka, C., Toya, H., Iwashige, Y., and Yamashita, K. (1951). *A.M.A. Arch. Ophthalmol.* **46**, 235.

Mitsui, Y., Yamashita, K., and Hanabusa, J. (1955). *Antibiot. Med. Clin. Therapy* **1**, 225.

Morgan, H. R. (1948). *J. Exptl. Med.* **88**, 285.

Moulder, J. W. (1962). "The Biochemistry of Intracellular Parasitism." Univ. of Chicago Press, Chicago, Illinois.

Moulder, J. W. (1964). "The psittacosis Group as Bacteria" "Ciba Lectures in Microbial Biochemistry" pp. 0–95. Wiley, New York. 95 pp.

Moulder, J. W. (1966). *Ann. Rev. Microbiol.* **20**, 107.

Moulder, J. W., McCormack, B. R. S., Gogolak, F. M., Zebovitz, M. M., and Itatani, M. K. (1955). *J. Infect. Diseases* **96**, 57.

Moulder, J. W., Novosel, D. L., and Officer, J. E. (1963). *J. Bacteriol.* **85**, 707.

Moulder, J. W., Novosel, D. L., and Tribby, I. I. E. (1965). *J. Bacteriol.* **89**, 17.

Nataf, R., Daghfous, T., and Tarizzo, M. L. (1963). *Rev. Intern. Trachome* **2**, 163.

Nema, H. V., Nath, K., Bal, A., Joshi, O. P., and Shukla, B. R. (1965). *Brit. J. Ophthalmol.* **49**, 330.

Page, L. A. (1966). *Intern. J. System. Bacteriol.* **16**, 223.

Page, L. A. (1968). *Intern. J. System. Bacteriol.* **18**, 51.

Perkins, H. R., and Allison, A. C. (1963). *J. Gen. Microbiol.* **30**, 469.

Perlman, L., and Milzer, A. (1954). *Arch. Internal Med.* **94**, 82.

Pijoan, M., Loe, F., and Payne, E. H. (1950). *J. Trop. Med. Hyg.* **53**, 193.

Pollard, M., and Sharon, N. (1963). *Proc. Soc. Exptl. Biol. Med.* **112**, 51.

Pollard, M., and Tanami, Y. (1961). *Proc. Soc. Exptl. Biol. Med.* **107**, 508.

Pollard, M., Bussell, R. H., Benedict, A. A., and Wilson, R. (1954). *Antibiot. Chemotherapy* **4**, 138.

Prouty, R. L., and Jordan, W. S., Jr. (1956). *Arch. Internal Med.* **98**, 365.

Reinhards, J., Weber, A., and Maxwell-Lyons, F. (1959). *Bull. World Health Organ.* **21**, 665.

Sarner, M., and Wilson, R. M. (1965). *Brit. Med. J.* **ii**, 1469.

Schachter, J. (1967). *Am. J. Ophthalmol.* **63**, 1049.

Schachter, J., Rose, L., and Meyer, K. F. (1967). *Am. J. Epidemiol.* **85**, 445.

Schachter, J., Arnstein, P., Dawson, C. R., Hanna, L., Thygeson, P., and Meyer, K. F. (1968). *Proc. Soc. Exptl. Biol. Med.* **127**, 292.

Schaffner, W., Drutz, D. J., Duncan, G. W., and Koenig, M. G. (1967). *Arch. Internal Med.* **119**, 433.

Shaffer, M. F., Jones, H., Grace, A. W., Hamre, D. M., and Rake, G. (1944). *J. Infect. Diseases* **75**, 109.

Shiao, L. C., Wang, S. P., and Grayston, J. T. (1967). *Am. J. Ophthalmol.* **63**, 1558.

Shukla, B. R., Nema, H. V., Mathur, J. S., and Nath, K. (1966). *Brit. J. Ophthalmol.* **50**, 218.

Sigel, M. M. (1962). "Lymphogranuloma Venereum—Epidemiological, Clinical, Surgical and Therapeutic Aspects Based on a Study in the Caribbean." Univ. of Miami Press, Miami, Florida.

Smadel, J. E., and Jackson, E. B. (1947). *Science* **106**, 418.

Sowa, S., Sowa, J., Collier, L. H., and Blyth, W. (1965). *Med. Res. Council, Spec. Rept. Ser.* **308**, 1.

T'ang, F. F., Chang, H. L., Huang, Y. T., and Wang, K. C. (1957). *Chinese Med. J.* **75**, 429.

Tarizzo, M. L., and Nabli, B. (1967). *Am. J. Opthalmol.* **63**, 1550.

Valasek, W. (1967). *Wien. Klin. Wochschr.* **79**, 810.

Weiss, E. (1950). *J. Infect. Diseases* **87**, 249.

Wells, E. B., and Finland, M. (1949). *Proc. Soc. Exptl. Biol. Med.* **72**, 365

Wiseman, R. W., Meiklejohn, G., Lackman, D. B., Wagner, J. C., and Beveridge, G. W. (1946). *J. Immunol.* **54**, 9.

Womack, C. R., Kass, E. H., and Finland, M. (1950). *J. Lab. Clin. Med.* **36**, 655.

Wong, S. C., and Cox, H. R. (1948). *Ann. N.Y. Acad. Sci.* **51**, 290.

Woodroofe, G. M., and Moulder, J. W. (1960). *J. Infect. Diseases* **107**, 195.

Woolridge, R. L., Cheng, K. H., Chang, I. H., Yang, C. Y., Hsu, T. C., and Grayston, J. T. (1967). *Am. J. Ophthalmol.* **63**, 1577.

Wright, L. T., Sanders, M., Logan, M. A., and Hill, L. M. (1948). *J. Am. Med. Assoc.* **138**, 408.

Composition of Bacterial Cell Walls in Relation to Antibiotic Action

H. R. Perkins

National Institute for Medical Research, London, England

I. Introduction

The cell walls of bacteria are generally regarded as the layers outside the cytoplasmic membrane that are responsible for the shape and rigidity of the organisms. They are composed of several chemically distinct types of component (Table I), and separate layers making up the wall can sometimes be recognized in electron micrographs (de Petris, 1967). Since the integrity of the cell wall is necessary to the survival of the organism in its usual vegetative form, it is not surprising that several antibiotics have been found either to interfere with its synthesis or to promote its breakdown. Such antibiotics are selectively toxic for bacteria as opposed to their mammalian hosts because the bacterial wall contains building blocks, such as muramic acid, diaminopimelic acid, and D-amino acids, not found as constituents of mammalian tissues. Furthermore, these components are linked together to form a dual polymer of polysaccharide and polypeptide (the murein, mucopeptide, or peptidoglycan), the synthesis of which is as specific to bacteria as the polymer itself.

At the moment there is no evidence for any bacterial cell wall that consists only of murein, and so it is not possible to say whether an antibiotic that effectively prevented the synthesis of one of the other polymers present (Table I) would or would not be bacteriostatic or bactericidal. In other words, we do

TABLE I

Components of Bacterial Cell Walls

1. Murein (mucopeptide, glycopeptide, peptidoglycan)
2. Teichoic acids (mainly in gram-positive species; may be linked to murein)
3. Polysaccharides (e.g., teichuronic acid in *B. licheniformis* or specific polysaccharides of streptococci; often linked to murein)
4. Protein (e.g. M protein of streptococci)
5. Lipoprotein (in gram-negative species)
6. Lipopolysaccharides (in gram-negative species; consist of specific polysaccharides linked to lipid A)

not yet know whether bacteria can exist and reproduce with murein as the sole structural component outside the cytoplasmic membrane. There is some evidence, at least in *Bacillus subtilis*, that when nutritional exigencies force the organism to give up making teichoic acid, it then proceeds instead to make another acidic polymer that lacks phosphorus (Tempest *et al.*, 1968). It seems possible that murein can only be polymerized and remodeled to suit the shape of dividing organisms, of which it remains the main rigid support, if it is bathed in other more elastic layers that can act as a sort of temporary dressing while alterations are taking place.

On the other hand there is no doubt that if murein synthesis is interrupted or its dissolution promoted, then the bacteria cannot continue to reproduce unchecked. The antibiotics that are considered below all interfere in some way or other with one of these processes. At this point, therefore, we shall consider briefly what is known about murein synthesis and breakdown.

II. Murein Biosynthesis

A. Muramic Acid-Nucleotide-Peptide Precursors

The first stage involves the serial addition of amino acids, and finally of a dipeptide of D-alanine, to the carboxyl end of uridinediphosphate-*N*-acetyl muramic acid (UDP-MurNAc). The stages are outlined in Scheme I. Each of the enzymes involved is specific for the appropriate substrate, that is, the next lower member of the series. The final product is a UDP-MurNAc-pentapeptide, the detail of which varies in different bacteria. In all such intermediates so far examined, D-glutamic acid at the second position and the terminal D-alanyl-D-alanine are always present. The other two positions can apparently be filled by a variety of amino acids, as shown in Table II. Most commonly the third position is occupied by a diamino acid, so important for cross-linking as described below, although the homoserine present in certain corynebacteria seems to be an exception to this rule (Chatterjee and Perkins, 1966a). So far the amino acid in the first position has never been found to have the D-configuration, and that in the third position has either been an L-amino acid, or has involved the L-center of a diaminopimelic acid molecule. Completed

(1) UDP-*N*-acetylmuramic acid + L-alanine

$$\xrightarrow[\text{Mn}^{++}]{\text{ATP}} \text{UDP-MurNAc-L-Ala}$$

(2) UDP-MurNAc-L-Ala + D-glutamic acid

$$\xrightarrow[\text{Mn}^{++}]{\text{ATP}} \text{UDP-MurNAc-L-Ala-D-Glu}$$

(3) UDP-MurNAc-L-Ala-D-Glu + L-Lysine

$$\xrightarrow[\text{Mn}^{++}]{\text{ATP}} \text{UDP-MurNAc-L-Ala-D-Glu-L-Lys}$$

(4) UDP-MurNAc-L-Ala-D-Glu-L-Lys + D-Ala-D-Ala

$$\longrightarrow \text{UDP-MurNAc-L-Ala-D-Glu-L-Lys-D-Ala-D-Ala}$$

SCHEME I. Biosynthesis of the murein precursor of *Staphylococcus aureus*. (Ito and Strominger, 1962a,b, 1964.)

murein has been found sometimes to contain a little DD-diaminopimelic acid [15% of the total in *Bacillus megaterium* KM, (Bricas *et al.* 1967) or large amounts of D-ornithine (Perkins and Cummins, 1964)], but there is no evidence that these molecules occurred in the precursor UDP-MurNAc-pentapeptide. It seems possible, therefore, that the amino acids of the pentapeptide chain may have the following sequence of configuration L(or glycine)-D-L-D-D.

A further feature of the pentapeptide chain is that the third amino acid is attached to the γ-carboxyl group of the D-glutamic acid residue (Ito and Strominger, 1964; Muñoz *et al.*, 1966b; Perkins, 1967). At a later stage in the biosynthesis of murein the α-COOH group of the glutamic acid is either amidated (Siewert and Strominger, 1968), or substituted by glycine (Katz *et al.*, 1967) or cross-linking amino acids (Miller *et al.*, 1966; Perkins, 1967; Guinand *et al.*, 1969).

B. FORMATION OF LIPID INTERMEDIATE AND COUPLING WITH *N*-ACETYLGLUCOSAMINE

The next stage in murein biosynthesis has been worked out by use of cell-free preparations, largely in the laboratories of J. L. Strominger. In the presence of membrane preparations from *Staphylococcus aureus*, *Micrococcus lysodeikticus*, or *Escherichia coli*, radioactivity of UDP-MurNAc-pentapeptide

TABLE II

Sequence of Amino Acids in the Primary Chain of Murein

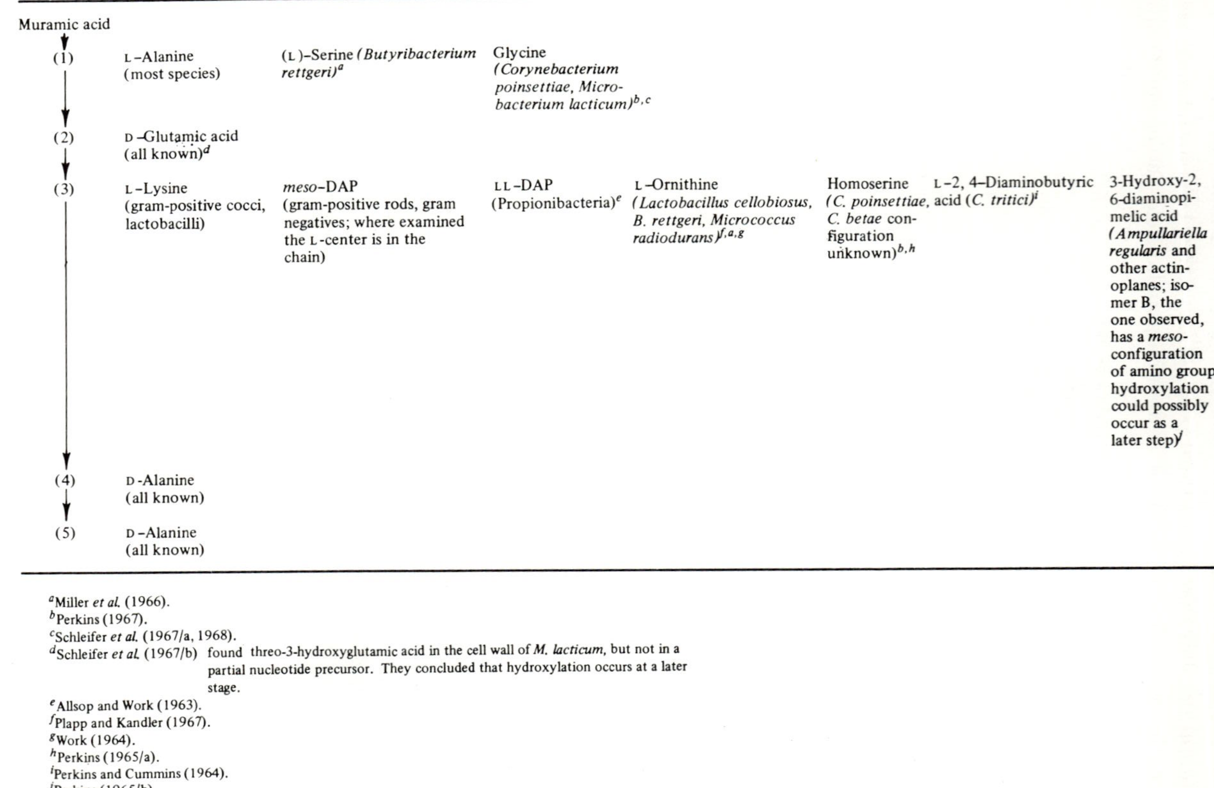

Muramic acid ↓							
(1)	L-Alanine (most species)	(L)-Serine *(Butyribacterium rettgeri)*[a]	Glycine *(Corynebacterium poinsettiae, Microbacterium lacticum)*[b,c]				
↓ (2)	D-Glutamic acid (all known)[d]						
↓ (3)	L-Lysine (gram-positive cocci, lactobacilli)	*meso*-DAP (gram-positive rods, gram negatives; where examined the L-center is in the chain)	LL-DAP (Propionibacteria)[e]	L-Ornithine *(Lactobacillus cellobiosus, B. rettgeri, Micrococcus radiodurans)*[f,a,g]	Homoserine *(C. poinsettiae, C. betae* configuration unknown)[b,h]	L-2, 4-Diaminobutyric acid *(C. tritici)*[i]	3-Hydroxy-2, 6-diaminopimelic acid *(Ampullariella regularis* and other actinoplanes; isomer B, the one observed, has a *meso*-configuration of amino groups; hydroxylation could possibly occur as a later step)[j]
↓ (4)	D-Alanine (all known)						
↓ (5)	D-Alanine (all known)						

[a] Miller *et al.* (1966).
[b] Perkins (1967).
[c] Schleifer *et al.* (1967/a, 1968).
[d] Schleifer *et al.* (1967/b) found threo-3-hydroxyglutamic acid in the cell wall of *M. lacticum*, but not in a partial nucleotide precursor. They concluded that hydroxylation occurs at a later stage.
[e] Allsop and Work (1963).
[f] Plapp and Kandler (1967).
[g] Work (1964).
[h] Perkins (1965/a).
[i] Perkins and Cummins (1964).
[j] Perkins (1965/b).

has been shown to be incorporated into some component that is extractable by lipid solvents and that has a high R_f on paper chromatograms developed in *iso*-butyric acid-ammonia as solvent (Anderson *et al.*, 1965, 1967; Izaki *et al.*, 1966). The reaction involves the elimination of uridine monophosphate (UMP) and the formation of a pyrophosphate bond between the muramic acid and the lipid (Struve *et al.*, 1966). This lipid is now thought to be a C_{55} polyisoprenoid alcohol (Higashi *et al.*, 1967).

While the *P*-MurNAc-pentapeptide is still attached to the lipid, *N*-acetylglucosamine (GlcNAc) is transferred from UDP-GlcNAc to the 4 position of the muramic acid, with elimination of UDP (Anderson *et al.*, 1965). At this point, in preparations from *S. aureus*, a pentaglycine chain is attached to the ε-amino group of the lysine residue. This process has been shown to require the presence of transfer RNA (tRNA); indeed the most recent evidence suggests that glycine transfer RNA isolated from *S. aureus* can be separated into three distinct fractions, only one of which is specific for the incorporation of glycine into murein, the other two also being active in protein synthesis (Bumsted *et al.*, 1968). Other organisms have different amino acid cross-links, and transfer RNA's have also been implicated in their biosynthesis. Thus, cross-bridge L-alanine incorporation into the murein of *Arthrobacter crystallopoietes* required L-alanyl-tRNA. A synthetic L-alanyl-tRNA made by reducing L-cysteinyl-tRNA with Raney nickel was not active in murein cross-linking (Roberts *et al.*, 1968a). Similarly, serine incorporation in *Staphylococcus epidermidis* (Petit *et al.*, 1968) and threonine incorporation in *Micrococcus roseus* (Roberts *et al.*, 1968b) also required the presence of specific tRNA.

C. Conversion of Lipid Intermediate to Murein Polymer

The completed disaccharide pentapeptide, still attached to lipid and in *S. aureus* adorned with a side chain of glycine molecules, is then transferred to an acceptor, presumably preformed murein polysaccharide chains, with loss of the phosphate residue hitherto present at C-1 of the muramic acid. Thus the process so far described allows for the continued growth of the polysaccharide chains of the murein.

The final step in murein synthesis involves the peptide cross-linking reaction, in which a transpeptidation takes place between the penultimate D-alanine molecule of the pentapeptide chain and the free amino group of another chain; this may belong to lysine (*M. lysodeikticus*), diaminopimelic acid (*E. coli*), side-chain glycine (*S. aureus*), or some other side-chain amino acid or peptide such as L-alanyl-L-alanyl-L-alanyl-L-threonine (*M. roseus*, Petit *et al.*, 1966), or D-*iso*-asparagine (*Streptococcus faecalis*, Ghuysen *et al.*, 1967). At the same time the C-terminal D-alanine residue of the original pentapeptide is eliminated (Tipper and Strominger, 1965; Wise and Park, 1965; Araki *et al.*,

1966a; Izaki *et al.*, 1966). The reactions just described are summarized in Scheme II.

The degree of peptide cross-linking finally achieved in whole bacteria is very variable. In many species only about a half of the available amino groups are used (e.g., *E. coli*, Weidel and Pelzer, 1964; *Bacillus licheniformis*, Hughes, 1968a,b); indeed it has been concluded that really high degrees of cross-linking such as those found in *S. aureus* are comparatively rare (Muñoz *et al.*, 1966a). There is evidence that in *M. lysodeikticus* a further type of cross-linking may occur, by which a whole primary pentapeptide chain becomes detached from a muramic acid carboxyl group and is transferred to the carboxyl group of a D-alanine molecule, presumably again the penultimate residue of another chain (Pickering, 1966; Schleifer and Kandler, 1967; Ghuysen *et al.*, 1968). A unified view of the structure and biosynthesis of the mureins has been presented by Ghuysen (1968).

It has become evident that many of the other polymers found in the cell walls of gram-positive bacteria (Table I) are in fact covalently linked to the murein, probably by a phosphodiester linkage on C-6 of a muramic acid residue (Liu and Gotschlich, 1967; Hall and Knox, 1965; Knox and Hall, 1965; Button *et al.*, 1966). At present it is not known how essential such links are for the integrity of the cell wall and the continued health of the bacteria. For instance, during the biosynthesis of cell walls other polymers could be attached after each piece of murein had been completed, but it is equally possible that murein is synthesized by addition of the new disaccharide-pentapeptide units described earlier to a disaccharide already joined by a phosphodiester bond to another type of polymer. If the second scheme were correct, then the interpolymer linkages would be essential primers for new chains of murein polysaccharide.

III. Connection between Antibiotic Action and Murein Synthesis

A. Penicillins and Cephalosporins

Since Park and Strominger (1957) first showed that compounds accumulating in penicillin-treated cultures of staphylococci were chemically related to the wall murein, ample evidence for such a connection has been obtained. Thus Mandelstam and Rogers (1959) showed that murein synthesis occurring during suppression of protein synthesis was inhibited by low concentrations of penicillin. Later, Rogers and Jeljasziewicz (1961) demonstrated that various penicillins differed in their antibiotic potency in the same proportion as they inhibited murein synthesis, and that the minimum concentration inhibitory for cell growth was also adequate to cause noticeable inhibition of incorporation of labeled amino acids into murein (Rogers and Perkins, 1968).

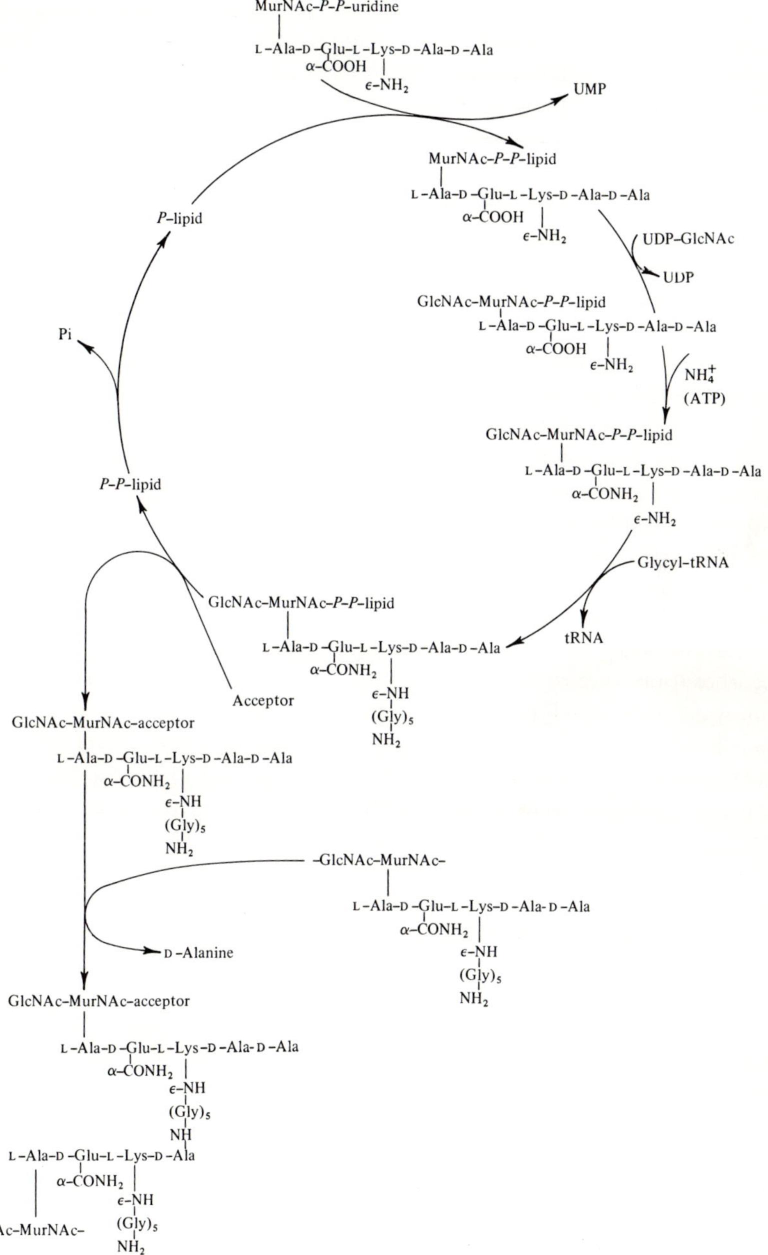

SCHEME II. Biosynthesis of cross-linked murein in *Staphylococcus aureus*. The order of addition of substituents to the lipid intermediate in the living cell is not known. (Siewert and Strominger, 1967.)

Although a general connection between penicillin action and murein synthesis was thus established, detailed understanding had to wait for developments in our knowledge of the synthesis itself. The stages now recognized in the biosynthesis of murein have been given in Scheme II (see Section II, C). In the first successful cell-free systems that showed incorporation of labeled material from UDP-MurNAc-pentapeptide precursor, no inhibition by added penicillin was observed (Chatterjee and Park, 1964; Meadow *et al.*, 1964). It was subsequently realized that the system of Chatterjee and Park (1964) was not capable of taking the process beyond the stage of the final lipid intermediate (the one including glycine). Later work showed that none of the processes up to and including extension of the murein polysaccharide chains was affected by the presence of penicillin, except to a small extent by very high concentrations (Anderson *et al.*, 1966).

One step remained for the completion of murein biosynthesis, namely, the cross-linking reaction, and it therefore seemed likely that penicillin must intervene at this point. Indeed, Martin (1964) had already suggested this idea to explain his results with stable and unstable L forms of *Proteus mirabilis*. Wise and Park (1965) studied the incorporation of labeled glycine and either alanine or lysine into the murein of whole *S. aureus*, under conditions in which murein synthesis was only partially inhibited by high concentrations of penicillin (10 μg/ml). They found that, in the presence of penicillin, lysine and glycine incorporation were reduced by the same amount, whereas alanine incorporation was less affected. On the assumption that glycine incorporation was not specifically altered by penicillin (in other words, that each chain synthesized had the same number of glycine residues as in the control) it could be calculated that penicillin at a concentration of 10 μg/ml caused the synthesis of 42% of new chains containing an extra alanine molecule. The proportion of free glycine amino groups increased at the same time. These results suggested that penicillin was indeed inhibiting the cross-linking step of murein synthesis.

As a mechanism for this reaction, Wise and Park (1965) suggested a structural analogy between the β-lactam ring of penicillin and the L-alanyl-γ-D-glutamyl part of the murein peptide chain, the presence of a free carboxyl group in both structures being a key feature of the similarity. They proposed that "when the reactive β-lactam ring of penicillin is in close contact with the enzyme, it would react specifically and covalently with the active site of this enzyme, thereby inactivating it."

In the same year, Tipper and Strominger (1965) also described experiments implicating the cross-linking reaction as the point of penicillin intervention. Early log-phase cultures of *S. aureus* were treated with penicillin G (0.08 to 1 μg/ml) for 10–40 minutes. Then labeled glycine was added and incorporation into murein proceeded for 30 minutes. The cell walls were isolated and degraded with an endoacetylmuramidase. From the digest disaccharide units

(N-acetylglucosaminyl-N-acetylmuramic acid) were isolated with peptide side chains, either cross-linked to a similar unit, or not. In the control cells only 7% of the low-molecular-weight fraction was uncross-linked (9% of the radioactivity in the fraction), whereas in the penicillin-treated cells the uncross-linked material contained 15–28% of the total reducing material and 40–60% of the radioactivity, that is, of the newly synthesized chains. Furthermore, the monomer units isolated in large amounts from the penicillin-treated cells and in small amounts from the control cells contained an extra molecule of D-alanine compared with the polymeric material from the same cells. Once more, therefore, penicillin was shown to have a direct inhibitory effect on cross-linking.

The mechanism suggested by Tipper and Strominger (1965) was different, however. They proposed, and supported with molecular models, the idea that N-acyl-6-aminopenicillanic acid (penicillin) is an analog of N-acyl-D-alanyl-D-alanine. The penicillin would be fixed to the transpeptidase in place of its natural substrate, and would then acylate the transfer site with production of a penicilloyl enzyme. Tipper and Strominger (1965) point out that the structural analogy proposed by Wise and Park (1965) requires a free carboxyl group on the glutamic acid residue, whereas they were able to show in their isolated monomer units that an amide group was already present, presumably on C-1 of the glutamic acid. Other work, quoted earlier, has shown that this group is indeed amidated in the completed murein.

The possibility that the proposed penicilloyl enzyme might succeed in transferring its penicilloyl residue to the end of a glycine chain, thereby blocking it, was also excluded by Tipper and Strominger (1965) by use of labeled penicillin. Such a mechanism might not seem very likely, since it would require a penicillin molecule for every nascent peptide chain in the murein, and would leave the enzyme free for further authentic transpeptidation. Nevertheless, Rogers (1967) has suggested that penicillin might indeed form a labile penicilloyl link with a free amino group in incomplete murein, rather than with a transpeptidase. The experiments that led him to this hypothesis were as follows. Staphylococci were saturated with benzylpenicillin, so that synthesis of murein ceased. They were then washed in penicillin-free medium, and reincubated in a phosphate buffer solution containing glucose, murein amino acids, and chloramphenicol. After a lag period, murein synthesis recommenced and soon attained the same rate as in control cells. Thus the presence of saturating penicillin (little of which was lost on washing, as shown by separate experiments) did not long inhibit murein synthesis. This escape from the grip of penicillin took place in the presence of chloramphenicol, an inhibitor of protein synthesis. Rogers (1967) therefore concluded that the renewed murein synthesis could not be due to the formation of new transpeptidase, and by the same token the old transpeptidase must still be free to act. A further striking feature of Rogers' system was that the renewed murein synthesis occurring in cells previously saturated with penicillin was hypersensitive to further addition of the drug. Significant inhibition was observed at a benzylpenicillin concentration of 1.5 mμM, about 50–100 times less than the concentration needed to produce the same effect in hitherto untreated cells.

In view of these results Rogers (1967) proposed that the part of the absorbed penicillin critical for inhibition of murein biosynthesis might indeed be bound to amino groups in growing murein chains. He proposed that when penicillin was withdrawn, the labile penicilloyl groups were lost, leaving fresh attachment points for the growing murein. If labile penicilloyl sites are to be postulated, however, it seems equally possible that the inhibited site may reside on the transpeptidase rather than on growing murein. As Rogers (1967) himself pointed out, his hypothesis does not account for the inhibition by penicillin of the D-alanine carboxypeptidase of *E. coli* B (Izaki *et al.*, 1966).

1. *Inhibition by Penicillin of Murein Biosynthesis in Gram-Negative Bacteria*

It is well known that gram-negative bacteria are less sensitive to penicillin than gram-positive species. Recently it has become possible to examine the penicillin sensitivity of murein biosynthesis in cell-free systems, and thus to see whether the process in gram-negative bacteria is intrinsically more resistant to the action of the drug. The system in *E. coli* has been examined by Araki *et al.* (1966b) and Izaki *et al.* (1966) with similar results. D-Alanine could be lost from the C-terminus of the primary pentapeptide chain involved in murein biosynthesis at three stages: (*a*) by the action of a carboxypeptidase on the precursor UDP-MurNAc-L-Ala-D-Glu-*meso*-DAP-D-Ala-D-Ala, (*b*) by the transpeptidation reaction of murein cross-linking, and (*c*) by the action of a carboxypeptidase after the murein polysaccharide chains had been synthesized (Fig. 1). All these reactions were inhibited by penicillin at low concentrations. Indeed Izaki *et al.* (1966) found that the action of the D-alanine carboxypeptidase of *E. coli* B upon the UDP-MurNAc-pentapeptide was 75% inhibited by as little as 0.04 μg/ml of penicillin G, whereas the cross-linking reaction in *E. coli* Y-10 required about 10 μg/ml to produce a 75% inhibition.

These results might suggest that UDP-MurNAc-tetrapeptide, lacking the terminal D-alanine residue, could also be a precursor for murein biosynthesis in *E. coli*. However, Araki *et al.* (1966b) examined this possibility and found that incorporation of the truncated precursor was only 20% of that observed with the complete molecule. It seems, therefore, that the biosynthesis in *E. coli* proceeds by the same sequence of reactions as in the cocci, any extra D-alanine residues not required for cross-linking being eliminated at a late stage. In the whole organism the UDP-MurNAc-pentapeptide may well be inaccessible to the D-alanine carboxypeptidase, since presumably, already deprived of UMP,

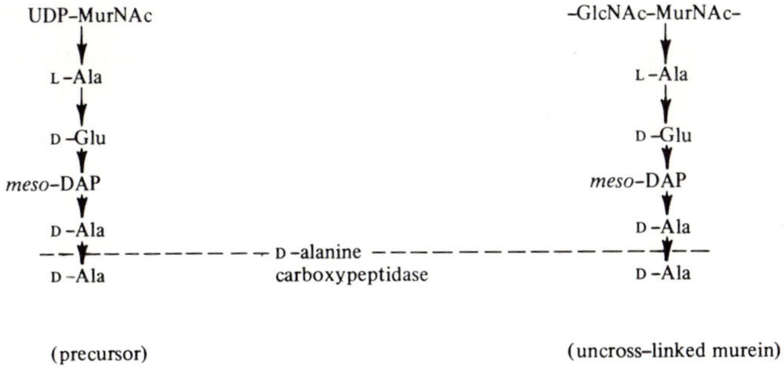

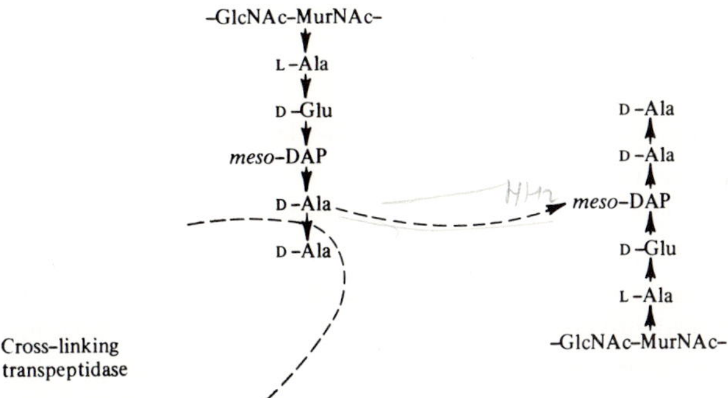

FIG. 1. Methods of loss of D-alanine in the synthesis of *Escherichia coli* murein. (Izaki *et al.*, 1966.)

it passes through the cytoplasmic membrane as a lipid intermediate, and any cross-linking occurs in the nascent murein on the outside. On the other hand, the D-alanine carboxypeptidase may serve as a regulator of cross-linking.

If D-alanine carboxypeptidase can regulate cross-linking in the living cell, as indeed it must if it is present together with the transpeptidase when murein is being synthesized, then a surprising result might ensue. Izaki *et al.* (1966) observed that, in *E. coli*, of the two enzymes the carboxypeptidase was the more sensitive to penicillin. It might be expected, therefore, that at low concentrations penicillin would lead to the synthesis of a murein more highly cross-linked than in the normal cell, because a higher proportion of the D-alanyl-D-alanine terminal groups would be spared from the action of the carboxypeptidase to be substrates for the transpeptidase.

The results of Araki *et al.* (1966b) and Izaki *et al.* (1966) show clearly that in particulate preparations from *E. coli* the cross-linking reaction of murein biosynthesis is sensitive to low concentrations of penicillin. The results of

TABLE III

INHIBITION BY PENICILLINS AND CEPHALOTHIN OF GROWTH AND MUREIN CROSS-LINKING IN *E. coli* Y-10[a]

Antibiotic	Concentration (μg/ml) to produce 50% inhibition: Liberation of D-alanine (cross-linking)	Growth
Penicillin G	3	30
Ampicillin	3	3
Methicillin	1000	1000
Cephalothin	50	50

[a] Results of Izaki *et al.* (1966).

Izaki *et el.* (1966) are summarized in Table III. They show that, for penicillin G at least, the cell-free system is more sensitive to the drug than is the growth of the organism. The concentrations required are still very large compared with those needed to prevent murein biosynthesis by intact staphylococci (e.g., 50% inhibition produced by 0.05–0.1 μg/ml of benzylpenicillin; Rogers, 1967).

A further hint of the relation between the structure of antibiotics and their action is to be found in the work of Izaki *et al.* (1966). Large concentrations of methicillin and ampicillin appeared to inhibit total synthesis of murein as well as to inhibit cross-linking. A smaller effect was observed when the benzylpenicillin concentration was raised to 1000 μg/ml (Table IV). Cephalothin, on the other hand, seemed to have no inhibitory effect at all on total incorporation

TABLE IV

EFFECTS OF PENICILLINS ON MUREIN SYNTHESIS IN *E. coli* Y-10[a]

Penicillin concentration (μg/ml)	Incorporation into murein of added UDP-MurNAc-pentapeptide (percentage of control without added antibiotic)			
	Benzylpenicillin	Cephalothin	Ampicillin	Methicillin
1	98	100	88	96
10	101	110	75	88
100	113	107	70	78
1000	82	104	76	69

[a] Calculated from the results of Izaki *et al.* (1966).

of MurNAc-peptide into murein, although it undoubtedly decreased liberation of free D-alanine and therefore inhibited cross-linking.

The relationship between penicillin and the transpeptidase of murein cross-linking is thus well established. At present, however, there is no evidence for its precise mode of action at a molecular level. Unless the transpeptidase can be purified in an active condition, the final details of penicillin action may be difficult to establish. Furthermore, it is not yet established that the transpeptidase is the only step of murein biosynthesis that is affected by penicillin in growing cells.

B. Bacitracin

The bacitracins are a group of related cyclic polypeptide antibiotics. The main component, bacitracin A, has the probable structure shown in Fig. 2 (Swallow and Abraham, 1959).

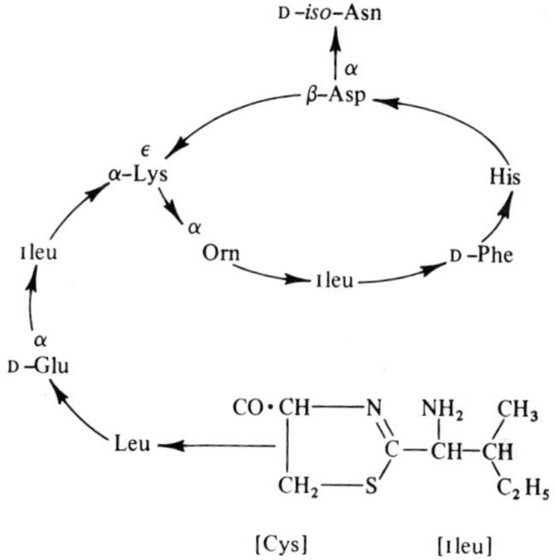

Fig. 2. Probable structure of bacitracin A.

Abraham and Newton (1959) showed that, like penicillin, bacitracin could cause the accumulation in staphylococci of UDP-MurNAc-pentapeptide, now known to be a murein precursor. They also commented on the fact that in bacitracin the ε-amino group of lysine was linked to aspartic acid, a structural feature then thought likely to occur in certain mureins (Cummins and Harris, 1958; Swallow and Abraham, 1958). The presence of such a link in the murein of *Streptococcus faecalis* has been shown conclusively by Ghuysen *et al.* (1967), who deduced the structure given in Fig. 3. The aspartic acid residue occurs as an *iso*-asparagine, as in the probable bacitracin structure given in Fig. 2. The apparent chemical similarity of bacitracin and some mureins may be mis-

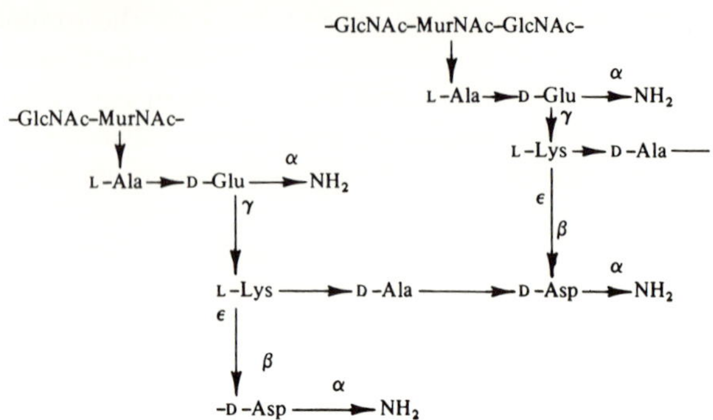

FIG. 3. Murein structure of *Streptococcus faecalis*. I thank the authors and copyright owners for permission to reprint this figure from p. 2609 of the article by J. M. Ghuysen, E. Bricas, M. Leyh-Bouille, M. Lache, and G. D. Shockman that appeared in *Biochemistry* **6**, No. 8, August, 1967. Copyright (1967) by the American Chemical Society.

leading, however, since recent work has suggested that bacitracin intervenes in the biosynthetic process at a stage independent of murein structure.

In the cycle of reactions for murein biosynthesis (see Scheme II, Section II, C), it will be observed that transfer of the GlcNAc-MurNAc peptide from the *P-P*-lipid to the acceptor (presumably growing chains of murein polysaccharide) means that *P-P*-lipid is set free. To accept another MurNAc-(peptide)-*P*-moiety, the *P-P*-lipid must first lose its terminal phosphate. Siewert and Strominger (1967) studied the influence of bacitracin on the biosynthesis of murein by membrane fractions of *M. lysodeikticus* and *S. aureus*. They found that bacitracin induced the accumulation of material containing phosphorus, of high chromatographic mobility, that was not radioactively labeled when UDP-MurNAc-^{14}C-pentapeptide was the substrate. This material was tentatively identified as *P-P*-lipid. At the same time bacitracin prevented the appearance of radioactive inorganic phosphate when ^{32}P-labeled lipid intermediate was used as substrate for murein synthesis.

Under conditions in which the enzyme system was not saturated, biosynthesis of murein from ^{32}P-UDP-MurNAc-^{14}C-pentapeptide was not inhibited by bacitracin, although ^{32}P-*P*-lipid accumulated, presumably because fresh molecules of *P*-lipid were available for continued synthesis. When, however, higher concentrations of substrate were used, then there was an inhibition of murein synthesis (75% decrease in the presence of 120 μg/ml of bacitracin). The results also suggested that in the absence of bacitracin the

P-P-lipid had undergone about 4 to 6 cycles of regeneration during 1 hour's incubation. The effect of various antibiotics on the hydrolysis of *P-P*-lipid by particulate enzyme from *M. lysodeikticus* is shown in Table V. It is clear that inhibition of phosphate release from *P-P*-lipid is specific to bacitracin.

TABLE V

HYDROLYSIS OF ^{32}*P-P*-LIPID BY PARTICULATE ENZYME FROM *M. lysodeikticus* IN THE PRESENCE OF DIFFERENT ANTIBIOTICS[a,b]

Antibiotic added	Concentration (μg/ml)	Inorganic ^{32}P (cpm)
None		1040
Bacitracin	153	361
Penicillin G	40	1030
Ristocetin A	40	1075
Vancomycin	40	1001
Novobiocin	40	1088

[a] Siewert and Strominger (1967).
[b] I thank the authors and the National Academy of Sciences for permission to reproduce this table from *Proceedings of the National Academy of Sciences* (1961) **57**, p. 772.

A question that arises from these results is whether the inhibitory effect of bacitracin is specific for the *P-P*-lipid concerned in murein biosynthesis. A similar lipid intermediate is known to be involved in the biosynthesis of lipopolysaccharides of enteric bacteria (Wright *et al.*, 1965, 1967; Weiner *et al.*, 1965). The lipid acceptor is thought to be a C_{55} isoprenoid alcohol phosphate, very like the one concerned in murein biosynthesis (Higashi *et al.*, 1967). It seems possible, therefore, that bacitracin might inhibit the biosynthesis of lipopolysaccharides, providing that the synthetic system were saturated with substrate so that the *P-P*-lipid needed to be recycled. Whether the specificity of bacitracin is directed against the lipid intermediate or the enzyme that dephosphorylates it is an open question.

C. D-CYCLOSERINE (OXAMYCIN, D-4-AMINO-3-ISOXAZOLIDONE)

The action of this antibiotic has long been known to be antagonized by D-alanine. Strominger *et al.* (1959) showed that in the presence of D-cycloserine, cultures of *Staphylococcus aureus* accumulated a nucleotide related to those found in the presence of penicillin, but lacking the final D-alanine dipeptide, namely, UDP-MurNAc-L-Ala-D-Glu-L-Lys. This action was antagonized by D-alanine, and much of the nucleotide that had accumulated in the presence of the antibiotic disappeared again when D-alanine was subsequently added to the medium.

The action of D-cycloserine was defined further by Strominger *et al.* (1960). The stages in the addition of the D-alanine residues to the murein precursor in *S. aureus* were as follows:

$$\text{(1) L-Alanine} \underset{\text{pyridoxal phosphate}}{\overset{\text{Racemase}}{\rightleftharpoons}} \text{D-alanine}$$

$$\text{(2) D-Alanine} \xrightarrow[\text{ATP}+\text{Mn}^{++}]{\text{synthetase}} \text{D-alanyl-D-alanine}$$

$$\text{(3) UDP-MurNAc-L-Ala-D-Glu-L-Lys} +$$

$$\text{D-Ala-D-Ala} \xrightarrow[\text{ATP}+\text{Mn}^{++}]{\text{ligase}} \text{UDP-MurNAc-L-Ala-D-Glu-L-Lys-D-Ala-D-Ala}$$

Reactions (1) and (2) were found to be inhibited by D-cycloserine. For reaction (1) the K_m for conversion in either direction was about 6.3×10^{-3} *M*, and the K_i for D-cycloserine was 0.6×10^{-4} *M* in the direction of D-alanine formation and 1.0×10^{-4} *M* for L-alanine formation. The synthetase of reaction (2) had $K_m = 3\text{–}5 \times 10^{-3}$ *M* and $K_i = 2\text{–}4 \times 10^{-5}$ *M*. Thus this stage was very sensitive to the presence of D-cycloserine and evidently lack of available dipeptide caused the accumulation of the UDP-MurNAc-tripeptide. Enzymatic addition of D-alanine dipeptide to this material (reaction 3) was not sensitive to the drug.

The structural analogy between D-cycloserine and D-alanine has been discussed by Strominger (1962) and molecular models have been compared. He suggested that in its combination with the enzyme D-alanine adopts the conformation in which it most closely resembles D-cycloserine.

The D-alanyl-D-alanine synthetase of *Streptococcus faecalis* R was studied in more detail by Neuhaus (1962a,b). Kinetic work showed that the enzyme had two sites, a "donor site" and an "acceptor site." The scheme proposed for the synthetase mechanism was as follows:

$$\text{Enzyme (E)} + \text{D-alanine (A)} \rightleftharpoons \text{EA ("donor" added)}$$

$$\text{EA} + \text{D-alanine} \rightleftharpoons \text{EAA ("acceptor" added)}$$

$$\text{EAA} \rightarrow \text{EA-A} \rightleftharpoons \text{E} + \text{A-A (D-alanyl-D-alanine)}$$

Neuhaus and Lynch (1964) showed that both D-alanine binding sites are sensitive to D-cycloserine (Table VI). It was also found that the 5-methyl derivatives of D-cycloserine, the D-cyclothreonines, inhibited the synthetase to a lesser extent (Table VI).

TABLE VI

INHIBITION OF D-ALANYL-D-ALANINE SYNTHETASE[a]

Inhibitor	K_i	
	Donor site	Acceptor site
D-Cycloserine	2.2×10^{-5} *M*	1.4×10^{-4} *M*
cis-D-Cyclothreonine	1.2×10^{-4} *M*	1.9×10^{-4} *M*
trans-D-Cyclothreonine	5.4×10^{-4} *M*	5.6×10^{-4} *M*

[a] I thank the authors and copyright owners for permission to reprint this table from p. 475 of the article by F. C. Neuhaus and T. L. Lynch that appeared in *Biochemistry* **3**, No. 1, April 10, 1964. Copyright (1964) by the American Chemical Society.

Other D-alanine analogs, such as β-aminoxy-D-alanine, inhibited the synthetase only very poorly, but were themselves converted into their D-alanyl derivatives; in other words, they took the place of the acceptor alanine. β-Aminoxy-D-alanine methyl ester, however, inhibited the synthetase.

It is evident that D-cycloserine and related antibiotics inhibit murein synthesis at an early stage by preventing the accumulation of the necessary nucleotide precursor. Again they fall into the category of drugs that are fairly specific for bacteria, because it is only in bacteria and closely related organisms (those containing murein) that the key intermediate, D-alanyl-D-alanine, requires to be synthesized.

D. *O*-CARBAMYL-D-SERINE

This antibiotic, obtained from a culture filtrate of a *Streptomyces* species, was shown to inhibit the synthesis of bacterial cell walls (Tanaka *et al.*, 1963). The antimicrobial activity of the drug was reversed by D-alanine, but was not greatly affected by glycine, L-alanine, L-serine, L-glutamic acid, L-lysine, or L-glutamine (Tanaka, 1963). The incorporation of radioactive glutamate into the cell wall fraction was also inhibited 58% (*B. subtilis*) and 35% (*S. aureus* 209P) by 0.4 mg/ml of *O*-carbamyl-D-serine. At the same time the drug caused intracellular accumulation of nucleotide-*N*-acetylamino sugar just as did D-cycloserine.

The site of action of *O*-carbamyl-D-serine was examined in more detail by Lynch and Neuhaus (1966). The minimal inhibitory concentration for *Streptococcus faecalis* R was found to be 5×10^{-3} *M*. The effect of a concentration of

7×10^{-3} *M* was completely reversed by 3×10^{-3} *M* D-alanine, or 3×10^{-2} *M* L-alanine, the latter result being different from the observation of Tanaka (1963), who used an agar plate method. Lynch and Neuhaus (1966) also showed that the major amino-sugar nucleotide accumulating in *S. faecalis* in the presence of *O*-carbamyl-D-serine was UDP-MurNAc-L-Ala-D-Glu-L-Lys, the same truncated murein precursor that would be obtained under the influence of D-cycloserine.

The drug was found to act upon the alanine racemase as a competitive inhibitor ($K_i = 4.8 \times 10^{-4}$ *M*) whether D-alanine or L-alanine was used as substrate. D-Alanyl-D-alanine synthetase caused *O*-carbamyl-D-serine to become incorporated into a new dipeptide, D-alanyl-*O*-carbamyl-D-serine. It had been shown earlier that other D-alanine analogs became acylated by D-alanine in exactly the same way (Neuhaus, 1962a; Neuhaus and Lynch, 1964). D-Alanyl-*O*-carbamyl-D-serine was not as effective an inhibitor of the synthetase as D-alanyl-D-alanine itself.

Just as *O*-carbamyl-D-serine could be incorporated into a dipeptide, so this dipeptide in turn was converted by UDP-MurNAc-L-Ala-D-Glu-L-Lys: D-Ala-D-Ala ligase (ADP) into UDP-MurNAc-L-Ala-D-Glu-L-Lys-D-Ala-*O*-carbamyl-D-Ser. The K_m value was 3.6×10^{-3} *M* compared with one of 1.6×10^{-4} *M* for D-alanyl-D-alanine as substrate. Furthermore, the enzyme is not inhibited even by 5×10^{-2} *M* *O*-carbamyl-D-serine.

The analog UDP-MurNAc-pentapeptide was also converted to the next stage of murein biosynthesis, the lipid intermediate described earlier, lipid-*P*-*P*-MurNAc-L-Ala-D-Glu-L-Lys-D-Ala-*O*-carbamyl-D-serine, at a rate equal to that for the natural substrate. Hence it may be concluded that the most important site of action of *O*-carbamyl-D-serine was upon the alanine racemase, since as Lynch and Neuhaus (1966) observed, inhibited cells did not contain intermediates in which D-alanine had been replaced by the analog.

E. Vancomycin and Ristocetin

These antibiotics appear to be similar in their action; both inhibit murein synthesis and cause the accumulation of precursors in sensitive bacteria (ristocetin, Wallas and Strominger, 1963; vancomycin, Reynolds, 1961, 1966; Jordan, 1961). The development of cell-free systems that synthesize murein has facilitated further pinpointing of the site of antibiotic action. Anderson *et al.* (1965, 1967) showed that cell-free murein syntheses by preparations from *S. aureus* and *M. lysodeikticus* were 50% inhibited by about the same concentrations of vancomycin and ristocetin as were required for 50% growth inhibition. The formation of lipid intermediate was not inhibited, and indeed was sometimes considerably enhanced by the presence of either antibiotic. This effect was further examined in *S. aureus* by Matsuhashi *et al.* (1967). While murein synthesis from either labeled UDP-MurNAc-pentapeptide or labeled glycine was inhibited even by the lowest concentrations of antibiotic used, over the range of about 10–100 μg/ml of ristocetin or 10–70 μg/ml of vancomycin, the incorporation into lipid intermediate was increased by as much as 50–70%. A similar effect of vancomycin at intermediate concentration was also observed during lipid-intermediate formation by the membranes of staphylococcal L forms (Chatterjee *et al.*, 1967).

Anderson *et al.* (1967) also examined the effect of antibiotics on the reversal of formation of MurNAc-(pentapeptide)-*P*-*P*-lipid, that is its reaction with UMP to form UDP-MurNAc-pentapeptide in the presence of a particulate preparation from *M. lysodeikticus*. They found that this reaction was inhibited only 30% by 55 μg/ml of ristocetin or 50 μg/ml of vancomycin, although at very high concentration (over 1 mg/ml) almost complete inhibition was observed. On the other hand, the forward conversion of purified GlcNAc MurNAc-(pentapeptide)-*P*-*P*-lipid to murein was 50% inhibited by only 20 μg/ml of either ristocetin or vancomycin. Hence it appeared that reactions before the glycan chain synthesis were relatively insensitive to these antibiotics.

As indicated earlier, the glycine residue in the murein of *M. lysodeikticus* is a C-terminal substituent on the α-carboxyl group of D-glutamic acid. The incorporation of glycine into this murein was studied in detail by Katz *et al.* 1967). In particular, the effect of antibiotics on the addition of glycine to GlcNAc-MurNAc-(pentapeptide)-*P*-*P*-lipid was examined. Low concentrations of ristocetin or vancomycin had no effect on incorporation to the lipid intermediate, but inhibited the formation of glycyl-murein. At higher concentration of antibiotic both processes were affected.

Another aspect of vancomycin and ristocetin action was first reported by Chatterjee and Perkins (1966b). They observed that these antibiotics not only caused the accumulation of UDP-MurNAc-pentapeptide in various gram-positive bacteria, but also led to the formation of a compound of the same precursor with a molecule of antibiotic. Subsequent work (Perkins, 1968) showed that the presence of cells or cell contents was not required for the formation of these antibiotic-murein precursor compounds. In fact, vancomycin combined *in vitro* with UDP-MurNAc-pentapeptides and related compounds so long as these terminated in a D-alanyl-D-alanine dipeptide (Table VII and Fig. 4).

In further work (Perkins, 1969) the smallest molecule found that would combine with vancomycin was acetyl-D-alanyl-D-alanine. The methyl ester of this compound was completely without action, as was acetyl-L-alanyl-L-alanine. Critical experiments showed that in forming these compounds ristocetin resembled vancomycin, once again indicating a close similarity between these two antibiotics.

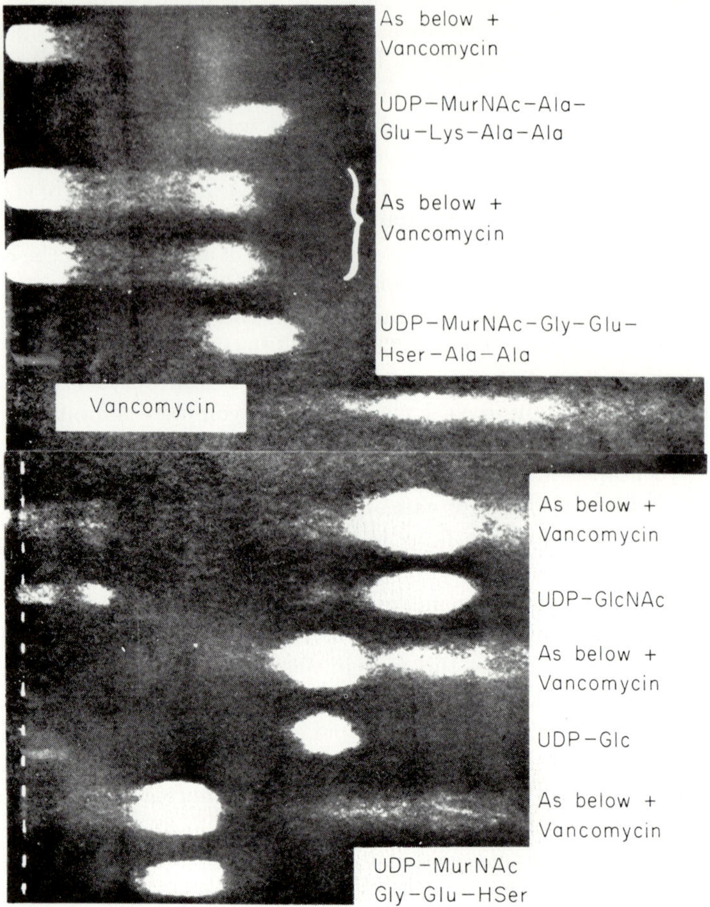

Fig. 4. Combination of nucleotide-muramic acid peptides with vancomycin. Approximately 0.1 μmole of each component was applied to the origin, and the chromatograms were developed overnight in ethanol-M-ammonium acetate, pH 7.5 (7.5:3 by volume) and photographed in UV light. Where combination occurred a new slow-running spot appeared. In the samples with UDP-MurNAc-Gly-Glu-Homoserine-Ala-Ala an excess of nucleotide over vancomycin was present and therefore some uncombined nucleotide can be seen (Perkins, 1968.)

The combination between vancomycin and the various peptides took place within seconds on mixing at room temperature and was not prevented by the presence of molar sodium chloride. The specificity for the acylated correct terminal dipeptide of the murein precursor was great, so that another group

TABLE VII

In vitro combination with vancomycin[a,b]

Combine with vancomycin							Do not combine with vancomycin				
UDP	UDP	UDP	UDP				UDP	UDP			
GlcNAc	GlcNAc	GlcNAc	GlcNAc	GlcNAc			GlcNAc	GlcNAc	GlcNAc		
Lactyl	Lactyl	Lactyl	Lactyl	Lactyl	Lactyl		Lactyl	Lactyl	Lactyl		
L-Ala	Gly	L-Ala	L-Ala	L-Ala	L-Ala		L-Ala	L-Ala	L-Ala	L-Ala	
D-Glu	Glu	D-Glu	D-Glu	D-Glu	D-Glu	L-Glu-NH_2 (α)	D-Glu	D-Glu	D-Glu	D-Glu-NH_2 (α)	
meso-DAP	H-Ser	L-Lys	L-Lys-ε-DNP	L-Lys	L-Lys	L-Lys	L-Lys	*meso*-DAP	*meso*-DAP	L-Lys	
D-Ala	D-Ala	D-Ala	D-Ala	D-Ala	D-Ala	D-Ala			D-Ala	D-Ala	D-Ala
D-Ala	D-Ala	D-Ala	D-Ala	D-Ala	D-Ala	D-Ala					D-Ala

[a] Combination was indicated by a reduction in R_f during chromatography in ethanol-*M*-ammonium acetate (7.5:3 by volume).
[b] Perkins (1968).

of antibiotics can be added to those already known to act in some way by recognition of, or resemblance to, this structure.

IV. Antibiotic Action and Murein Breakdown

A. Lysostaphin

A completely different type of antibiotic from those described above is lysostaphin. Schindler and Schuhardt (1964) isolated a strain of *Staphylococcus* that produced extracellularly a substance capable of lysing other strains of staphylococci. The substance was partially purified and shown to be a basic enzyme protein (Schindler and Schuhardt, 1965). This enzyme was surprisingly specific for staphylococci, and was shown to have two actions upon their murein, a major one of hydrolyzing bonds to the amino groups of alanine and of glycine, and a minor one of acting as an endohexosaminidase, splitting the polysaccharide backbone (Browder *et al.*, 1965). These two activities could be separated. Evidence was obtained that one enzyme split the glycosidic bond between *N*-acetyl-glucosamine and *N*-acetylmuramic acid, since the digest after reduction with sodium borohydride contained glucosaminitol in the place of glucosamine.

This result was amply confirmed by Tipper and Strominger (1966), who also succeeded in isolating the disaccharide 4-*O*-*N*-acetylmuramyl-*N*-acetylglucosamine, as well as its derivative *O*-acetylated on C-6 of the muramic acid residue, from digests of staphyloccocal cell walls. Nuclear magnetic resonance studies suggested that the link was of the β-configuration. This disaccharide is different from the one derived from lysozyme digests of murein polysaccharide, namely, 4-*O*-β-*N*-acetyl-glucosaminyl-*N*-acetylmuramic acid. It is, nevertheless, not a substrate for egg-white lysozyme or other similar enzymes. The work of Tipper and Strominger (1966) also showed that the peptidase of lysostaphin removed all the side chains from the polysaccharide, as well as splitting some glycine cross-links.

It was observed by Browder *et al.* (1965) that the glycosidase of lysostaphin is not lytic for staphylococci, but presumably it must hydrolyze the polysaccharide from all mureins, since so far as is known their composition is always the same—a chitin substituted on every alternate residue by a 3-*O*-D-lactyl ether to make a muramic acid moiety. Hence the specificity of lysostaphin for staphylococci must reside in its peptidase. At present, however, the precise chemical limits of its specificity have not been defined.

Lysostaphin has been shown to have considerable potency as an antibiotic against staphylococci, and has been proposed for topical application in cases of staphylococcal infection, or for the treatment of nasal carriers. Its minimum inhibitory concentration for certain hospital isolates of staphylococci is lower than that of penicillins or cephalosporins (Zygmunt *et al.*, 1966a,b).

V. Conclusion

The observations described above suggest that three important groups of antibiotics exert their specific action against bacteria through some involvement with the D-alanyl-D-alanine sequence that is first synthesized and then broken down during the buildup of the cross-linked murein of bacterial cell walls. Thus D-cycloserine and related compounds act by inhibiting alanine racemase to some extent but chiefly D-alanyl-D-alanine synthetase. The penicillins and cephalosporins inhibit the transpeptidation reaction, in which the terminal D-alanine residue is split from a free pentapeptide chain in the nascent murein and a cross-link is formed. Vancomycin and ristocetin have an affinity for the terminal D-alanine dipeptide of the murein precursor, and they seem to allow the synthesis of lipid intermediate to continue, but to prevent any further advance in the biosynthesis of murein.

REFERENCES

Abraham, E. P., and Newton, G. G. F. (1959). *Ciba Founda. Symp. Amino Acids Peptides Antimetab. Activity* p. 205.

Allsop, J., and Work, E. (1963). *Biochem. J.* **87**, 512.

Anderson, J. S., Matsuhashi, M., Haskin, M. A., and Strominger, J. L. (1965). *Proc. Natl. Acad. Sci. U.S.* **53**, 881.

Anderson, J. S., Meadow, P. M., Haskin, M. A., and Strominger, J. L. (1966). *Arch. Biochem. Biophys.* **116**, 487.

Anderson, J. S., Matsuhashi, M., Haskin, M. A., and Strominger, J. L. (1967). *J. Biol. Chem.* **242**, 3180.

Araki, Y., Shirai, R., Shimada, A., Ishimoto, N., and Ito, E. (1966a). *Biochem. Biophys. Res. Commun.* **23**, 466.

Araki, Y., Shimada, A., and Ito, E. (1966b). *Biochem. Biophys. Res. Commun.* **23**, 518.

Bricas, E., Ghuysen, J.-M., and Dezélée, P. (1967). *Biochemistry* **6**, 2598.

Browder, H. P., Zygmunt, W. A., Young, J. R., and Tavormina, P. A. (1965). *Biochem. Biophys. Res. Commun.* **19**, 383.

Bumsted, R. M., Dahl, J. L., Söll, D., and Strominger, J. L. (1968). *J. Biol. Chem.* **243**, 779.

Button, D., Archibald, A. R., and Baddiley, J. (1966). *Biochem. J.* **99**, 11C.

Chatterjee, A. N., and Park, J. T. (1964). *Proc. Natl. Acad. Sci. U.S.* **51**, 9.

Chatterjee, A. N., and Perkins, H. R. (1966a). *Biochem. J.* **100**, 32P.

Chatterjee, A. N., and Perkins, H. R. (1966b). *Biochem. Biophys. Res. Commun.* **24**, 489.

Chatterjee, A. N., Ward, J. B., and Perkins, H. R. (1967). *Nature* **214**, 1311.

Cummins, C. S., and Harris, H. (1958). *J. Gen. Microbiol.* **18**, 173.

de Petris, S. (1967). *J. Ultrastruct. Res.* **19**, 45.

Ghuysen, J.-M. (1968). *Bacteriol. Rev.* **32**, 425.

Ghuysen, J.-M., Bricas, E., Leyh-Bouille, M., Lache, M., and Shockman, G. D. (1967). *Biochemistry* **6**, 2607.

Ghuysen, J.-M., Bricas, E., Lache, M., and Leyh-Bouille, M. (1968). *Biochemistry* **7**, 1450.

Guinand, M., Ghuysen, J.-M., Schleifer, K. H., and Kandler, O. (1969). *Biochemistry* **8**, 200.

Hall, E. A., and Knox, K. W. (1965). *Biochem. J.* **96**, 310.

Higashi, Y., Strominger, J. L., and Sweeley, C. C. (1967). *Proc. Natl. Acad. Sci. U.S.* **57**, 1878.

Hughes, R. C. (1968a). *Biochem. J.* **106**, 41.
Hughes, R. C. (1968b). *Biochem. J.* **106**, 49.
Ito, E., and Strominger, J. L. (1962a). *J. Biol. Chem.* **237**, 2689.
Ito, E., and Strominger, J. L. (1962b). *J. Biol. Chem.* **237**, 2696.
Ito, E., and Strominger, J. L. (1964). *J. Biol. Chem.* **239**, 210.
Izaki, K., Matsuhashi, M., and Strominger, J. L. (1966). *Proc. Natl. Acad. Sci. U.S.* **55**, 656.
Jordan, D. C. (1961). *Biochem. Biophys. Res. Commun.* **6**, 167.
Katz, W., Matsuhashi, M., Dietrich, C. P., and Strominger, J. L. (1967). *J. Biol. Chem.* **242**, 3207.
Knox, K. W., and Hall, E. A. (1965). *Biochem. J.* **96**, 302.
Liu, T.-Y., and Gotschlich, E. C. (1967). *J. Biol. Chem.* **242**, 471.
Lynch, J. L., and Neuhaus, F. C. (1966). *J. Bacteriol.* **91**, 449.
Mandelstam, J., and Rogers, H. J. (1959). *Biochem. J.* **72**, 654.
Martin, H. H. (1964). *J. Gen. Microbiol.* **36**, 441.
Matsuhashi, M., Dietrich, C. P., and Strominger, J. L. (1967). *J. Biol. Chem.* **242**, 3191.
Meadow, P. M., Anderson, J. S., and Strominger, J. L. (1964). *Biochem. Biophys. Res. Commun.* **14**, 382.
Miller, I., Plapp, R., and Kandler, O. (1966). *Biochem. Biophys. Res. Commun.* **25**, 415.
Muñoz, E., Ghuysen, J.-M., Leyh-Bouille, M., Petit, J.-F., and Tinelli, R. (1966a). *Biochemistry* **5**, 3091.
Muñoz, E., Ghuysen, J.-M., Leyh-Bouille, M., Petit, J.-F., Heymann, H., Bricas, E., and Lefrancier, P. (1966b). *Biochemistry* **5**, 3748.
Neuhaus, F. C. (1962a). *J. Biol. Chem.* **237**, 778.
Neuhaus, F. C. (1962b). *J. Biol. Chem.* **237**, 3128.
Neuhaus, F. C., and Lynch, J. L. (1964). *Biochemistry* **3**, 471.
Park, J. T., and Strominger, J. L. (1957). *Science* **125**, 99.
Perkins, H. R. (1965a). *Biochem. J.* **97**, 3C.
Perkins, H. R. (1965b). *Nature* **208**, 872.
Perkins, H. R. (1967). *Biochem. J.* **102**, 29C.
Perkins, H. R. (1968). *Biochem. J.* **106**, 35P.
Perkins, H. R. (1969). *Biochem. J.* **111**, 195.
Perkins, H. R., and Cummins, C. S. (1964). *Nature* **201**, 1105.
Petit, J.-F., Muñoz, E., and Ghuysen, J.-M. (1966). *Biochemistry* **5**, 2764.
Petit, J.-F., Strominger, J. L., and Söll, D. (1968). *J. Biol. Chem.* **243**, 757.
Pickering, B. T. (1966). *Biochem. J.* **100**, 430.
Plapp, R., and Kandler, O. (1967). *Z. Naturforsch.* **22b**, 1062.
Reynolds, P. E. (1961). *Biochim. Biophys. Acta* **52**, 403.
Reynolds, P. E. (1966). *Symp. Soc. Gen. Microbiol.* **16**, 47.
Roberts, W. S. L., Petit, J.-F., and Strominger, J. L. (1968a). *J. Biol. Chem.* **243**, 768.
Roberts, W. S. L., Strominger, J. L., and Söll, D. (1968b). *J. Biol. Chem.* **243**, 749.
Rogers, H. J. (1967). *Biochem. J.* **103**, 90.
Rogers, H. J., and Jeljasziewicz, J. (1961). *Biochem. J.* **81**, 576.
Rogers, H. J., and Perkins, H. R. (1968). "Cell Walls and Membranes," p. 295. Spon, London.
Schindler, C. A., and Schuhardt, V. T. (1964). *Proc. Natl. Acad. Sci. U.S.* **51**, 414.
Schindler, C. A., and Schuhardt, V. T. (1965). *Biochim. Biophys. Acta* **97**, 242.
Schleifer, K. H., and Kandler, O. (1967). *Biochem. Biophys. Res. Commun.* **28**, 965.
Schleifer, K. H., Plapp, R., and Kandler, O. (1967a). *Biochem. Biophys. Res. Commun.* **26**, 492.

Schleifer, K. H., Plapp, R., and Kandler, O. (1967b). *Biochem. Biophys. Res. Commun.* **28**, 566.

Schleifer, K. H., Plapp, R., and Kandler, O. (1968). *Biochim. Biophys. Acta* **154**, 573.

Siewert, G., and Strominger, J. L. (1967). *Proc. Natl. Acad. Sci. U.S.* **57**, 767.

Siewert, G., and Strominger, J. L. (1968). *J. Biol. Chem.* **243**, 783.

Strominger, J. L. (1962). *In* "The Bacteria" (I. C. Gunsalus and R. Y. Stanier, eds.), Vol. 3, p. 413. Academic Press, New York.

Strominger, J. L., Threnn, R. H., and Scott, S. S. (1959). *J. Am. Chem. Soc.* **81**, 3803.

Strominger, J. L., Ito, E., and Threnn, R. H. (1960). *J. Am. Chem. Soc.* **82**, 998.

Struve, W. G., Sinha, R. K., and Neuhaus, F. C. (1966). *Biochemistry* **5**, 82.

Swallow, D. L., and Abraham, E. P. (1958). *Biochem. J.* **70**, 364.

Swallow, D. L., and Abraham, E. P. (1959). *Biochem. J.* **72**, 326.

Tanaka, N. (1963). *Biochem. Biophys. Res. Commun.* **12**, 68.

Tanaka, N., Sashikata, K., Wade, T., Sugawara, S., and Umezawa, H. (1963). *J. Antibiot. (Tokyo)* **A16**, 217.

Tempest, D. W., Dicks, J. W., and Ellwood, D. C. (1968). *Biochem. J.* **106**, 237.

Tipper, D. J., and Strominger, J. L. (1965). *Proc. Natl. Acad. Sci. U.S.* **54**, 1133.

Tipper, D. J., and Strominger, J. L. (1966). *Biochem. Biophys. Res. Commun.* **22**, 48.

Wallas, C. H., and Strominger, J. L. (1963). *J. Biol. Chem.* **238**, 2264.

Weidel, W., and Pelzer, H. (1964). *Advan. Enzymol.* **26**, 193.

Weiner, I. M., Higuchi, T., Rothfield, L., Saltmarsh-Andrew, M., Osborn, M. J., and Horecker, B. L. (1965). *Proc. Natl. Acad. Sci. U.S.* **54**, 228.

Wise, E. M., and Park, J. T. (1965). *Proc. Natl. Acad. Sci. U.S.* **54**, 75.

Work, E. (1964). *Nature* **201**, 1107.

Wright, A., Dankert, M., and Robbins, P. W. (1965). *Proc. Natl. Acad. Sci. U.S.* **54**, 235.

Wright, A., Dankert, M., Fennessey, P., and Robbins, P. W. (1967). *Proc. Natl. Acad. Sci. U.S.* **57**, 1798.

Zygmunt, W. A., Browder, H. P., and Tavormina, P. A. (1966a). *Can. J. Microbiol.* **12**, 204.

Zygmunt, W. A., Browder, H. P., and Tavormina, P. A. (1966b). *Can. J. Microbiol.* **12**, 341.

Advances in the Chemotherapy of Viral Diseases

JAMES A. MCFADZEAN

The Research Laboratories,
May & Baker Ltd.,
Dagenham, Essex, England

I. Introduction

There are several previous reviews of the progress made in the chemotherapy of viral diseases, for example, those by Prusoff (1967), Bock (1967), Kaufman (1965), O'Sullivan (1965), Pienta and Groupé (1964), Pienta (1966), and Thompson (1964), and they should be consulted for detailed bibliographies on this subject. Other reviews with less extensive bibliographies are those by Appleyard (1967) and Bauer (1966a, 1967).

Much of the literature on antiviral chemotherapy describes the results of testing a compound or a series of compounds in an experimental virus system in the laboratory. In many instances, the reader is left to speculate on the reasons why the activity which has been described was not pursued in other systems against the same virus, or against other viruses, and why the compound was not developed further as a potential therapeutic agent. The absence of reasons for not pursuing what might have been a promising lead is the most perplexing aspect of the literature. Certainly there would appear to be an abundance of diverse chemical structures showing some degree of antiviral activity in a variety of systems and the more enthusiastic reader may well agree with an enthusiastic author, who has succeeded in demonstrating an antiviral effect in a particular system, that rapid progress is being made in the attempts to develop antiviral drugs. The many meetings held to discuss antiviral chemotherapy probably help to support this impression. Nevertheless, the ultimate goal, and the only yardstick of success in the field of chemotherapy, is the demonstration that a compound can control mortality or morbidity in man or, secondarily, in animals, usually those of economic importance. Compounds active only in tissue culture can be useful tools for the study of viruses but, as has already been said, there are plenty of compounds which have been shown to be active in the laboratory and which are available for detailed studies of this type. There is an almost open field in clinical medicine and at times one has the impression that the aim of chemotherapy has somehow been forgotten. In actual fact, there has been remarkably little success in making available practical antiviral chemotherapeutic or chemoprophylactic agents. All the same, and this is important, the modicum of success that has been attained in man, with the definite activity of the thiosemicarbazones against poxviruses and the activity of idoxuridine against herpes simplex virus, should be sufficient to convince those who doubted that a clinically effective chemotherapeutic agent could be found. Antiviral chemotherapy is an established fact but it is still in its infancy. On the other hand, the little that has been achieved gives some measure of confidence for the future. Bauer (1966a) believes that "we can confidently expect a series of developments which will parallel the rise of the sulfonamides after the initiation of the era of antibacterial chemotherapy."

It is proposed in this chapter to review the real achievements to date in antiviral chemotherapy and chemoprophylaxis in man. This will permit us to make an assessment of the practical outcome of the laboratory work. A comparison of the results obtained in man with those in the laboratory will also enable the laboratory tests to be evaluated.

We shall examine the possible reasons for the failure to make available to physicians larger numbers of useful drugs from the apparent wealth of active substances. It might be argued that any activity of a compound against any pathogenic virus is of potential interest and it has been standard practice in many laboratories to employ a range of viruses using representatives from different groups in screening programs. The stage probably has now been reached, having established the feasibility of antiviral chemotherapy in man, when a more concentrated effort should be made to uncover compounds active against the viruses which are the most important in man from the point of view of mortality and morbidity and where the epidemiology and clinical course are such that chemotherapeutic or chemoprophylactic intervention with an active drug is feasible. We shall try to define from existing knowledge the avenues of approach which would seem to offer the greatest chance of success in the future. It is difficult, and possibly dangerous, in the early stages of the development of a new field to forecast future developments, but an attempt will be made to outline the possible ways in which antiviral chemotherapy may develop. Mention has been made above of the frequent meetings held to discuss the subject of antiviral chemotherapy and, from the more recent of these, one can say that there is reason to believe that there will be important new developments published in the near future—possibly before this article appears in print.

The subjects of interferon and interferon inducers will not be dealt with in this chapter, nor will the question of vaccines and serum therapy.

II. The Current Status of the Chemotherapy of Viral Diseases

There are at present only three substances available for use as chemotherapeutic or chemoprophylactic agents in man. These are *N*-methylisatin *β*-thiosemicarbazone (methisazone), 5-iodo-2′-deoxyuridine (idoxuridine), and 1-adamantanamine hydrochloride (amantadine).

The efficacy of methisazone in the chemoprophylaxis of variola major and variola minor and in the therapy of the complications of vaccination in man has been established. Idoxuridine has been clearly shown to be of value in the topical treatment of herpes simplex keratitis in man. The real value of amantadine in the chemoprophylaxis of influenza A virus infections in man has yet to be determined.

A. *N*-Methylisatin *β*-Thiosemicarbazone (Methisazone)

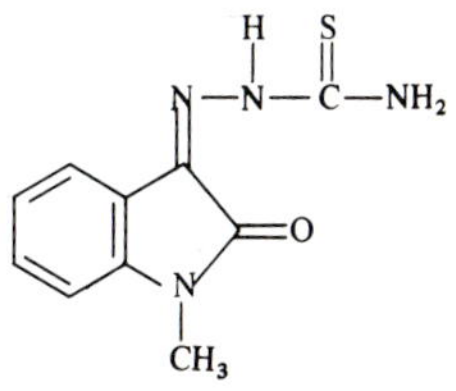

(I)

The history of the development of the thiosemicarbazones as antiviral agents dates from Hamré *et al.* (1950), who demonstrated the protective effect of benzaldehydethiosemicarbazone against vaccinia infections in mice, and the subject has been reviewed a number of times: Bauer (1965a, 1966a, 1967) and Thompson (1964). The successful development of methisazone (I) for use in man has been due largely to the efforts of Bauer in having the compound studied intensively against viral diseases in man.

In the laboratory, methisazone, or the closely related ethylisatin thiosemicarbazone, was found to be active in mice against neurovaccinia (Bauer and Sadler, 1960a), variola minor (Bauer and Sadler, 1960b), rabbit pox (Bauer and Sheffield, 1959), and variola major virus (Bauer *et al.*, 1962).

In clinical trials, the value of methisazone as a prophylactic agent, when given to contacts of patients with variola major, was demonstrated by Bauer *et al.* (1963) and Bauer (1965a); 2297 close contacts of patients with variola major were dosed with methisazone, and 2842 contacts were left untreated. The incidence of smallpox in the treated group was 6 cases with 2 deaths, compared with 114 cases of smallpox and 20 deaths in the untreated group. Bauer believes that some of the treated group were, in fact, not given sufficient drug. do Valle *et al.* (1965) reported the results of a prophylactic trial with methisazone against variola minor (alastrim). In this trial, considering only the unvaccinated contacts, 187 were dosed with methisazone and 219 were left untreated; 7 cases of alastrim occurred in the contacts treated with the drug and 38 cases occurred among the control contacts.

Various dose schedules of methisazone have been employed, but that currently recommended for the prophylaxis of variola infections is 2 doses of 3 gm at an interval of 8–10 hours. The compound has not been described as having any effects on established variola infections.

Another thiosemicarbazone, 4-bromo-3-methylisothiazole-5-carboxaldehydethiosemicarbazone, was also shown to be active in the laboratory against neurovaccinia and variola major viruses in mice, and rabbit pox in rabbits (Rao *et al.*, 1965). This compound has undergone extensive controlled clinical trials and has been shown to have a significant prophylactic effect when given to contacts of variola major infections but to a lesser degree than methisazone (Rao *et al.*, 1966b). An extended therapeutic trial involving 1293 patients with variola major infections showed no definite activity, although there was some evidence of lower virus titers in scabs from treated patients as compared with the titers in scabs from control patients (Rao *et al.*, 1966a).

The other proved indications for the use of methisazone are for the treatment of eczema vaccinatum and vaccinia gangrenosa. Bauer (1965a) reported that 22 cases of eczema vaccinatum had been treated with methisazone. Treatment was assessed as being effective in 12 patients, of doubtful value in 6 patients, and ineffective in 4 patients. He also reported on 10 patients with vaccinia gangrenosa but the results obtained were difficult to assess. Kempe *et al.* (1967) summarized their results up to that time as follows: 7 patients with "life threatening progressive eczema vaccinatum" showed a clinical response which was "prompt and seemingly specific"; 5 out of 9 patients with progressive vaccinia gangrenosa showed "prompt clinical response and virologic cure."

The currently recommended dose schedule for the treatment of the complications of vaccination is an initial dose of 200 mg/kg followed by 50 mg/kg every 6 hours for a total of 8 doses.

Methisazone has also been shown to have other interesting activities. In particular, it inhibited the multiplication in the laboratory of various types of adenovirus (Apostolov, 1967; Bauer and Apostolov, 1966). It is of interest that the structure activity relationships against poxviruses and against adenoviruses are similar. Caunt (1967) also described methisazone as producing a reduced titer of virus in primary human thyroid cell culture infected with varicella virus. Bauer (1967) described methisazone as showing activity in 15 patients with varicella pneumonia in man. Sandeman (1966) reported beneficial effects using methisazone in 6 patients with advanced malignant lymphoma.

1. *Side Effects*

The principal side effect of methisazone is vomiting, which occurs in up to 50% of patients. Other side effects have been reported, but these are certainly acceptable when dealing with the life-threatening conditions described above.

2. *Mode of Action*

The thiosemicarbazones affect a late stage in the growth cycle of poxviruses and inhibit the production of antigens which appear late in the growth cycle (Appleyard *et al.*, 1965). Pollikoff *et al.* (1965), using ethylisatin thiosemicarbazone, showed that the compound when administered to mice which were then infected intracerebrally with vaccinia virus, produced a 1–2 log decrease in plaque-forming units in extracts of the brains of the treated mice. Bauer (1955) reported similar findings with isatin thiosemicarbazone. Rao *et al.* (1965) reported similar results with 4-bromo-3-methylisothiazole-5-carboxaldehyde-thiosemicarbazone against neurovaccinia in mice. The experiments of Westwood and Bowen, quoted by Rao *et al.* (1965), showed a similar effect with the same compound against variola major virus in baby mice. Pollikoff and his colleagues (1965) found that no antibody or interferon was produced in the brains of the drug-treated mice prior to day 10. They deduced that protection was due solely to the action of the drug. On the other hand, the presence of an interfering substance in the brains of mice infected with neurovaccinia virus and treated with 4-bromo-3-methylisothiazole-5-carboxaldehydethiosemicarbazone was demonstrated by Squires and McFadzean (1966). In a series of experiments they showed that the protective effect of this compound against neurovaccinia was almost certainly associated with the production of an interfering substance. The protective action of the compound was abolished if the animals were maintained in an atmosphere of high oxygen tension or when the animals were given cortisone. Both of these sets of conditions reduce the production of interferon.

Appleyard and Way (1966) demonstrated the induction of increased resistance of rabbit poxvirus to the thiosemicarbazones when the virus was passed repeatedly in tissue culture or in mice in the presence of the compounds. These observations may have serious implications for the use of thiosemicarbazones in man.

B. 5-Iodo-2′-deoxyuridine (Idoxuridine)

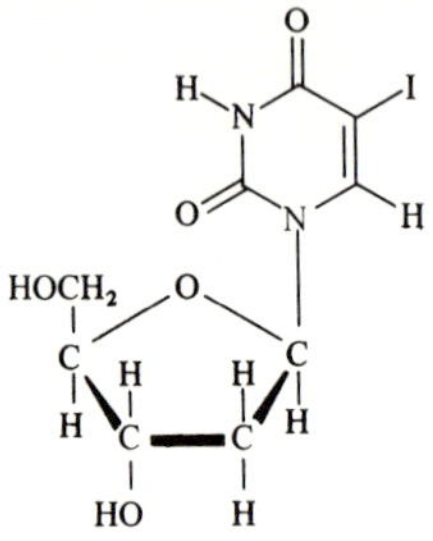

(II)

In the laboratory, idoxuridine (II), commonly known as IUdR or IDU, is active principally against DNA viruses. Herrmann (1961) showed that it, or the bromo analog, inhibited vaccinia and herpes simplex viruses *in vitro*. The frequent application of either of these compounds in solution to the corneas of rabbits suppressed keratitis due either to vaccinia or herpes simplex virus (Kaufman, 1962; Kaufman *et al.*, 1962a). Kaufman and his colleagues also demonstrated the activity of these compounds against herpes simplex infections of the corneal epithelium in man (Kaufman *et al.*, 1962b). Since then, these results have been amply confirmed and have been reviewed by Jones (1967). Patterson (1967) reviewed the management of ocular herpes simplex infections and gave details of dosage.

The effect against herpes lesions elsewhere appears to be variable. MacCallum and Juel-Jensen (1966) applied the compound in solution in dimethylsulfoxide to herpes simplex lesions of the skin of man and obtained a 63% reduction in the duration of the lesions compared with a 43% reduction in duration in patients treated with the solvent alone. Corbett *et al.* (1966) treated 111 patients with recurrent cutaneous herpes simplex with the drug in three different bases, and claimed that polyvinyl alcohol was the most effective base and that the best concentration of the drug was 0.1%. They concluded that the compound is highly effective but its action is dependent on such parameters as the time of commencement of treatment, the base used, and the regime employed.

Herpes-varicella virus is inhibited by idoxuridine *in vitro* (Rawls *et al.*, 1964) but the topical application of the compound seems to have little effect on clinical infections. McCallum *et al.* (1964) reported the results of a trial involving 52 patients suffering from herpes zoster when a 0.1% solution of idoxuridine in saline was shown to be without any therapeutic effect.

It was originally thought that the toxicity of this compound prohibited its systemic use in man. All the same, it has been administered intravenously and perhaps it might have an effect on established variola major infections (personal communication in Prusoff, 1967).

Breeden *et al.* (1966) described a patient suffering from acute necrotizing temporal lobe encephalitis due to herpes simplex who was treated with idoxuridine by intravenous infusion, and decompression craniotomy. The total dose given was 550 mg/kg. Severe side effects, marrow depression, and possible hepatotoxicity were encountered but these rapidly subsided. The authors stated that it was not possible to say conclusively whether or not the drug played any part in the patient's recovery, but initiation of treatment was followed by considerable improvement. An unsuccessful attempt was made with this patient to demonstrate uptake by the brain using a dose of 460 μC ^{131}I idoxuridine. Evans *et al.* (1967) treated another patient suffering from herpes simplex encephalitis—an 8-year-old girl—with an intravenous infusion of 1.5 gm of idoxuridine, given over 8 hours and repeated 4 times more on alternate days. The outcome suggested that the compound may have had antiviral activity within the central nervous system. Buckley and MacCallum (1967) reported on a further case in a 41-year-old patient, in whom there was little evidence of a therapeutic response. Marshall (1967) reported on another single patient treated with intravenous idoxuridine. There was no immediate improvement on decompression. The author believes that the subsequent speed and extent of recovery were more complete than could have been accounted for by decompression alone. With this patient it was difficult to assess the role of the drug. Clarkson *et al.* (1967) reported work in animals which showed that no significant quantities of idoxuridine reached the cerebrospinal fluid after intravenous injections and that the drug was rapidly metabolized after intravenous administration or injection into the ventricles.

Mode of Action

Idoxuridine behaves as an analog of thymidine and is incorporated into DNA as the triphosphate in place of thymidine. A detailed review of the mode of action of the halogenated deoxyribonucleosides is given by Prusoff (1967). Kaplan and Ben-Porat (1967) stated that idoxuridine can be classified as a selective antiviral agent because of the difference between the degree of incorporation of the compound into the DNA of infected cells compared with control cells when low concentrations of the drug are employed. With concentrations of the drug up to 1 μg/ml there was a decrease of 95% in virus infectivity and there was no apparent decrease in cell multiplication. This large difference, however, disappeared when higher concentrations of the drug were used. Diwan and Prusoff (1968) described the effect of 5-iodo-2′-deoxyuridine 5′-triphosphate in inhibiting deoxycytidylate deaminase "induced" by herpes simplex virus in monkey kidney cells. The importance of this observation in relationship to the action of idoxuridine remains to be elucidated.

Prusoff (1967) reviewed the question of resistance of herpes simplex to idoxuridine. A small percentage of the herpes simplex population is resistant to the drug, and resistant strains can be selected *in vitro*. Strains of herpes simplex and vaccinia viruses have been isolated which are resistant because they are unable to induce formation of thymidine kinase and therefore cannot phosphorylate idoxuridine, although this is not necessarily the mechanism in all cases of resistance.

C. 1-Adamantanamine Hydrochloride (Amantadine)

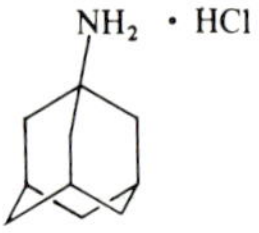

$NH_2 \cdot HCl$

(III)

There is no doubt about the activity of amantadine (III) against certain influenza viruses in the laboratory. It has been shown (Davies *et al.*, 1964; Wood, 1965) to be active in tissue culture and *in ovo* against influenza A, A1, and A2 viruses. It was also active in tissue culture against parainfluenza 1/Sendai and pseudorabies viruses. Maassab and Cochran (1964) demonstrated activity in cell culture against rubella virus. The compound in general has to be added prior to infection of the cells with a virus to show its activity. Activity in mice has been shown against influenza A/swine/S15, A/WS, A1/FM-1/47, A2/AA/2/60, A/equine 2/Lexington/3/63, and parainfluenza 1/Sendai (Davies *et al.*, 1964; Grunert *et al.*, 1964; Wood, 1965). Some strains have responded well to treatment begun a considerable time after infection (Wood, 1965). Oxford and Schild (1967) reported that the compound had no activity against rubella infections in the ferret, rabbit, or hamster.

Sabin (1967) analyzed the data, both published and unpublished, related to the proposed use of amantadine in the prevention of A2 influenza virus disease in man. He states that the most significant study carried out in volunteers was that by Hornick *et al.* (1966) in prison volunteers who had little or no neutralizing antibodies to the strain used. The challenge was by Rockville/1/65 strain which was susceptible to the drug in tissue culture. In the 29 volunteers given a placebo, 6 developed severe illnesses and 7 developed moderate febrile illnesses. The group treated with amantadine was given the standard dose schedule of

100 mg twice a day and only 5 out of 29 showed what was described as a moderate febrile illness. All the drug-treated volunteers became infected as judged by the development of antibodies, although the titers were significantly lower than those in the placebo group. Tyrrell *et al.* (1965) used a less virulent strain of A2 influenza virus (Scot/49/57) which had previously been shown in tissue culture to be the strain most susceptible to the drug. No effect was found in adult volunteers, although larger quantities of drug were used than those normally recommended. Other trials in volunteers discussed by Sabin (1967), for example, Jackson *et al.* (1963), and Stanley *et al.* (1965), showed "a significant but relatively slight reduction in subclinical infection."

In describing what he called the one valid trial of the drug in man exposed to natural infection with influenza A2 virus (personal communication to Sabin), Sabin (1967) stated that there was no significant effect on the number of clinical illnesses but a definite reduction in the subclinical infections. Sabin concluded that the general use of the drug was not warranted until careful trials had been conducted in an open community with an extensive outbreak of A2 influenza.

The results of a clinical evaluation in a rubella epidemic, quoted by Sabin, showed the failure of the compound to protect; possibly in this study the compound had an aggravating effect. Plotkin *et al.* (1966) described the failure of amantadine to stop virus excretion in a patient with rubella and hypogammaglobulinaemia.

Smith *et al.* (1967) described a trial in adult male volunteers infected with type 1 parainfluenza virus. The three parameters of illness, of virus isolation, and of serological response were the same for the drug-treated and for the placebo groups. The amount of drug found in the serum and in the nasal secretions was less than that required for the inhibition of parainfluenza virus in tissue culture.

1. *Side Effects*

The incidence of side effects is low (1–2%) at the recommended dosage. The daily dose of 200 mg/day for an adult should not be exceeded (statement from Council on Drugs, 1967). The most common side effects are hyperexcitability, tremors, slurred speech, ataxia, psychic depression, insomnia, lethargy, and dizziness.

2. *Mode of Action Studies*

The evidence available suggests that the compound interferes with the penetration of the virus into the cell (Davies *et al.*, 1964). Cochran *et al.* (1965) demonstrated the development of resistance of influenza A2/Japan 305 after one passage of the virus in tissue culture in the presence of the drug.

D. Other Compounds

1. *Floxuridine*

Cangir and Sullivan (1966) reported the transient improvement of a child suffering from cytomegalic inclusion disease following treatment with floxuridine (2′-deoxy-5-fluorouridine), commonly known as FUdR. Cangir *et al.* (1967) reported on a further 5 possible cases of cytomegalic inclusion disease responding to treatment with this compound.

2. *UK2371*

Beare *et al.* (1968) described the results of a prophylactic clinical trial with an isoquinoline, UK 2371 (IV), against influenza viruses in volunteers.

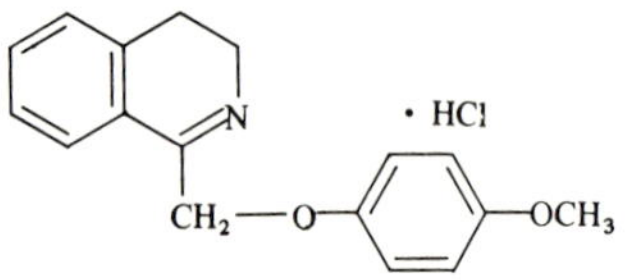

N
· HCl
CH_2—O—⟨benzene ring⟩—OCH_3

(IV)

The publication of these results offers a sharp contrast to the usual pattern in the literature on antiviral chemotherapy insofar as the results of a sound clinical assessment have appeared before any data have been published on the behavior of this compound in experimental systems. The series of compounds is said to inactivate influenza A and B viruses and some paramyxoviruses after a period of direct contact; they were synthesized as potential inhibitors of viral neuraminidase. A dose of 1.5 gm of the drug was given daily in divided dosage for 24 hours before infection and thereafter, for a total of 7 days. Five trials were undertaken with influenza B (B/England/101/62) which was sensitive to the drug *in vitro* and two trials were undertaken with A2/Leningrad/4/65 for which no *in vitro* data were available. In each of the trials with influenza B virus there was a reduction of infection by clinical or laboratory evidence, or by both, in the drug-treated group. Of 34 patients who were given the drug, 7 had symptoms and 9 had laboratory evidence of infection. Of 33 in the placebo group, 13 had symptoms and 17 had laboratory evidence of infection. With the influenza A2 virus trials, the numbers were too small to permit analysis but the drug appeared to have some effect.

This is the first evidence of activity in man against an influenza B virus, although the protection rate was only 50%. The authors point out that much further work is required to demonstrate a protective effect against a natural infection with a virulent virus.

III. The Reasons for the Limited Progress Made to Date and Suggestions for Improved Approaches

For many years it has been apparent that the majority of large pharmaceutical organizations and a number of academic institutes have been putting varying degrees of effort into the field of antiviral chemotherapy. The preceding section makes it clear how little success has been achieved to date. Appleyard (1967) suggested that "the specific treatment of viral disease is no further advanced than was that of bacterial infections in pre-sulphonamide days." This point is arguable but certainly little more than a modest beginning has been obtained.

What is important and somewhat surprising is that compounds with antiviral activity in experimental systems are remarkably easy to find, and a careful search of the literature would probably reveal that some experimental activity with a compound has been recorded against most of the viruses which can be conveniently handled in the laboratory. The question which is very difficult to answer is why so few compounds have been presented to clinicians for assessment in man. The possible factors responsible for this might be listed as follows: lack of satisfactory experimental models; use of the wrong viruses in the laboratory; inadequate activity of the compounds; toxicity of the active compounds; cost of developing the compounds, and difficulties of clinical assessment.

A. Lack of Satisfactory Experimental Models

In certain fields, the absence of any experimental system is the obvious reason for the absence of the assessment of the activities of compounds against a particular virus. On the other hand, there cannot be many instances where some sort of assessment could not be made in the laboratory against the more important viruses.

In general, there have been two approaches to the problem of testing compounds. Some laboratories have established a range of viruses in tissue culture which enables a large number of compounds to be screened for activity. The compounds found to be active in tissue culture are then subjected to evaluation by *in vivo* tests. While the examination of compounds in tissue culture is a somewhat more advanced technique for the assessment of activity than the standard *in vitro* test system used against bacteria, it is still far removed from the demonstration of activity in an animal system. Buthala (1965) reported on the evaluation of 6405 compounds *in vitro* for antiviral activity. Approximately 6% of these compounds showed some degree of activity. When 4230 compounds were tested *in vivo* only 0.33% were found to be active. It is of interest that Buthala reported that of 14 compounds which were active *in vivo*, 12 had *in vitro* activity but 2 had no *in vitro* activity.

Other laboratories prefer to test fewer compounds and to examine them directly in an *in vivo* system using a smaller number of different viruses. On the whole, it would seem to be preferable, where possible, to examine compounds initially *in vivo*. Where a rational approach is being pursued, or where analogs of compounds known to be active *in vivo* are being tested in large numbers, evaluation in tissue culture has its merits.

Other approaches have also been suggested. Trown *et al.* (1967) described a technique for the rapid assessment of antiviral activity by measuring the effect of compounds on the synthesis of viral nucleic acids using radioactive precursors.

Clearly it is not going to be possible to have ideal experimental systems for antiviral chemotherapy for some time to come. An ideal system could be defined as one in which all the compounds active against the disease in man showed parallel activities in the animal system. A comparison of the laboratory results with the clinical results obtained with the thiosemicarbazones suggests that neurovaccinia in mice is a valid screening test for activity against variola in man. One cannot at this stage, however, say much about relative activities of compounds, since only two thiosemicarbazones have been tested against variola major in man and they have not been tested in direct comparison. Activity against variola major and variola minor viruses in mice, and against rabbit poxvirus in mice and in rabbits, also seems to correlate with activity in variola infections in man. It is of interest that isatin thiosemicarbazone is inactive against ectromelia in mice [Bauer and Sadler (1960a), but the same authors (Bauer and Sadler, 1961) later found highly active derivatives of methisazone]. In the case of idoxuridine, the experimental model of herpes simplex in the cornea of rabbits is so closely allied to the clinical condition in man that little need be said about this experimental system.

The position with experimental influenza remains obscure. The activity of amantadine in cell systems and in mice against influenza is undoubted; but in ferrets the compound appears to cause an exacerbation of the disease (Cochran *et al.*, 1965). The last infection is favored by many virologists as being closer to influenza infections in man. In view of the fact that the activity of amantadine in man has not yet been established clearly, it is not yet possible to pass judgement on the laboratory models available for influenza.

In the absence of much information on the behavior of compounds in man, the next best approach is to try to develop an animal infection in which the disease process parallels that of man pathologically and, preferably, clinically. A less satisfactory procedure would be to infect an animal with a particular virus which caused either signs of disease that could be used as parameters, or, possibly, death of the animal. On the other hand, it is completely artificial to induce death of an animal with a virus such as influenza which is usually non-lethal to man. If even this is not possible, the use of an *in vitro* system in parallel with an *in vivo* study of the distribution of the compound in question, as suggested by Acornley *et al.* (1967), will have to suffice. Preferably the *in vivo* distribution studies should be combined with *in vivo/in vitro* assays of the compound. It was gratifying to see the report of the clinical trial, albeit with negative results, of sodium fusidate against Coxsackie A21 virus (Acornley *et al.*, 1967) in spite of the fact that the only evidence of activity which could be produced in the laboratory was activity in tissue culture against the virus.

It is obvious that in most viral infections the models available are far from ideal; this fact may well have been a contributing factor in the inhibition of the development of promising compounds. Probably the most important antiviral agent available today is methisazone. While the experimental systems used to develop this compound have been fully justified by the achievements recorded, the models, except for rabbit pox in rabbits, bear little relationship to the human disease of smallpox. Vaccinia and variola virus, given intracerebrally, respond to methisazone but the infections have little resemblance per se to variola major in man.

Efforts should constantly be made to improve the experimental models available. Bauer (1967) believes that high challenges should be employed in experimental systems. On the other hand, it may be possible to give too great a challenge and to render the experimental system quite unrealistic. It is difficult to be dogmatic about this point, as little is known of the magnitude of challenge in natural viral infections in man.

B. Use of the Wrong Viruses in the Laboratory

It has been the usual practice of those setting up a chemotherapeutic program to try to establish a range of viruses representative of the main groups.

In the very early stages of the development of antiviral chemotherapy, this was a reasonable approach, as any activity against any virus was of interest. Having now established the feasibility of antiviral chemotherapy, however, it is opportune to give further thought to the viruses being used, for two main reasons. First, active compounds must be followed through to clinical trial, provided they pass each of the hurdles of assessment and toxicity; it takes much expertise to do this and many units are not big enough to undertake thorough detailed evaluation within each virus group. Second, a greater degree of selection should be exercised to ensure that an active product has a chance of being assessed clinically; therefore the viruses to be included in the screening test should be chosen to ensure that there is, first, a need for an active product against that particular virus and, second, that facilities could be made available for clinical evaluation.

In general, where effective vaccination procedures are available, there is clearly less need for a chemotherapeutic agent; a pertinent example is poliomyelitis. There will certainly continue to be cases of poliomyelitis but the incidence has decreased so dramatically with the introduction of vaccination that there are other diseases against which effort would be better directed. A short list of the more important viruses in man, could be:

RNA viruses	DNA viruses
Rhinoviruses	Herpesviruses—herpes simplex and cytomegalo viruses
Influenza	
Rubella	Poxviruses

A secondary objective for the chemoprophylaxis and chemotherapy of viral disease are the diseases of veterinary importance. There are a number of them which are of great economic importance in their own right. Substantial losses are suffered in the poultry industry from such conditions as Newcastle disease and the avian-leukosis complex. Active compounds against the viruses responsible for these conditions would be welcomed. Another sound reason for evaluating compounds against veterinary viruses is that one would be dealing with a natural host-parasite system and selection of viruses related to those causing disease in man could yield valuable results indirectly. Thus, Newcastle disease might be of value as a screening system for compounds active against influenza in man. A short list of veterinary viruses that might be employed could be:

RNA viruses	DNA viruses
Picornaviruses—foot-and-mouth disease	Herpesviruses—infectious laryngotracheitis
Paramyxoviruses—Newcastle disease	
Avian-leukosis complex	
Infectious bronchitis	

C. Inadequate Activity of the Compounds

While it is true that there are many compounds with antiviral activity in experimental systems, the activity recorded is usually of a modest order. Sabin (1967) described the effect of amantadine against influenza viruses *in ovo* and in mice as significant though minimal. Protection of 100% against lethal experimental viral infections in animals has certainly been achieved, but high levels of protection using a fraction of the maximum tolerated dose are unusual. Few papers describing active compounds in the laboratory give details of the therapeutic ratios for antiviral substances, and while the therapeutic ratio is by no means the only factor to be taken into consideration, it most certainly gives a guide to the possible usefulness of a compound in man. It seems to be a possibility that nearly all of the compounds that have been examined in the laboratory were just not sufficiently active for further development. This would explain the frequency of papers describing activity with no subsequent follow-up in the literature. There is no particular reason to be despondent about this; although there seems to be a vast armamentarium of compounds for the control of bacterial diseases in man, there are, in fact, very few compounds of value in clinical therapeutics outside the two groups of the sulfonamides and the antibiotics. In the field of mycology there are few effective systemic agents. It is also true that there is no field of chemotherapy where there is a surfeit of effective drugs, and in some important areas our margins of protection are all too narrow, for example, in the cases of malaria and tuberculosis.

D. Toxicity of the Active Compounds

It may well be that the majority of compounds which have been found to be active in the laboratory have also been shown to have undesirable toxic effects. It is difficult to generalize on this point from the literature, but from one's own experience, antiviral activity and toxicity by no means run parallel, as is the case, for example, with antineoplastic substances. What is obvious is that when a tissue culture test system is used many compounds will be found where the cytotoxic level and the apparent antiviral level are close together. This is one of the strongest arguments against the use of tissue culture, unless one uses a sufficiently wide margin between apparent cytotoxic and antiviral levels, before suggesting that a compound has antiviral properties. A compound can damage a cell sufficiently to prevent the support of viral replication at a dose level just below that required to destroy the cell. The reports of activity based on this mechanism may account for the incorrect impression that toxicity and antiviral activity go hand in hand.

E. Cost of Developing the Compounds

The cost of studying the toxiciology of a promising substance for use in man greatly outweighs the possible future financial return in many fields of antiviral chemotherapy. This would apply particularly if we assume that specific activity against a single virus will be the likely event in the future. The pharmaceutical industry, like any other industry, is required to make a profit to be viable. It must, and does, support much fundamental work and can occasionally be philanthropic, but few companies can afford to spend very often the vast sum of money required to develop a drug to the stage of administration to man, knowing that the financial return could well be negligible, even with a "successful" product. This stresses the need to give much careful thought to the question as to which viruses should be employed in the laboratory in the search for active compounds. It would seem reasonable, in the first instance, to concentrate on viruses where a successful compound would command wide usage and a reasonable financial return. Such a return could then support future work against viruses of lesser importance but possibly of more dramatic significance in their behavior in man.

F. Difficulties of Clinical Assessment

These are so obvious that they need little comment. Many virus diseases occur in epidemic form, and it is difficult to be ready with a potential compound and to act sufficiently quickly to obtain meaningful results from sporadic outbreaks of infection. In addition it is difficult to be sure sufficiently early of the identity of the virus with which one is dealing. Volunteer studies are permissible with some respiratory viral infections but the majority of viruses could certainly not be given to volunteers. In the past, skepticism by physicians may have partly accounted for the failure to have compounds assessed.

If one had to underline the most likely explanation for our failure to develop compounds for use in clinical medicine, the answer would be that we have not yet found sufficiently active agents. It is worthwhile, however, to reflect on the fact that the thiosemicarbazones, which are now probably the most active compounds available for viral diseases of man, remained in the laboratory for a very long time before being taken to clinical trial.

Considering on more general lines the possible ways of enhancing the chances of success in this field, one remembers that the major discoveries in most aspects of chemotherapy have stemmed from chance observations. It is the belief of many workers in the field of chemotherapy that chance observations from random screening will continue to be the most fruitful approach for some time to come. This would suggest that the more compounds that are tested, the greater the chance of success. Bauer (1966a) rejects this view and suggests that the most effective approach is to test compounds which have shown interesting activities in some other biological system. Methisazone and idoxuridine were developed on this basis, the former from the use of thiosemicarbazones against tuberculosis and the latter from attempts to develop nucleic acid antagonists for the chemotherapy of tumors. It is of interest that the latest compound that has been reported as showing activity in man, the isoquinoline derivative UK 2371, was synthesized as a potential inhibitor of viral neuraminidase and probably represents a successful outcome from a rational chemical approach.

Consequently, it is important to develop new and better experimental systems for carefully selected viruses, and to try to have ready facilities and defined parameters for the evaluation of compounds in the clinical disease in man.

IV. The Future of the Chemotherapy of Viral Diseases

A forecast at this stage about the possible future developments in the field of antiviral chemotherapy is difficult and probably dangerous, but a number of points can be made. It is wrong to generalize and to say that the future use of chemical agents lies in their use as prophylactics. Each virus disease requires to be assessed separately. For the therapeutic use of drugs the most important factor is the time in the disease process at which a reasonably certain diagnosis can be made. Bauer (1965b) described three classes of viral infections which should be amenable to a therapeutic approach:

1. Those with a prodromal period, e.g., smallpox
2. Those with a protracted course, e.g., chickenpox
3. Those with a biphasic course, e.g., enterovirus meningitis

In each of these groups a diagnosis may be made at a stage when the administration of an active compound could well interrupt the virus cycle with resulting beneficial results to the host.

Two groups of virus diseases probably not amenable to treatment are those in which the pathological processes are near maximal when the diagnosis can be made with certainty, e.g., influenza, and those in which the diagnosis can only be made after "cumbersome laboratory investigations." The latter category, of course, would be amenable to treatment if wide spectrum agents became available and the diagnosis could then be made in retrospect.

Chemoprophylaxis would appear to be much easier. One can certainly envisage the mass medication prophylactically of certain groups of animals against certain viral diseases, for example, Newcastle disease and infectious bronchitis in chickens. The prophylactic use of drugs in the poultry industry against such conditions as coccidiosis is widespread but there must be a limit to the amount of foreign substances which can be incorporated into animal feeds. One can also envisage the mass chemoprophylaxis of man in a pandemic of influenza such as that which occurred in 1958, or the administration of a drug like methisazone to a nonimmune population in the event of an outbreak of smallpox. On the other hand, one wonders if the administration of a drug throughout each winter to prevent the "common cold" would be justified.

Nevertheless, there are examples of the prolonged administration of prophylactic agents in man: probably the best known being the malarial prophylactics —proguanil, chloroquine, and pyrimethamine. More feasible would be the use of long-acting prophylactic agents, an approach which was restricted until recent years to the prophylaxis of trypanosomiasis. More recently, however, long-acting antimalarials have been developed. Study of the basic mechanisms involved in prolonged drug prophylaxis has been largely neglected and this is an aspect which may well be worthy of consideration in the development of antiviral prophylactic agents.

In general, the use of active immunization has much to commend it over chemoprophylaxis; on the other hand, the antigenic variations in many viruses and the multiplicity of viruses causing a syndrome such as the common cold rule out this approach. It is also true that it is difficult to immunize an entire population and to maintain a high level of immunity. It would greatly enhance the value of a prophylactic drug if the individual were rendered immune following a natural challenge while protected by the compound. Mice protected by thiosemicarbazones against neurovaccinia are, in fact, rendered immune.

Another aspect for future consideration is the spectrum of activity which might be expected from drugs. The evidence just now suggests a narrow range of activity but there are few data available from which to argue. The increasing range of viruses against which methisazone is now being shown to be active tends to change one's views on this problem.

As soon as any measure of success is achieved in any field of chemotherapy, the problem of the development of resistance has to be considered. There is evidence with methisazone, idoxuridine, and amantadine that resistant strains can occur naturally or can be induced by exposure to the compound. In some cases this has been demonstrated *in vitro* and in others *in vivo*. It would seem, therefore, that as this field develops it is unlikely that it will be free from the unending difficulties posed by the emergence of resistant strains.

Bauer (1966b) pointed out that the successes achieved in antiviral chemotherapy have been with the larger viruses; he questioned if there was any relationship between the size of the virus particles and the activity of chemotherapeutic agents. He examined the hypothesis that a therapeutic agent has a maximum effect if one molecule of the agent inhibits the maturation of one virus particle and that for maximum activity each volume of cytoplasm of an infected cell equivalent to the volume of the virus particle should contain one molecule of the drug. He calculated that of the known active drugs, methisazone is 15% efficient against rabbit pox, idoxuridine is 4.6% efficient against herpes simplex, and amantadine is 2.5% efficient against influenza. Against poliomyelitis 5-chloro-2(α-hydroxybenzyl)-benzimidazole is 100% efficient. He forecast the minimal inhibitory concentrations for compounds against viruses for which there is yet no therapy and the dosages which would, theoretically, be required to be administered to man to produce a significant effect. For the larger viruses (and he draws the line at the verruca virus), his calculations would suggest that therapy is feasible, but for the smaller viruses, treatment might be impracticable. For these he suggested that the search should be made for compounds of high water solubility and low molecular weight.

In a general concept of antiviral chemotherapy, one should remember that a direct antiviral effect is not absolutely necessary for a drug to be of value in man. Thompson (1964) stresses this point and stated that "the logical objective of therapy should be to assist the natural body defences of the patient to overcome his illness."

A. Tumor Viruses

As yet there is no proof that any malignant neoplasm of man is caused by a virus, although evidence is accumulating to suggest that a viral etiology is likely in at least some instances. Viruses are certainly the causal agents in a number of tumors of animals, but the field of oncogenic virology is indeed complex and it is difficult to foresee at this stage the potential role of a compound active against the viruses implicated in human tumor production. Westwood (1966) gave his views on the theoretical basis of the chemotherapy of viruses and the possible relationship to the chemotherapy of cancer.

The isolation of a cytopathogenic agent from chickens with Marek's disease, suggestive of a member of the herpes B virus group (Churchill and Biggs, 1967), should aid the investigation of possible chemotherapeutic approaches to this widespread and economically important disease.

B. Slow Viruses

A developing field which is of great interest is the study of the "slow" virus infections—in particular, the chronic human infectious neuropathic agents (CHINA). Gibbs (1967) reviews the search for infective agents in the chronic and subacute degenerative diseases of the central nervous system. The passage of the infectious agent from Kuru in man to chimpanzees (Gajdusek *et al.*, 1966) marks a step forward in the elucidation of chronic degenerative diseases of the central nervous system. Brody (1967) stated that "leukodystrophies and subacute encephalitides" are the leading candidates for having a viral etiology, and lists the following conditions—amyotrophic lateral sclerosis, peroneal muscular atrophy, myasthenia gravis, the presenile dementias of Alzheimer and Pick, and other central nervous system degenerative diseases—as those where there is speculation as to a viral origin. Further, he stated that the concentration on Guam of amyotrophic lateral sclerosis and Parkinsonism dementia is suggestive of viral etiology.

It is of interest that Thormar (1965) has described the inhibition, in cell culture, of visna virus, a slow virus of sheep, by 5-bromodeoxyuridine added 1 to 2 hours after inoculation with the virus. Idoxuridine was not as effective. Actinomycin D also interfered with the replication of visna virus.

V. Conclusions

The belief that the close association of a virus with its host cell would not permit of a differential toxicity of foreign chemical agents against the virus, leaving the cells of the host untouched, has been shown to be invalid. There are now drugs available for the treatment and prevention of viral diseases in man.

The activity of idoxuridine against herpes simplex virus has demonstrated that a topical therapeutic approach in viral disease is possible. The activity of methisazone against the complications of vaccination has shown that a systemic therapeutic approach is also possible. The activity of methisazone in preventing variola major and variola minor in contacts has demonstrated the feasibility of a systemic chemoprophylactic approach. These are all contributions in their own right in this field, but they are small achievements compared to the vast morbidity and mortality caused by viruses in man and in animals.

The field of antiviral chemotherapy is one in which the moral rewards to be obtained are high; but, with a few notable exceptions the financial returns for large expenditures are, in general, not great, particularly if a narrow range of activity is anticipated with chemotherapeutic or chemoprophylactic agents in the future. It is to be hoped that financial considerations will not be an insuperable barrier to the development of potentially active agents. To help overcome this difficulty, greater care should be exercised in the selection of the viruses against which compounds are tested, bearing in mind such factors as the epidemiology of the virus disease in the natural host, the disease pattern, the incidence of the disease, and the feasibility of obtaining meaningful results in the clinical assessment of the compound. Influenza viruses have always been rated high in the list of viruses against which compounds should be assessed. Nonetheless, the failure to evaluate satisfactorily the prophylactic activity of amantadine against influenza A infections in man has underlined one of the great difficulties of working with this undoubtedly important group of viruses. Facilities must be developed for the proper clinical evaluation of the increasing number of active agents which it is to be hoped will come forward in the future. It is to be hoped too that skepticism will not hinder in any way the development of facilities for clinical evaluation.

Attempts must be made constantly to evolve more satisfactory experimental laboratory systems, particularly to mimic more closely the disease as it occurs in the natural host. Newly isolated strains should be introduced to the laboratory at intervals to avoid working continually with strains antigenically different from those existing currently and which have changed in other ways by their being maintained for long periods in experimental animals. Consideration should also be given to the use of natural host-parasite systems.

Some believe that we have yet to find a really active compound and that when we do so its activity will be so clear-cut that it will be possible to demonstrate its value without the detailed statistical analysis which seems to be required at present.

There is already evidence from the histories of the development of compounds active in man that a rational chemical approach to the chemotherapy of viruses may prove to be more fruitful than it has been against other parasites. Further developments in the basic study of viruses may well facilitate the development of such a rational approach. This would be most satisfying intellectually to those engaged in this field.

The possible implications of viruses in neoplastic diseases of man and the elucidation of a viral origin in other major groups of disease broaden the potential field for the possible application of antiviral agents in the future.

REFERENCES

Acornley, J. E., Bessell, C. J., Bynoe, M. L., Godtfredsen, W. O., and Knoyle, J. M. (1967). *Brit. J. Pharmacol.* **31**, 210.

Apostolov, K. (1967). *Proc. 5th Intern. Congr. Chemotherapy, Vienna,* 1967 **4**, 319.

Appleyard, G. (1967). *Brit. Med. Bull.* **23**, 114.

Appleyard, G., and Way, H. J. (1966). *Brit. J. Exptl. Pathol.* **47**, 144.

Appleyard, G., Hume, V. M. B., and Westwood, J. C. N. (1965). *Ann. N.Y. Acad. Sci.* **130**, 92.

Bauer, D. J. (1955). *Brit. J. Exptl. Pathol.* **36**, 105.

Bauer, D. J. (1965a). *Ann. N.Y. Acad. Sci.* **130**, 110.

Bauer, D. J. (1965b). *Ann. N.Y. Acad. Sci.* **130**, 324.

Bauer, D. J. (1966a). *Sci. Basis Med. Ann. Rev.* p. 174.

Bauer, D. J. (1966b). *Nature* **209**, 639.

Bauer, D. J. (1967). *In* "Modern Trends in Medical Virology," (R. B. Heath and A. P. Waterson, eds.), Vol. 1, p. 49. Butterworth, London and Washington, D.C.

Bauer, D. J. (1967). Personal communication.

Bauer, D. J., and Apostolov, K. (1966). *Science* **154**, 796.

Bauer, D. J., and Sadler, P. W. (1960a). *Brit. J. Pharmacol.* **15**, 101.

Bauer, D. J., and Sadler, P. W. (1960b). *Lancet* **i**, 1110.

Bauer, D. J., and Sadler, P. W. (1961). *Nature* **190**, 1167.

Bauer, D. J., and Sheffield, F. W. (1959). *Nature* **184**, 1496.

Bauer, D. J., Dumbell, K. R., Fox-Hulme, P., and Sadler, P. W. (1962). *Bull. World Health Organ.* **26**, 727.

Bauer, D. J., St. Vincent, L., Kempe, C. H., and Downie, A. W. (1963). *Lancet* **ii**, 494.

Beare, A. S., Bynoe, M. L., and Tyrrell, D. A. J. (1968). *Lancet* **i**, 843.

Bock, M. (1967). *Current Topics Microbiol. Immunol.* **41**, 100.

Breeden, C. J., Hall, T. C., and Tyler, H. R. (1966). *Ann. Intern. Med.* **65**, 1050.

Brody, J. A. (1967). *Current Topics Microbiol. Immunol.* **40**, 64.

Buckley, T. F., and MacCallum, F. O. (1967). *Brit. Med. J.* **ii**, 419.

Buthala, D. A. (1965). *Ann. N.Y. Acad. Sci.* **130**, 17.
Cangir, A., and Sullivan, M. P. (1966). *J. Am. Med. Assoc.* **195**, 616.
Cangir, A., Sullivan, M. P., Sutow, W. W., and Taylor, G. (1967). *J. Am. Med. Assoc.* **201**, 612.
Caunt, A. E. (1967). *Proc. 5th Intern. Congr. Chemotherapy, Vienna,* 1967 **4**, 313.
Churchill, A. E., and Biggs, P. M. (1967). *Nature* **215**, 528.
Clarkson, D. R., Oppelt, W. W., and Byvoet, P. (1967). *J. Pharmacol. Exptl. Therap.* **157**, 581.
Cochran, K. W., Maassab, H. F., Tsunoda, A., and Berlin, B. S. (1965). *Ann. N.Y. Acad. Sci.* **130**, 432.
Corbett, M. B., Sidell, C. M., and Zimmerman, M. (1966). *J. Am. Med. Assoc.* **196**, 441.
Council on Drugs Statement (1967). *J. Am. Med. Assoc.* **201**, 374.
Davies, W. L., Grunert, R. R., Haff, R. F., McGahen, J. W., Neumayer, E. M., Paulshock, M., Watts, J. C., Wood, T. R., Herrmann, E. C., and Hoffmann, C. E. (1964). *Science* **144**, 862.
Diwan, A., and Prusoff, W. H. (1968). *Virology* **34**, 184.
do Valle, L. A. R., de Melo, P. R., de Salles Gomes, L. F., and Proença, L. M. (1965). *Lancet* **ii**, 976.
Evans, A. D., Gray, O. P., Miller, M. H., Jones, E. R. V., Weeks, R. D., and Wells, C. E. C. (1967). *Brit. Med. J.* **ii**, 407.
Gajdusek, D. C., Gibbs, C. J., and Alpers, M. (1966). *Nature* **209**, 794.
Gibbs, C. J. (1967). *Current Topics Microbiol. Immunol.* **40**, 44.
Grunert, R. R., McGahen, J. W., and Davies, W. L. (1964). *Federation Proc.* **23**, 387.
Hamré, D., Bernstein, J., and Donovick, R. (1950). *Proc. Soc. Exptl. Biol. Med.* **73**, 275.
Herrmann, E. C., Jr. (1961). *Proc. Soc. Exptl. Biol. Med.* **107**, 142.
Hornick, R. B., Togo, Y., and Dawkins, A. T. (1966). *Bacteriol. Proc.* p. 131. (Abstr.)
Jackson, G. G., Muldoon, R. L., and Akers, L. W. (1963). *Antimicrobial Agents Chemotherapy* p. 703.
Jones, B. R. (1967). *Trans. Ophthalmol. Soc. U.K.* **87**, 537.
Kaplan, A. S., and Ben-Porat, T. (1967). *Virology* **31**, 734.
Kaufman, H. E. (1962). *Proc. Soc. Exptl. Biol. Med.* **109**, 251.
Kaufman, H. E. (1965). *Progr. Med. Virol.* **7**, 116.
Kaufman, H. E., Nesburn, A. B., and Maloney, E. D. (1962a). *Virology* **18**, 567.
Kaufman, H. E., Martola, E. L., and Dohlman, C. (1962b). *Arch. Ophthalmol.* (*Chicago*) **68**, 235.
Kempe, C. H., Fulginiti, V., and Sieber, O. (1967). *Proc. 5th Intern. Congr. Chemotherapy, Vienna,* 1967 In abstracts p. 1233.
Maassab, H. F., and Cochran, K. W. (1964). *Science* **145**, 1443.
McCallum, D. I., Johnston, E. N. M., and Raju, B. H. (1964). *Brit. J. Dermatol.* **76**, 459.
MacCallum, F. O., and Juel-Jensen, B. E. (1966). *Brit. Med. J.* **ii**, 805.
Marshall, W. J. S. (1967). *Lancet* **ii**, 579.
O'Sullivan, D. G. (1965). The Royal Institute of Chemistry, Lecture Series No. 2.
Oxford, J. S., and Schild, G. C. (1967). *Proc. 5th Intern. Congr. Chemotherapy, Vienna,* 1967 **2** (1), 23.
Patterson, A. (1967). *Brit. J. Ophthalmol.* **51**, 494.
Pienta, R. J. (1966). *In* "Experimental Chemotherapy" (R. J. Schnitzer and F. Hawking, eds.), Vol. 4, p. 592. Academic Press, New York.
Pienta, R. J., and Groupé, V. (1964). *In* "Experimental Chemotherapy" (R. J. Schnitzer and F. Hawking, eds.), Vol. 3, p. 525. Academic Press, New York.
Plotkin, S. A., Klaus, R. M., and Whitely, J. P. (1966). *J. Pediat.* **69**, 1085.

Pollikoff, R., Lieberman, M., Lem, N. E., and Foley, E. J. (1965). *J. Immunol.* **94**, 794.

Prusoff, W. H. (1967). *Pharmacol. Rev.* **19**, 209.

Rao, A. R., McFadzean, J. A., and Squires, S. (1965). *Ann. N.Y. Acad. Sci.* **130**, 118.

Rao, A. R., McFadzean, J. A., and Kamalakshi, K. (1966a). *Lancet* **i**, 1068.

Rao, A. R., McKendrick, G. D. W., Velayudhan, L., and Kamalakshi, K. (1966b). *Lancet* **i**, 1072.

Rawls, W. E., Cohen, R. A., and Herrmann, E. C., Jr. (1964). *Proc. Soc. Exptl. Biol. Med.* **115**, 123.

Sabin, A. B. (1967). *J. Am. Med. Assoc.* **200**, 943.

Sandeman, T. F. (1966). *Brit. Med. J.* **ii**, 625.

Smith, C. B., Purcell, R. H., and Chanock, R. M. (1967). *Am. Rev. Respirat. Diseases* **95**, 689.

Squires, S. L., and McFadzean, J. A. (1966). *Trans. Roy. Soc. Trop. Med. Hyg.* **60**, 419.

Stanley, E. D., Muldoon, R. E., Akers, L. W., and Jackson, G. G. (1965). *Ann. N.Y. Acad. Sci.* **130**, 44.

Thompson, R. L. (1964). *Advan. Chemotherapy* **1**, 85.

Thormar, H. (1965). *Virology* **26**, 36.

Trown, P. W., Brindley, K. P., and Miller, P. A. (1967). *Proc. 5th Intern. Congr. Chemotherapy, Vienna,* 1967 **2** (1), 7.

Tyrrell, D. A. J., Bynoe, M. L., and Hoorn, B. (1965). *Brit. J. Exptl. Pathol.* **46**, 370.

Westwood, J. C. N. (1966). *Chemotherapia* **11**, 192.

Wood, T. R. (1965). *Ann. N.Y. Acad. Sci.* **130**, 419.

A Pharmacological Analysis of Aspirin

H. O. J. Collier*

Department of Pharmacological Research, Division of Medical and Scientific Affairs, Parke-Davis and Company, Hounslow, Middlesex, England

I. Introduction

Modern drugs are discovered in laboratories and are given to man only later in their development; but the traditional drugs, such as opium and cinchona, were taken by man long before they were studied in laboratories. We therefore ask, in the case of a modern drug, how far the animal experiments

* Present address: Miles Laboratories Limited, Stoke Poges, Buckinghamshire, England

predict the clinical findings; with a traditional drug, how far they reproduce them.

The salicylates are old enough, in the form of willow bark and other herbal preparations, for their therapeutic effects to have been reported in man first. Thus, when Stone (1763) describes, in the *Philosophical Transactions of the Royal Society*, the febrifugal effect of willow bark in agues, he probably used it first in man, since he does not mention animal experiments. Although there is little doubt of this, there is much uncertainty whether Stone's first name was Edward or Edmund, since the printer has allotted him one name at the beginning and the other at the end of his paper (Collier, 1963a). The active principle of willow bark is salicin; and, a century after Stone's report, Maclagan (1876) observed the efficacy of salicin in acute rheumatism without testing it first in animals, although he took large doses of the drug himself before giving it to his patients.

According to Domenjoz (1966a), salicylic acid was first used clinically in place of carbolic acid to disinfect wounds. Thiersch (1875) introduced this practice after Bertagnini (1856) and Kolbe (1874) had shown by experiments in man, presumably on themselves, that large doses could safely be taken. The first paper on the antipyretic use of salicylic acid (Buss, 1875) appeared in the same issue of the *Zentralblatt des Medizinschen Wissenschaft* that contained a paper by Fürbringer (1875) describing its antipyretic effect in animals. In the same year Zimmermann (1875) also described the antipyretic effect in rabbits.

When aspirin was introduced as a more palatable and less topically toxic form of salicylic acid, the therapeutic properties of the parent compound were already well known. Although, at its introduction, Dreser (1899) reported some scanty toxicity tests on fishes and frogs, as well as experiments on himself, aspirin was soon used clinically and seems to belong essentially to the traditional drugs, in which animal experiments come as an afterthought, dotting the i's and crossing the t's of the clinical findings.

Since aspirin is probably the most widely used medicinal drug in the world (Collier, 1963a), it is the mainstay of several pharmaceutical manufacturers. The wish to find an even better drug has therefore impelled much research on aspirin. From this wish spring laboratory models of the drug's therapeutic and toxic effects in man, by means of which new compounds can be screened for aspirin-like effects. The amount of fruit that directly utilitarian experiments of the screening type can bear, however, is probably limited, and greater improvements in drugs may depend on understanding how they act. Thus, the desire to replace aspirin has also provided a part of the motive for studies on the mechanism by which it exerts its therapeutic effects.

Any scientific investigation may be regarded as the product of certain questions, which may or may not have been consciously formulated. If the main questions that appear to have guided laboratory experiments on aspirin are formulated, they seem to be the following. (1) In experimental systems, how far can the therapeutic and toxic effects of aspirin in man be reproduced, and what other effects can be observed? (2) Using these models of its clinical effects, can better drugs of the same type be found? (3) What are the pharmacologic relatives of aspirin, where do the boundaries of this group of drugs lie, and does aspirin differ from sodium salicylate in its quantitative profile of actions? (4) How does aspirin exert its pharmacologic (including toxic) effects, and can these be attributed to a few underlying actions on living cells? (5) How is aspirin absorbed, distributed, metabolized, and excreted, and how do these processes affect its action? Such questions have yielded the material upon which the present analysis is based. This analysis is based on the literature up to mid-1968.

A. In What Chemical Form Does Aspirin Act?

At the introduction of aspirin, Dreser (1899) showed that it was converted to salicylate in the body, and he expressed no doubt but that this salicylate was responsible for the therapeutic effect. Nearly half a century later, however, Lester *et al.* (1946) suggested that aspirin acts in its own right as acetylsalicylate. Before embarking on an account of the pharmacology of aspirin, therefore, we should try to decide whether we are considering the action of aspirin itself or of the salicylate to which it is converted.

Whereas aspirin and sodium salicylate are probably qualitatively alike in their actions, there is today good evidence that aspirin is the more potent, particularly in the tests summarized in Table I. Even in antipyretic and anti-inflammatory tests, when aspirin and sodium salicylate have been compared, the advantage, if any, lies with aspirin.

When the blood levels of acetylsalicylate and salicylate are measured soon after administration of aspirin, both compounds are present, about one quarter of the total being in the acetyl form (Lester *et al.*, 1946; Smith, 1951). Since a dose of aspirin produces a lower blood level of unsubstituted salicylate than does an equivalent dose of sodium salicylate (Smith *et al.*, 1946) and yet aspirin is several times more active in antinociceptive tests, we can infer that aspirin acts as an analgetic in its own right, as Lester *et al.* (1946) suggested, although the salicylate into which it is converted presumably supplements the activity of aspirin itself. The same argument would apply with still more force to the other effects of aspirin listed in Table I. If aspirin thus acts in these ways without having first to be converted to sodium salicylate, there seems good reason to suppose that it also has antipyretic and anti-inflammatory activity of its own, which accounts for at least a part of these effects of administered aspirin.

We should not overlook the possibility that aspirin might act through conversion to a metabolite other than salicylate. To explain the findings in Table I, however, this metabolite would have to be produced in larger amounts by the

TABLE I

EXAMPLES OF THE GREATER POTENCY OF ASPIRIN THAN OF SODIUM SALICYLATE AGAINST SOME INDUCED RESPONSES[a]

Response		Inhibitory dose (mg/kg) and route		
Type	Induced by	Aspirin	Na salicylate	Reference
Abdominal constriction in mouse	Phenylquinone i.p.	68 (53–86) s.c.	250 (217–287) s.c.	Hendershot and Forsaith (1959)
	Acetic acid i.p.	49 (35–67) p.o.	190 (134–268) p.o.	Whittle (1964)
	Acetylcholine i.p.	26 (17–40) s.c.	151 (97–235) s.c.	Collier *et al.* (1964)
Nociception in dog	Bradykinin i.a.	38 ± 12 i.v.	167 ± 13 i.v.	Guzman *et al.* (1964)
Broncho-constriction in guinea pig	Bradykinin i.v.	2 i.v.	64 i.v.	Collier and Shorley (1960)
Skin erythema in man	Thurfyl nicotinate p.c.	3 p.o.	> 8 p.o.	Adams and Cobb (1963)
Platelet clumping in shed plasma of man	Collagen adrenaline	2 p.o.	> 27 p.o.	O'Brien (1968a, b)

[a] Key to abbreviations: i.p., intraperitoneal; in parentheses, fiducial limits; s.c., subcutaneous; p.o., by mouth; i.a., intra-arterial; i.v., intravenous; p.c., percutaneous.

breakdown of aspirin than by that of salicylate. Such a possibility seems remote.

Taking the view that aspirin is effective in its own right, the present analysis concerns the pharmacology of aspirin rather than that of salicylate in general, unlike most previous books or reviews in this field. Results obtained with salicylates other than aspirin will only be included, therefore, insofar as they help to throw light on the pharmacology of aspirin.

B. The Pharmacologic Character of Aspirin

The most important effects of a drug are those that occur at low doses, for these are likely to be used in therapy or to be the commonest causes of poisoning. Among such effects of aspirin in man are the lessening of fever, pain, and inflammation induced by microbial toxins, by antigens, or by other chemical challenges. Since fever, pain, and inflammation may be regarded as some of the body's natural defensive mechanisms, the therapeutic effects for which aspirin is so widely taken—antipyresis, analgesia, and antiphlogosis—may therefore be characterized as antidefensive.

We may also regard as defensive reactions, designed to exclude or expel noxious materials, the contraction of smooth muscle and the secretion of fluid that occur in the bronchial tree (Collier, 1968) and in the bowels, in response to toxins, antigens, or irritants. In the laboratory, aspirin readily antagonizes contractions of some smooth muscles, and it has been reported to inhibit the gastric secretion of mucus (Menguy and Masters, 1965). Again, hemostasis at the rupture of a blood vessel is a defensive reaction that aspirin to some extent antagonizes. Aspirin and sodium salicylate also inhibit the rise in free fatty acids in the blood induced by cold, fasting, or other challenges, which has been considered a reaction to emergency (Bizzi *et al.*, 1965). Yet again, the multiplication of epithelial cells in mucous membranes and the production of keratin in the skin may be regarded as defensive processes, and so the destruction by salicylates of mucous epithelia and keratin might also be regarded as antidefensive. For many reasons, therefore, aspirin may be characterized as an antidefensive drug.

C. Experimental Models of Defensive Reactions

Insofar as laboratory conditions are more favorable than clinical for an analysis of the mode of action of a drug, the present review will concentrate on those antidefensive effects of aspirin that are reproducible in the laboratory. In many, although not all, a defensive reaction is induced by an experimental challenge. Such a challenge is often, though not always, the application of a noxious stimulus (or noxa).

Noxae may be mechanical, thermal, electrical, radiant, or chemical. Chemical noxae may be abnormal osmotic or hydrogen-hydroxyl ion concentrations, or they may be particular substances, either those of low molecular weight, or macromolecules such as antigens and the toxins of parasites. Included below among noxae are substances, naturally present on occasions in the body, such as histamine and bradykinin, that can elicit local defensive reactions. These have been called "nocisimulant" (Collier, 1964) or "nocistimulant" (Jacob, 1967), rather than noxious, but they form part of the armory of challenges used by the experimental pharmacologist.

According to the noxa used, the defensive reactions differ in pattern. Some occur at a distance from the site of injury. One such systemic reaction is fever; another is the complex of responses, including vocalization, avoiding movements, hyperpnea, and a rise in blood pressure, that we take to indicate pain and may conveniently call nociception. Some defensive reactions to local noxae themselves remain local. These include hyperemia, edema, diapedesis, coagulation of blood or exudate, necrosis, phagocytosis, and granulation.

Where smooth muscle is present, as in the walls of arterioles and bronchioles, its contraction may also be part of the local response to challenge. Although the reactions of living material to noxae can be classified into a few main categories, responses within each category vary in detail according to the particular challenge and the circumstances of the experiment.

In the analysis that follows of the antidefensive action of aspirin, we shall consider responses to noxae under various heads—antipyresis, antinociception, anti-inflammation, antagonism of smooth muscle responses, and antihemostasis. We shall also consider other effects of aspirin that might be deemed antidefensive, such as damage to epithelia. When these pharmacologic effects of aspirin have been considered separately, an attempt will be made to assess how aspirin exerts these effects and to what extent a common mechanism underlying defensive responses may be identified as the target of this drug.

II. Antipyresis

Aspirin lowers body temperature arising from various natural pathologic states in man (Rénon, 1900; Barbour, 1919); but it does not appreciably lower normal body temperature, and it tends to enhance rather than reduce fever owing to heatstroke or to drugs that stimulate metabolism (von Euler, 1961; Woodbury, 1965; Cranston and Rosendorff, 1968). In contrast with aspirin, chlorpromazine lowers body temperature from a normal level or when elevated by a high environmental temperature, as well as that raised by natural pathologic processes (Courvoisier *et al.*, 1953; Decourt *et al.*, 1953). These facts conform with the concept that aspirin acts by moderating natural defensive reactions of the body.

A. Antipyretic Effects in Animals

The potency of aspirin in lowering fever in experimental animals is measured fairly often because aspirin may be used for reference when new methods of evaluating antipyretic potency or when new drugs against pain or rheumatism are sought. To measure antipyretic potency, rats or rabbits usually are kept in a constant environmental temperature, rectal temperature is recorded, and fever is induced by injecting pyrogenic microbes or microbial pyrogens. Table II summarizes some tests of the antipyretic effect of aspirin in experimental animals. This table shows that aspirin, at doses of 22–200 mg/kg, lowered fevers induced by microbial toxins in every animal species in which it was tested. In mouse, rat, and guinea pig, aspirin was less effective in lowering normal body temperature than in lessening fever induced with yeast (Bianchi *et al.*, 1967).

TABLE II

ANTIPYRETIC EFFECT OF ASPIRIN IN EXPERIMENTAL FEVERS

Species	Fever induced by	Effective dose of aspirin (mg/kg) and route[a]	Approx. relative potency of other antipyretics[b] (aspirin = 1)	Reference
Mouse	Yeast	300 p.o.	Am, 4; In, 10; Pb, 1	Bianchi *et al.* (1967)
Rat	Yeast	40 p.o.	Am, 1.8; Pa, 1.45	Brownlee (1937) Brownlee and Gaddum (1939)
		50 i.p.	—	Bavin *et al.* (1952)
		100 p.o.	—	Smith *et al.* (1963)
		50 p.o.	Fl, Mc, Me, 1 or more	Winder *et al.* (1962, 1963, 1965)
		200 p.o.	Am, > 1; In, 10	Bianchi *et al.* (1967)
	Witte peptone after incubation	100 p.o.	—	Buller *et al.* (1957)
	Escherichia coli lipopolysaccharide	25 i.p.	Am, 2.13; In, 16; Pb, 2.15	Winter and Nuss (1963) Winter *et al.* (1962)
		25 p.o.	—	Winter *et al.* (1963)
Rabbit	Piqure	16–26 s.c.	Sa, < 0.6	Bondi and Katz (1911)
	Typhoid toxin	100 p.o.	—	Climenko (1936)
	Proteus pyrogen	200 p.o.	—	Warren and Werner (1946)
		22 i.p.	—	Collier and Chesher (1956)
Guinea pig	*Salmonella* lipopolysaccharide	100 p.o.	—	Smith *et al.* (1963)
	Yeast	100 i.p.	Am, > 1	Bianchi *et al.* (1967)
Cat	*E. coli* culture	54 p.o.	Am, 2.5; Pa, 1.67	Brownlee (1937) Brownlee and Gaddum (1939)
Dog	Hay infusion	100 p.o.	—	Winter and Barbour (1928)
Monkey	Yeast	100 p.o.	—	Guerra and Barbour (1943)

[a] Routes of administration abbreviated as in Table I.

[b] Am, amidopyrine; Fl, flufenamic acid; In, indomethacin; Mc, meclofenamic acid; Me, mefenamic acid; Pa, phenacetin; Pb, phenylbutazone; Sa, sodium salicylate.

In some of the experiments in Table II, aspirin was compared in potency with amidopyrine, phenacetin, phenylbutazone, or sodium salicylate. In such comparisons, aspirin was probably slightly more potent than sodium salicylate and less potent than the other drugs. In clinical fevers, also, aspirin is reported to be slightly more effective than sodium salicylate (Seed, 1965).

Table II includes some of the main established drugs of the group of which aspirin is the most widely used member. The presence of antipyretic action in all members of this group that have been tested justifies the continued use of the early term antipyretic as a convenient group name.

B. Site of Antipyretic Action

It is generally agreed that the temperature-regulating center lies in the hypothalamus (Hardy, 1961); a small amount of pyrogen injected into the anterior part of the hypothalamus induced fever in the cat (Villablanca and Myers, 1965) and rabbit (Cooper *et al.*, 1965). Many findings support the view that microbial infections and antigens induce fever by liberating endogenous pyrogen (Wood, 1958; Atkins, 1960). Thus, there was an appreciable delay before fever began after microbial pyrogen was injected into the blood (Grant and Whalen, 1953) or a lateral ventricle of the brain (Sheth and Borison, 1960; Villablanca and Myers, 1965; Cooper, 1965); after injection of leukocyte pyrogen intravenously (Bennett and Beeson, 1953a,b) or into the anterior hypothalamus (Cooper *et al.*, 1967), fever began sooner than after injecting bacterial pyrogen into the same site. Again, an endogenous pyrogen has been extracted from leukocytes (Bennett and Beeson, 1953a,b; Fessler *et al.*, 1961) and has been demonstrated in the blood of rabbits acutely infected with bacteria (King and Wood, 1958). Such a pyrogen has also been obtained from tissues in which an Arthus or Shwartzmann reaction has been induced (Bennett and Beeson, 1953a).

The signal given to the temperature-regulating center in the hypothalamus by endogenous pyrogen may be translated into action by a change there in the balance of mediating amines. From the effects of injecting amines into the cerebral ventricles of the cat, Feldberg and Myers (1963, 1964) have suggested that 5-hydroxytryptamine (5-HT) mediates a rise and noradrenaline a fall of body temperature. The effects of these amines, however, differ in different species. Whereas in the monkey and dog, as in the cat, 5-HT raised and noradrenaline lowered body temperature (Feldberg and Myers, 1965; Feldberg *et al.*, 1966, 1967), 5-HT lowered temperature in the goat (Andersson *et al.*, 1966) and ox (Findlay and Robertshaw, 1967), and noradrenaline raised it in the rabbit (Cooper *et al.*, 1965) and sheep (Bligh, 1966). In the rat, when monoamines were injected into the cerebral ventricles, low doses of noradrenaline raised body temperature. On the contrary, higher doses of noradrenaline and 5-HT lowered the temperature (Feldberg and Lotti, 1967).

How antipyretic drugs affect the mechanism by which toxins induce fever has not been fully established. Earlier workers thought that aspirin acted in the hypothalamus (Guerra and Brobeck, 1944; Guerra, 1944), but so little aspirin penetrated into the brain of dogs after parenteral administration that Lim *et al.* (1967a) concluded that it acts outside the brain. The latter belief is supported by the recent finding of Cooper *et al.* (1968) that intravenous sodium salicylate lessened fever in the rabbit when endogenous pyrogen was injected intravenously, but not when it was injected into a cerebral ventricle.

Aspirin does not greatly lower normal body temperature. It is an effective antipyretic in the rat, in which 5-HT lowers temperature, and in the cat, dog, and monkey, in which 5-HT is pyrogenic (Table II). Aspirin likewise is effective where noradrenaline lowers body temperature (cat, dog, and monkey) and where noradrenaline raises it (rabbit). These conclusions seem to exclude the possibility that aspirin acts by releasing or blocking in the hypothalamus either of the amines that may mediate temperature changes.

The recent findings summarized above suggest that salicylates exert their antipyretic action outside the hypothalamus. If so, they might do so either by inhibiting the release of endogenous pyrogen from leukocytes or by obstructing its passage into the brain. Which of these mechanisms operates is uncertain. Gander *et al.* (1967) have reported that, in the rabbit, sodium salicylate did not reduce fever induced by endogenous pyrogen, but lessened the amount of that pyrogen released from leukocytes. Cooper *et al.* (1968), on the contrary, found that salicylate lowered fever induced by endogenous pyrogen and that its interference with the liberation of that pyrogen from leukocytes was relatively unimportant. They suggested that salicylate acts by blocking the entry of endogenous pyrogen into the brain.

Although pyrogenic processes have lately been very actively studied, until quite recently antipyretic mechanisms have been neglected as a subject of pharmacologic research. This neglect probably reflects the unfashionableness of the symptomatic treatment of fever, which has been encouraged by the introduction of antimicrobial drugs that lower fever causally and by the finding that fever is sometimes therapeutically useful, as in the treatment of late syphilis.

III. Antinociception

In a second paper on aspirin, published a year after he had helped to launch the drug, Witthauer (1900) recorded its ability to relieve pain in many clinical conditions. At the same time, others also reported its powerful analgetic effect (Rénon, 1900; Comby, 1900). Since aspirin was supposed to be merely a form of sodium salicylate that was pleasanter to take, its analgetic effectiveness was unexpectedly high (Gross and Greenberg, 1948), as patients taking the drug were probably the first to notice (H. H. Dale, personal communication).

In spite of its practical efficacy against pain, aspirin long resisted critical attempts to prove that it had analgetic action in man. In 1953, however, recognition of the placebo effect and the use of double-blind technique enabled Beecher *et al.* (1953) to demonstrate that it relieved postoperative pain and to estimate that 600 mg of aspirin was more effective than 60 mg of codeine or 10 mg of morphine when each was given by mouth.

A. Effectiveness in the Laboratory

To show that aspirin relieves experimental nociception was still harder than to show that it relieves pathologic pain (Beecher, 1957). In man, aspirin has proved effective against experimentally induced pain in muscles (Deneau *et al.*, 1953; Benjamin, 1958; Williams, 1959; Williams *et al.*, 1965); Table III summarizes the tests in which aspirin was more effective than placebo against experimental muscle pain.

TABLE III

Analgetic Effect of Aspirin against Experimental Muscle Pain in Man

Pain induced by	Dose of aspirin significantly more effective than placebo[a]	Effective dose of other analgetics[a,b]	Reference
Pressure on calf	1296 mg	Co, 32 mg; Pe, 107 mg	Deneau *et al.* (1953)
Ischemia of arm	648 mg	—	Benjamin (1958)
	648 mg	—	Williams (1959)
	8.5 mg/kg	Me, 8.5 mg/kg	Williams *et al.* (1965)

[a] Administered orally.
[b] Co, codeine; Pe, pethidine; Me, mefenamic acid.

In a few tests based on thermal or electrical stimulation, aspirin has shown detectable activity in experimental animals (Smith *et al.*, 1943; Hart, 1947; Winder, 1947; Bonnycastle and Leonard, 1950; Gibson *et al.*, 1955; Nilsen, 1961; Weiss and Laties, 1961; Smith *et al.*, 1963). Irritants, however, may themselves exert an antinociceptive effect (Jacob and Szerb, 1951, 1952; Winter and Flataker, 1965; Hitchens *et al.*, 1967). Therefore the question arises of how far the activity seen in these tests was due to an irritant effect of aspirin, especially when the drug was given parenterally, as it was by some of the workers referred to above. This question was recently tested by injecting aspirin into the peritoneal cavity of conscious mice (Collier *et al.*, 1968a). This procedure elicited no abdominal constriction (writhing) response, which is taken to indicate nociception. No evidence was obtained, therefore, that, in this situation, aspirin exerted an irritant effect likely to suppress nociception, although Jori and Bernardi (1966) have obtained evidence that aspirin may exert such an effect when given by mouth to rats.

Aspirin is ineffective, although morphine is effective, against nociception induced by pinching the tail or toes of mouse, rat, or guinea pig (Collier and Chesher, 1956; Collier *et al.*, 1961; Collier, 1964; Winter and Flataker, 1965). Aspirin, however, lessens nociceptive responses elicited by mechanical stimuli applied to an inflamed site. In an early test of this type, Hesse *et al.* (1930) observed that 400 mg of aspirin lessened the tenderness that had been produced by injecting croton oil under guinea-pig skin. In such tests, aspirin is not always outstandingly potent, nor is its potency against the nociception induced by pressure or movement at an inflamed site the same as that against the accompanying edema (Table IV). For example, when inflammation was induced by injecting silver nitrate into the foot joint of a rat and a nociceptive response was elicited by moving the swollen joint, aspirin was more effective against the swelling than it was against the nociception (Margolin, 1965). On the contrary, in the inflammation resulting from injecting yeast under the skin of the plantar surface of the rat foot, aspirin was more active against the nociception than against the swelling (Gilfoil *et al.*, 1963; Winter, 1965; Winter and Flataker, 1965). Although aspirin suppressed nociception induced by pressure on the rat foot inflamed with yeast or bradykinin, it was ineffective when turpentine, dextran, or 5-HT was used as noxa (Gilfoil *et al.*, 1964).

In antinociceptive tests not involving previous induction of inflammation, aspirin is more often effective when nociception is elicited chemically than mechanically. Table V gives the performance of aspirin and other analgetics in some antinociceptive tests based on chemical challenges.[1]

Table V shows that even against responses to chemical stimuli, however, the potency of aspirin depends on the chemical applied. For example, when the antinociceptive potency of aspirin in mice was measured by its ability to suppress the abdominal constriction responses occurring within 2 minutes of intraperitoneal injection of various substances, aspirin was highly effective against challenge by acetylcholine, moderately effective against adenosine triphosphate, less effective against bradykinin, and still less effective against tryptamine (Collier *et al.*, 1968a). Likewise, in the dog, analysis of the published records of Guzman *et al.* (1964) shows that aspirin suppressed nociceptive responses induced by intra-arterial acetylcholine in 8 of 10 animals, whereas, in corresponding doses, it suppressed responses to bradykinin in 27 of 43 animals and those to potassium in only 9 of 23 animals. Morphine, on the contrary,

[1] H. Helfer and R. Jaques (1968, *Helv. Physiol. Pharmacol. Acta* **26**, 137) have used arachidonic acid intraperitoneally as a challenge in the mouse. Against this, sodium salicylate had an ED 50 value of 200 (45–950) mg/kg p.o.

TABLE IV

ANTIEXUDATIVE AND ANTINOCICEPTIVE ACTIVITIES OF ASPIRIN, TESTED IN THE SAME EXPERIMENT

Species and site	Exudation induced by	Nociception induced by	Effective oral dose (mg/kg) Antiexudation	Effective oral dose (mg/kg) Antinociception	Reference
Mouse peritoneum	Acetic acid	Acetic acid	104 (61–176)	49 (35–67)	Whittle (1964)
Rat foot	Yeast, bradykinin	Pressure	> 200	50	Gilfoil *et al.* (1963, 1964)
	Turpentine, 5-HT,[a] dextran		> 200	> 200	
	Yeast		> 270	30	Winter (1965); Winter and Flataker (1965)
Rat ankle	Silver nitrate	Flexion	70 ± 7	415 ± 38	Margolin (1965)

[a] 5-HT, 5-hydroxytryptamine.

TABLE V

SOME TESTS OF ASPIRIN AGAINST CHEMICALLY INDUCED NOCICEPTION[a]

Species	Nociceptive response	Induced by	Effective dose of aspirin (mg/kg) and route	Approx. relative potency of other antipyretics (aspirin = 1)	Effective dose of morphine (mg/kg) and route	Reference
Mouse	Abdominal constriction (writhing)	Phenylquinone i.p.	165(133–204) p.o.	Am, 1.7; Pa, 0.60	1.15(0.88–1.5) s.c.	Siegmund *et al.* (1957)
			38 s.c.	Am, 0.25; Pb, 0.1; Sa, 0.15	1.5 s.c.	Keith (1960)
						Randall (1963)
			100(74–135) s.c.	Pa, 0.52; Pb, 1.61; Pm, 0.31; Sa, 0.28	—	Hendershot and Forsaith (1959)
			50(36–70) s.c.	—	—	Silvestrini *et al.* (1966)
			150(129–174) p.o.	Am, 2.1; Pb, 1.0	—	Emele and Shanaman (1963)
		Bradykinin i.p.	21(12–37) p.o.	Am, 0.30; Pb, 0.34	—	
		Acetic acid i.p.	190 p.o.	Am, 1.7; Sa, < 0.19	1.5 s.c.	Koster *et al.* (1959)
			49(35–67) p.o.	Am, 1.9; Pb, 0.79; Pm, 0.36; Sa, 0.26	1.3(0.9–1.8) p.o.	Whittle (1964)
		Acetylcholine i.p.	26(17–40) s.c.	Sa, 0.17	0.43(0.29–0.64) s.c.	Collier *et al.* (1964)
			30(25–37) s.c.	Fl, 1.2; Mc, 3.2; Me, 2.1; Pm, 0.43	0.52(0.46–0.95) s.c.	Collier *et al.* (1968a)
		Adenosine triphosphate i.p.	87(69–109) s.c.	Fl, 2.7; Mc, 13; Me, 3.5	0.30(0.20–0.43) s.c.	
		Bradykinin i.p.	268(135–531) s.c.	Fl, 3.3; Mc, 15; Me, 16	< 0.2 s.c.	
		Tryptamine i.p.	484(351–666) s.c.	Fl, 2.7; Mc, 13; Me, 6.4	0.40(0.29–0.55) s.c.	
		KCl i.p.	188(65–543) s.c.	—	0.18(0.12–0.29) s.c.	
Rat	Avoiding movements, squeak	Bradykinin, i.a.	88(67–101) i.p.	Am, 4.9; Pa, 0.81; Pb, 0.52	—	Deffenu *et al.* (1966)
			125 i.p.			Blane (1967)

TABLE V—*continued*

SOME TESTS OF ASPIRIN AGAINST CHEMICALLY INDUCED NOCICEPTION[a]

Species	Nociceptive response	Induced by	Effective dose of aspirin (mg/kg) and route	Approx. relative potency of other antipyretics (aspirin = 1)	Effective dose of morphine (mg/kg) and route	Reference
	Abdominal constriction	Iodomethamate i.p.	Ineffective	—	4.8 s.c.	Vander Wende and Margolin (1956)
Guinea-pig	Movement, behaviour	Bradykinin, i.v.	10–40 i.v.	Pb, 1	10–40 i.v.	Gjuris *et al.* (1964b)
		Bradykinin, i.d.	Ineffective	—	5 s.c.	Collier and Lee (1963)
Dog	Vocalization	Bradykinin, i.a.	50 ± 16 i.v.	Am, < 0.9; Pb, 1.6; Pm, 0.46; Sa, 0.26	1.1 ± 0.24 i.v.	Guzman *et al.* (1964)
		Bradykinin, i.p.	56 ± 12 i.v.	—	1.5 ± 0.13 i.v.	Dickerson *et al.* (1965)
	Impaired locomotion	Formalin i.ar.	100 p.o.	—	—	Pardo and Rodriguez (1966)
Man	Subjective	Bradykinin, b.b.	> 1.2[b] p.o.	—	—	Lewis (1963)
		Bradykinin, i.a.	6[b] p.o.	—	—	Coffman (1964)
		Bradykinin, i.p.	0.65[b] p.o.	—	—	Lim *et al.* (1967b)

[a] Key to abbreviations: Pm, paracetamol (other drugs abbreviated as in Table II); i.d., intradermal; i.ar., intra-articular; b.b., onto exposed blister base (other routes of administration abbreviated as in Table I).

[b] Dose in gm/man.

suppressed responses to acetylcholine, to bradykinin, or to potassium with about equal effectiveness.

Within one species, using the same challenge substance, the effectiveness of aspirin differs also with the site of challenge. Thus, in the guinea pig, aspirin suppressed nociceptive responses to intra-arterial bradykinin (Gjuris *et al.*, 1964b); but it was completely ineffective against intradermal bradykinin (Collier and Lee, 1963). In man, aspirin failed to suppress pain caused by applying bradykinin to the exposed base of a blister (Lewis, 1963); although a very large oral dose was effective against intra-arterial bradykinin (Coffman, 1964), and a small dose was effective against intraperitoneal bradykinin (Lim *et al.*, 1967b).

Table V shows that other antipyretic drugs also are usually effective in tests in which aspirin is effective and that each drug has its own potency over a range of tests. In all tests in which aspirin was compared with sodium salicylate, aspirin was distinctly the more potent.

Unlike aspirin, morphine has proved effective in any antinociceptive test in mammals in which it has been tried (Collier, 1964). The contrast between aspirin and morphine in the field of analgesia resembles that between aspirin and chlorpromazine as antipyretics. It suggests that pain, like fever, is of various types, against only some of which aspirin is effective. Just as aspirin is a clinically useful antipyretic because the types of fever against which it acts are those that often arise in illness, so we may suppose that aspirin is a useful analgetic because the types of pain that respond to it are common. These are mainly slow, aching pains, as in rheumatism and headache, rather than the sharp, stabbing pains arising from mechanical or direct nerve stimulation. This contrast is probably expressed in Table IV, in which aspirin was more effective against nociception induced by pressure on the yeast-inflamed foot (Gilfoil *et al.*, 1963, 1964; Winter and Flataker, 1965) than against that induced by manual flexion of an inflamed joint (Margolin, 1965).

B. Site of Antinociceptive Action

That morphine, which is known to depress pain perception in the central nervous system, exerts an antinociceptive effect in a wide variety of tests, whereas aspirin is selective, raises doubts whether aspirin can exert the whole of its effect upon pain perception in the CNS, as, for example, Woodbury (1965) has claimed, or even a small part of its analgetic effect there, as Winder (1959) has proposed.

The suspicion that aspirin acts at or near the site of painful stimulation is strengthened by the experiments of Lim *et al.* (1964). In one group of experiments, these workers established cross-circulation between pairs of dogs, so that the splenic circulation of a recipient dog was connected with the systemic circulation of a donor dog, while the splenic nerve supply of the recipient remained unchanged. Injection of bradykinin into the splenic artery of the recipient elicited nociceptive responses, such as vocalization, withdrawal movements, biting, struggling, increased amplitude of respiration, and a rise in blood pressure. Intravenous administration of aspirin, sodium salicylate, paracetamol, or phenylbutazone to the donor blocked the nociceptive responses of the recipient, but the same drugs were ineffective when given to the recipient itself. Morphine produced the opposite effect to aspirin. Administered to the donor, morphine was ineffective, but to the recipient it blocked nociception.

In another series of experiments in single dogs, nociception was again induced by injecting bradykinin into the splenic artery (Lim *et al.*, 1964). In these experiments, aspirin was more effective as an antinociceptive when injected into the splenic than when injected into the cerebral blood supply, whereas the reverse was true of morphine.

In a third series of experiments, Lim *et al.* (1964) showed that aspirin prevented, but morphine did not, the appearance of action potentials in the splanchnic nerve after injecting bradykinin into the spleen of dogs. Experiments of the three types described above are taken to mean that aspirin and related drugs act at or near the site of noxious stimulation, whereas morphine and other narcotics act in the central nervous system.

In the lightly anesthetized guinea pig or rabbit, high intravenous doses of bradykinin elicited an arousal reaction, which was inhibited by relatively large intravenous doses of aspirin, phenylbutazone, or morphine (Gjuris *et al.*, 1964b). This reaction to bradykinin and its suppression seem comparable to those described by Guzman *et al.* (1962, 1964) in the dog. Gjuris and co-workers have distinguished, from this arousal response, an apnea, which was readily elicited by injecting bradykinin into a carotid artery. This apneic response was significantly inhibited by small intravenous doses of aspirin (1–2 mg/kg) or of phenylbutazone (5 mg/kg). Marquardt (1966) has confirmed these observations. Gjuris and co-workers believe that the apnea is due to a direct effect of bradykinin on the respiratory center within the CNS. If so, bradykinin presumably passes from the blood into the brain and aspirin either blocks this passage or antagonizes aspirin at the respiratory center; but, to sustain this explanation, evidence is needed that bradykinin and possibly also aspirin enter the brain in appreciable amounts.

If aspirin acts as an antinociceptive near the peripheral site where a pain originates, how does it exert its effect there? Several investigators have suggested that aspirin acts locally against pain by reducing the edema that raises pain sensitivity (Harris and Fosdick, 1952; Randall and Selitto, 1957; Smith, 1960; Randall, 1963). This supposition does not explain the experiments of Lim *et al.* (1964) outlined above. It also fails to explain the findings that aspirin inhibited abdominal constriction responses to acetylcholine in the mouse before much edema was likely to have developed (Collier *et al.*, 1964, 1968a) and that it inhibited nociception, in several tests in Table IV, at doses lower than those required to lessen exudation (Gilfoil *et al.*, 1963, 1964; Whittle, 1964; Winter, 1965).

Winder (1959) has suggested the more satisfying explanation that aspirin mainly acts on an "early process—a preinflammatory process—in the course of reaction by tissue to injury. The same process could lead both to stimulation of pain endings and, eventually, to frank inflammation."

Yet a third possibility remains—that aspirin acts against a local process leading to pain, but not necessarily leading to inflammatory changes in blood vessels. If so, aspirin could have a peripheral antinociceptive action in situations where exudation and hyperemia were slight or absent. Aspirin might well act by more than one of these peripheral mechanisms.

The failure of some early attempts to find, among the chemical relatives of aspirin, analgetics that are clinically more effective, provides further evidence upon the site of the antinociceptive action of aspirin. One of the best-known attempted improvements on aspirin is salicylamide, which was more effective than aspirin in antinociceptive tests in the rat, based on thermal (Hart, 1947; Bavin *et al.*, 1952) or mechanical (Collier and Chesher, 1956) stimuli. Controlled clinical trials of salicylamide as an analgetic, however, suggest that its clinical efficacy is doubtful (Wallenstein and Houde, 1954; Batterman and Grossman, 1955; Winder, 1959; Woodbury, 1965; Hook, 1966). In keeping with this lack of clinical efficacy, salicylamide was inactive, in the guinea pig, both against erythema of skin induced by ultraviolet radiation (Winder *et al.*, 1958; Adams, 1960) and against bronchoconstriction elicited by bradykinin (Collier and Shorley, 1960). Against this bronchoconstriction, on the contrary, aspirin was highly effective, even after destruction of the brain and spinal cord (Collier *et al.*, 1966) or adrenalectomy (Collier *et al.*, 1965).

4-Hydroxyisophthalic acid, an impurity produced in the manufacture of aspirin, provides a like example. This acid was effective as an antipyretic in the rabbit and as an antinociceptive in the tail-pressure test in the rat (Collier and Chesher, 1956); but it was less effective than aspirin in rheumatoid arthritis (Hajnal *et al.*, 1959). In keeping with these properties, 4-hydroxyisophthalic acid inhibited neither UV erythema of skin (Adams, 1960) nor bradykinin-induced bronchoconstriction (Collier and Shorley, 1960) in the guinea pig.

Winder (1959) cites two other compounds that were active in mechanical and thermal antinociceptive tests, but inactive against UV erythema of skin, in the laboratory, and proved ineffective as analgetics in man. These experiences reinforce the conclusion that aspirin acts against pain at or near the site of stimulation, by inhibiting at some point the sequence of events by which injury produces pain.

C. Aspirin and Clinical Pain

That pain can be suppressed by mental influences in man is well shown by the existence of the placebo effect (Beecher, 1957) and by the analgetic effect of music and white noise (Gardner *et al.*, 1960). That a corresponding central inhibition of pain can occur in the dog is suggested by the observations that nalorphine increased the proportion of animals in which intra-arterial bradykinin elicited nociception (Rodgers, 1964; Lim, 1966). Morphine has been supposed to increase this inhibition in the CNS (Lim, 1966), either by blocking pain impulses directly or by reinforcing inhibitory influences. The evidence, summarized above and discussed in greater detail by Lim (1966), that aspirin, on the contrary, blocks pain at a peripheral site, is now very strong.

Since aspirin probably acts peripherally, it can be expected to relieve pain without eliciting euphoria, sedation, or dependence. Clinical experience agrees with this expectation. Nonetheless, possibly because of a continuing background of pain or discomfort, individuals who take large doses of aspirin daily over many years are encountered (Wilson, 1965; Prescott, 1966b).

The statement is sometimes made that, in clinical use, aspirin is effective against pain of low or moderate intensity, but not against pain of high intensity (Woodbury, 1965; Lim, 1966). This statement contrasts with the laboratory findings described above, in which aspirin almost completely suppressed some kinds of nociception, such as that induced by injecting acetylcholine into the peritoneal cavity of a mouse or into the artery of a dog, but was quite ineffective against other kinds of nociception, such as that induced by pinching the tail of the same mouse, by injecting bradykinin into the skin of a guinea pig, or by applying it to an exposed blister base in human skin. The conflict between the clinical and the laboratory observations may be resolved by supposing that the analgetic effect of aspirin in the clinic depends on the way the pain is engendered, rather than upon its intensity, and that pains arising from processes susceptible to antagonism by aspirin also happen to be those usually felt as of low or moderate intensity.

Pain may be supposed to arise in at least two different ways. First, it may be elicited by direct stimulation of nociceptive nerve endings or fibers. Second, pain may be engendered by a humoral mechanism, in which injury liberates a mediating substance that, in turn, excites the pain endings. Pains arising in these two ways may further be supposed to differ in quality, that arising by direct stimulation of nerves being sharp and stabbing and that mediated humorally being dull and aching.

Clinical experience shows that aspirin is effective against aching pain, as in early cancer (Houde and Wallenstein, 1953; Perese, 1961), headache, postoperative states, osteoarthritis, rheumatoid arthritis, and ankylosing spondylitis (Lim, 1966), rather than against stabbing pains, arising from muscular spasm, from noxious stimulation of skin, or from nerve injury. Such experience therefore is consistent with the view that aspirin acts as an analgetic by blocking in some way the humoral mechanism by which injury elicits pain.

Phenylbutazone clearly shows antinociceptive activity in several animal tests (Table V), and this is consistent with its well-established analgetic action in man (von Rechenberg, 1962; British Pharmaceutical Codex, 1963; Balme, 1967). Since phenylbutazone, however, is not much more potent than aspirin in any antinociceptive test in Table V, and since it is more toxic than aspirin in man, the relative rarity of its clinical use as an analgetic is understandable. Paracetamol was effective in some of the same tests as aspirin, but was less potent (Table V). The low toxicity of paracetamol, however, helps to explain its widespread clinical use against pain.

IV. Anti-Inflammation

The terms anti-inflammatory and antiphlogistic are common and convenient, but they can be confusing, since they may not be meant to include depression of the nociception and of the coagulation of blood and exudate occurring in inflammation. In this chapter, anti-inflammatory and antiphlogistic are used to cover the delay or reduction of hyperemia, of exudation of fluid through the walls of blood vessels, of the infiltration and proliferation of cells, and of phagocytosis, but not the depression of nociception or of hemostasis.

Many drugs, including antipyretics, corticosteroids, catecholamines, immune suppressants, and chlorpromazine inhibit inflammatory responses (Garattini *et al.*, 1965; Silvestrini, 1965; Rosenthale and Nagra, 1967; Trnavsky, 1967). Below, the anti-inflammatory effects in the laboratory of aspirin will be particularly considered, but those of other antipyretics and of drugs of other groups will also be discussed insofar as they illustrate the principle that the profile of activity of each drug differs from that of others in the same group and still more from that of drugs in other groups.

The critical bibliographic review of the salicylates by Gross and Greenberg (1948), published about twenty years ago with some four thousand references, contained no section on the anti-inflammatory effects of these drugs, although it recorded the isolated observation of Hagebush and Kinsella (1930) that salicylate inhibited a skin reaction induced with streptococcal antigen in the infected rabbit. Yet in the recent symposium on nonsteroidal anti-inflammatory drugs in Milan (Garattini and Dukes, 1965) and in the recent review of the mode of action of these drugs (Domenjoz, 1966a), salicylates occupied a central position as reference compounds.

This revolution in the experimental pharmacology of the salicylates began soon after the publication of the monograph of Gross and Greenberg (1948), when Smith and Humphrey (1949) showed that sodium salicylate inhibited some local hypersensitivity reactions more effectively than did antihistamine drugs, and Wilhelmi (1949) reported that phenylbutazone delayed the erythema of guinea-pig skin exposed to ultraviolet radiation. This revolution in testing methods was promoted by the failure of new drugs that were effective in conventional antipyretic and antinociceptive tests in animals to show analgetic efficacy in man, which has been discussed above.

A. Laboratory Models

Pharmacologists devising laboratory models of inflammation have concentrated on sites readily accessible to stimulation and measurement—the skin, the limbs, the body cavities, and the subcutaneous tissue. They have mainly used, as stimuli, ultraviolet radiation, noxious or nocisimulant chemicals, antigens, infective microbes, or foreign bodies. They have used hyperemia, exudation of fluid (sometimes colored with protein-bound dye), or granulation as indicators of response.

The variety of tests arising from such a multiplicity of sites, stimuli, and responses is made more bewildering by the inadequacy of many of the measurements recorded. Most studies on aspirin establish that it significantly depresses the particular form of inflammation under test, but few are full enough to give the potency and limits of confidence that can be placed in the value given. Table VI summarizes some of the investigations that give these values. This table shows clearly that the relative potencies of different drugs, and even the presence or absence of activity in some of them, depends on the test used.

In most anti-inflammatory tests, glucocorticoids, salicylates, or phenylbutazone have been used for reference. The fact that sodium salicylate is not markedly less potent than aspirin in most anti-inflammatory tests has led to aspirin being omitted, in favor of sodium salicylate, as a reference compound in many of them. If the potencies of aspirin and sodium salicylate had been farther apart, aspirin might have been used more often and the present section on anti-inflammation would have been longer.

Table VI shows the main sites in which the effects of aspirin upon inflammation have been satisfactorily measured. Tables VII, VIII, and IX summarize the results of some antiphlogistic tests of aspirin in these sites—skin, limbs, and body cavities, respectively. In these tables, very approximate potencies of other drugs relative to aspirin are given, where these could be assessed.

1. *Skin*

Table VII shows that aspirin inhibited the inflammatory response of mouse and guinea pig to ultraviolet radiation and of guinea pig and human skin to thurfyl nicotinate. Aspirin delayed, but did not abolish, the inflammatory response (Winder *et al.*, 1958; Truelove and Duthie, 1959; Adams and Cobb, 1963; Sim, 1965); yet aspirin exerted this retardation for several days after its

TABLE VI

SOME ESTIMATES OF THE ANTI-INFLAMMATORY POTENCY OF ASPIRIN AND OTHER DRUGS

Drug[a]	Skin erythema,[b] relative potency	Edema of paw[c]			Peritoneal exudate,[d] ED_{50} (mg/kg)
		ED_{50} (mg/kg)	Relative potency		
Aspirin	0.1(0.079–0.13)	72(50–104)	1[e]	—	104(61–176)
Sodium salicylate	—	98(65–148)	—	—	270(155–470)
Amidopyrine	0.14(0.094–0.20)	31(20–49)	—	—	200
Phenylbutazone	1[e]	25(14–47)	2(1.3–2.9)	1[e]	200
Mefenamic acid	0.51(0.37–0.71)	9(4.3–19)	—	2.6(1.1–5.9)	—
Flufenamic acid	1.6(0.99–2.7)	10(4.8–21)	—	9.3(4.0–21)	—
Meclofenamic acid	15(9.6–23)	—	—	—	—
Indomethacin	3.1(1.8–5.8)	2.2(1.2–3.8)	—	21(9.3–52)	—
Cortisone	Inactive	40(28–57)	—	—	Inactive
Hydrocortisone	Inactive	30(16–57)	16(11–24)	4.8(2.1–11)	—

[a] All drugs were administered orally.

[b] Skin erythema was induced by UV-irradiation in the guinea pig (Winder *et al.*, 1958, 1962, 1963, 1965).

[c] Edema of paw was induced by carrageenin in the rat (ED_{50} values, Niemegeers *et al.*, 1964; relative potencies, Winter *et al.*, 1962; Winter, 1965).

[d] Peritoneal exudate was induced by acetic acid in the mouse (Whittle, 1964).

[e] Reference drug in terms of which relative potencies are expressed.

TABLE VII

SOME TESTS OF ASPIRIN AGAINST EXPERIMENTAL INFLAMMATION OF SKIN

Species	Noxa and route[a]	Effective dose of aspirin (mg/kg) and route[a]	Approx. relative potency of other antipyretics[b] (aspirin = 1)	Reference
Mouse	UV-radiation	100–300 p.o.	Am, 2; In, 266; Me, 4; Pa, 1; Pb, 3; Pm, 1; Sa, 1	Sim (1965)
	Xylol, p.c.	Versus bluing 220 p.o.	Pb, 3.4	Brown and Robson (1964)
		Versus ear weight 370 p.o.	Pb, <0.9	
Rat	Hyaluronidase, i.d.	500 s.c.	—	Mathies (1958)
	Bradykinin, i.d.	500 i.p.	Fl, >5; Mc, >5; Me, 5; Pb, >2.5	Starr and West (1967)
Guinea pig	UV-radiation	100–200 p.o.	Am, 1.4; Fl, 16; In, 31; Mc, 150; Me, 5.1; Pa, <0.05; Pb, 10	Winder *et al.* (1958, 1962, 1963, 1965)
		80 p.o.	Am, 1; Pa, <0.33; Pb, 8; Pm, <0.33; Sa, 0.67	Adams (1960)
		139 p.o.	Am, 1.3; Pb, 13; Sa, 0.57	Brittain and Spencer (1965)
		80 p.o.	Sa, 0.53	Smith *et al.* (1963)
		100 p.o.	Pb, 10; Sa, 0.3	Haining (1963)
	Thurfyl nicotinate, p.c.	50 p.o.	Pb, 10; Sa, 0.3	
	Bradykinin, i.d.	Inactive at 200 i.p.	—	Collier and Shorley (1960)
		Inactive at 100 i.v.	—	Lewis (1963)
Rabbit	Bradykinin, i.d.	75 s.c.	Pn, <1	Lish and McKinney (1963)
Man	Thurfyl nicotinate, p.c.	10 p.o.	—	Truelove and Duthie (1959)
		3 p.o.	Pb, <0.38; Sa, <0.35	Adams and Cobb, (1963)

[a] Routes of administration abbreviated as in Tables 1 and V.

[b] Drugs abbreviated as in Tables II and V.

administration (Adams and Cobb, 1963; Smith *et al.*, 1963). These facts suggest that the response involves at least two processes, one of which is affected by aspirin.

When bradykinin was injected intradermally into guinea pigs previously treated intravenously with a protein-binding blue dye, fairly large parenteral doses of aspirin or of sodium salicylate did not reduce the resulting area of skin bluing (Collier and Shorley, 1960; Lewis, 1963; Willoughby *et al.*, 1965). In the rabbit, however, Lish and McKinney (1963) found that aspirin and, to a lesser degree, phenylbutazone, significantly diminished the area of bluing induced by intradermal injection of bradykinin (Table VII), but not of histamine. In this species, also, phenylbutazone delayed the onset of wealing induced by intradermal bradykinin (Lecomte and Troquet, 1960). In the rat, calcium aspirin and other antipyretics inhibited the wealing induced by intradermal injection of bradykinin (Table VII), histamine, or 5-hydroxytryptamine (Starr and West, 1967). In these experiments, phenylbutazone was more effective than aspirin and fenamates more effective than phenylbutazone. In the experiments of Brown and Robson (1964) aspirin and phenylbutazone inhibited the bluing of mouse ear induced by xylol. Aspirin also inhibited the concomitant increase in weight of the ear, but phenylbutazone did not (Table VII).

As well as delaying inflammation of the skin induced by UV-radiation or thurfyl nicotinate in mouse, guinea pig, or man, salicylates inhibit inflammation induced by some hypersensitivity reactions of the skin in guinea pig and rabbit. Thus sodium salicylate inhibited the reaction to intradermal injection of streptococcal culture filtrates in rabbits experimentally injected with the same organism (Hagebush and Kinsella, 1930). Salicylate also inhibited the reaction of guinea pig or rabbit to intradermal injection of antibody provoked by subsequent intravenous injection of antigen (Smith and Humphrey, 1949; Marks *et al.*, 1961). Aspirin and sodium salicylate likewise depressed the skin reaction to bacterial antigen provoked by subsequent intravenous injection of that antigen (Smith and Humphrey, 1949; Shwartzman *et al.*, 1950; Shwartzman and Schneierson, 1953), but salicylate failed to depress the response of sensitized guinea pig or rabbit to intradermal injection of antigen (Smith and Humphrey, 1949; Long, 1955; Floersheim, 1965). In short, salicylates inhibit the passive reverse Arthus and the Shwartzman reactions and fail to inhibit the tuberculin reaction.[1]

Against UV erythema of guinea-pig skin, phenylbutazone was about 10 times as potent as aspirin; but paracetamol and salicylamide were inactive

[1] A. Somogyi, I. Berczi, and H. Selye (1969, *Arch. Intern. Pharmacodyn.* **177**, 211) have reported that aspirin or sodium salicylate inhibited several forms of local calcification induced by various chemical challenges in the rat. For example, 45 mg/kg orally of either salicylate inhibited subcutaneous calcification induced by local injection of potassium permanganate, but not that induced by lead acetate.

TABLE VIII

Inhibition by Aspirin and other Anti-inflammatory Drugs of Experimental Inflammation of the Foot or Ankle

Species	Noxa	Effective dose of aspirin(mg/kg) and route[a]	Approx. relative potency of other antipyretics[b] (aspirin = 1)	Effective dose of glucocorticoids[c] or catecholamines[d] (mg/kg) and route	Reference
Mouse	Yeast	675 p.o.	Am, 4; Pb, 5.4; Sa, 1	Co, 2×50 s.c.	Weis (1963)
	5-HT[e]	675 p.o.		Co, 2×6 s.c.	
		100 p.o.	Pb, 1; Sa, 1–2	—	Vogin and Rossi (1963)
	Formalin	675 p.o.	Am, 4; Sa, 1	Co, 2×50 s.c.	Weis (1963)
		2×160 s.c. and 3×150 s.c.	Am, 1–2; Pb, > 2; Sa, 1	Co, > 3×40; Is, 0.4; NA, 0.4 s.c.	Northover and Subramanian (1961a, (1962)
Rat	Yeast	100 p.o.	—	Hc, 6 p.o.	Winter (1965)
	5-HT	Inactive at 300 p.o.	—	—	
		500 s.c.	Am, 2.5; Pb, 2.5; Sa, 1	Co, 2×50 s.c.	Theobald and Domenjoz (1958)
	Formalin	500 s.c.	Am, 2.5; Pb, 5	Co, 2×20 s.c.	Domenjoz (1955)
		500 p.o.	Pb, 1; Sa, 1	—	Domenjoz and Morsdorf (1965)
		100 p.o.	Pb, 1	Hc, 2 p.o.	Winter (1965)
	Dextran	500 s.c.	Am, 2.5; Pb, 2.5; Sa, 1	Co, 2×10 s.c.	Domenjoz (1955)
		100–300 p.o.	In, 100	Hc, 2 p.o.	Winter (1965)
	Trypsin	500 p.o.	Pb, 1.25; Sa, 1	—	Domenjoz and Morsdorf (1965)
	Carrageenin	33.3 p.o.	Pb, 2	Hc, 2 p.o.	Winter *et al.* (1962)
			Fl, 18; In, 40; Me, 5		Winter (1965)
		72 (50–104) p.o.	Am, 2.3; Fl, 7.2; In, 33; Pa, 0.82; Pb, 2.9; Sa, 0.73	Co, 40(28–57) p.o. Hc, 30 (16–57) p.o.	Niemegeers *et al.* (1964)
	Bradykinin	250 i.p. twice daily for 5 days	Pb, 25; Sa, 1	—	Lisin and Leclerq (1963)
		400 i.p.	Sa. 1	—	Martelli (1967)

Rat	Dead mycobacterium	100–200 p.o. daily for 14 days	Pb, 2; Sa, 1	Co, 50–100 p.o. × 14 Pl, 10–20 p.o. × 14	Newbould, (1963)
		70 p.o. daily for 21 days	In, 70; Pb, 2.3	Pl, 0.4 p.o. × 21	Ward and Cloud (1966)
		36 p.o. daily for 14 days	Pb, > 1	Co, 8.5 s.c. × 14	Rosenthale and Nagra (1967)
	Heat (46.5°C)	500 i.p.	Fl, 5; Mc, 5; Pn, 2.5	—	Starr and West (1967)
Guinea pig	Antigen after intravenous antibody	250 p.o.	—	—	Ungar *et al.* (1952).

[a] Routes of administration abbreviated as in Table I.
[b] Antipyretic drugs abbreviated as in Table II.
[c] Co, cortisone; Hc, hydrocortisone; Pl, prednisolone.
[d] Is, isoprenaline; NA, noradrenaline.
[e] 5-HT, 5-hydroxytryptamine.

TABLE IX

INHIBITION BY ASPIRIN AND OTHER ANTI-INFLAMMATORY DRUGS OF EXPERIMENTAL PERITONITIS AND PLEURISY

Species and site	Noxa	Effective dose of aspirin (mg/kg) and route[a]	Approx. relative potency of other antipyretics (aspirin = 1)	Effective doses of glucocorticoids[b] (mg/kg) and route	Reference
Mouse peritoneum	0.9% NaCl	83 s.c.	Am, 1.1; Pb, 1.2;	Inactive	Northover (1963)
	Acetic acid	104(61–176) p.o.	Am, 0.5; Pb, 0.5; Sa, 0.4	Inactive	Whittle (1964)
Rat peritoneum	Formalin	250 p.o.	Am, 1.3; In, 13; Pn, 1.3	Pr, 2 × 4 p.o.	Wilhelmi (1965)
Rat pleura	$AgNO_3$	250 p.o.	In, 13; Pb, 1.3	Pr, 2 × 50 p.o.	
	Evans blue and carrageenin	50 p.o.	Fl, 5; In, 50; Me, 5; Pb, 1.7	Hc, 50 p.o.	Sancilio and Rodriguez (1965)
	Evans blue	50–150 p.o.	In, 150; Me, 5; Pb, 5	—	Sancilio and Rodriguez (1966)

[a] Results are based on the volume of exudate; routes of administration abbreviated as in Table I.

[b] Pr, prednisone; other drugs abbreviated as in Tables II and VIII.

(Winder *et al.*, 1958, 1962; Adams, 1960). In the parallel test in mouse skin, however, phenylbutazone was only 2–3 times as potent as aspirin, paracetamol was about as potent as aspirin, and even salicylamide was detectably effective (Sim, 1965).

Where they have been tested against inflammation of skin elicited by UV-irradiation or by antigen, neither the quinoline antimalarials nor antagonists of histamine or of 5-HT have shown much activity (Smith and Humphrey, 1949; Wilhelmi and Domenjoz, 1951; Winder *et al.*, 1958; Sim, 1965).

Against the skin inflammation induced by UV-radiation in guinea pig or mouse, glucocorticoids were ineffective (Winder *et al.*, 1958; Sim, 1965). Unlike glucocorticoids, adrenaline and other catecholamines were effective against UV erythema in the mouse (Sim, 1965). In the inflammation of rabbit skin induced by chloroform, sodium salicylate was effective but cortisone was not (van Cauwenberge and Lecomte, 1952); in the inflammation of mouse ear induced by xylol, hydrocortisone inhibited the increase in weight, but not the intensity of bluing (Brown and Robson, 1964).

In skin reactions induced by antigen in sensitized animals, in which salicylates were ineffective, glucocorticoids were effective (Humphrey, 1951; Shwartzman and Schneierson, 1953; Ungar *et al.*, 1959). For example, glucocorticoids reduced the tuberculin reaction of guinea-pig or rabbit skin (Long and Miles, 1950; Harris and Harris, 1950; Winder *et al.*, 1957; Floersheim, 1965).

2. *Limbs*

The edema of the rat or mouse paw that follows injection of a noxa has provided a model of inflammation with a bewilderingly large number of varieties. Winter (1965) has scanned this scene of confusion by comparing the effects of seven drugs against the edema induced by seven noxae (Fig. 1). The profiles of activity in Fig. 1 show that only hydrocortisone was effective against every noxa, and only inflammations induced by mustard and yeast were susceptible to inhibition by every drug.

Table VIII gives some representative tests of aspirin against inflammation of the foot or ankle in experimental animals. In these tests, aspirin was effective at oral or subcutaneous doses between 33 and 675 mg/kg and sodium salicylate was usually of roughly similar potency. Phenylbutazone, being 2–6 times as potent as aspirin, was relatively less active than against the UV erythema of guinea-pig skin. Amidopyrine was intermediate in potency between aspirin and phenylbutazone.

Although aspirin was effective against the arthritis induced by injecting dead tubercle bacilli in the rat, it was ineffective against the paw swelling of allergic encephalomyelitis (Rosenthale and Nagra, 1967). Cortisone and 6-mercaptopurine, however, were effective in both conditions.

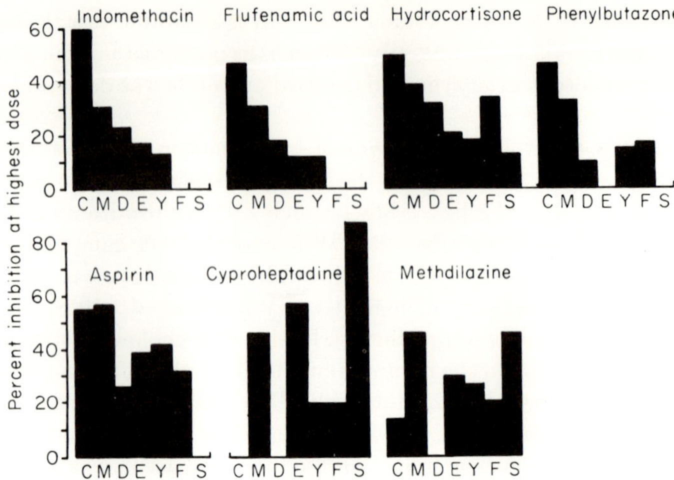

FIG. 1. Antiphlogistic profiles of various agents in different types of foot edema in the rat. The doses in mg/kg orally were: indomethacin, 9; flufenamic acid, 9; hydrocortisone, 18; phenylbutazone, 90; aspirin, 300; cyproheptadine, 9; methdilazine, 18. C, carrageenin; M, mustard; D, dextran; E, egg white; Y, yeast; F, formalin; S, serotonin. (Winter, 1965).

Cortisone or hydrocortisone was usually more effective than salicylates against foot edemas induced by various noxae in mouse or rat (Domenjoz, 1955; Winter *et al.*, 1962; Newbould, 1963; Weis, 1963; Niemegeers *et al.*, 1964; Garattini *et al.*, 1965; Winter, 1965; Rosenthale and Nagra, 1967). In the inflammation of limb joints in the rat induced by *Mycoplasma arthritidis*, however, hydrocortisone was not more effective than sodium salicylate (Wiesinger, 1965).

Many workers have found that catecholamines are effective against limb edemas. In the rat, adrenaline or noradrenaline inhibited edema induced by formalin, dextran, kaolin, yeast, 5-hydroxytryptamine, compound 48/80, or mild heat (Geschikter *et al.*, 1960; Schmidt, 1963; Garattini *et al.*, 1965; Kellett, 1965; Fearn *et al.*, 1965; Starr and West, 1967). In the mouse, adrenaline, noradrenaline, or isoprenaline inhibited formalin-induced edema of the foot and this inhibition was antagonized by appropriate adrenergic blockade (Northover and Subramanian, 1962).

3. *Body Cavities*

Another reaction used for testing antiphlogistic activity is the effusion provoked by injecting a noxa into the pleural or peritoneal cavity. Table IX summarizes values obtained with aspirin and other drugs against exudation into a body cavity induced by this means. In tests of this type, the patterns of activity of antipyretics, glucocorticoids, and catecholamines differ from their patterns against skin inflammation. Thus, aspirin, sodium salicylate, phenylbutazone, and amidopyrine were effective against peritoneal exudation in mice induced by saline or acetic acid, but their potencies were not sharply distinguished (Northover, 1963; Whittle, 1964). In the same test, paracetamol, glucocorticoids, and catecholamines were ineffective. Against pleural or peritoneal effusion in the rat, aspirin, sodium salicylate, phenylbutazone, and mepyramine showed activity; but glucocorticoids were relatively ineffective (Spector and Willoughby, 1959; Sancilio and Rodriguez, 1965; Wilhelmi, 1965).

4. *Phagocytosis and Granulation*

Antweiler (1957) tested the effect of antipyretics on the ability of polymorphonuclear leukocytes to take up grains of rice starch. Rats were treated subcutaneously with aspirin or other drug. Blood was withdrawn 1 hour later by heart puncture and the phagocytic activity of the leukocytes tested. By this method, aspirin or amidopyrine (250 mg/kg), or phenylbutazone (50 or 100 mg/kg) significantly inhibited phagocytosis. Sodium salicylate (500 mg/kg) was ineffective.

Antipyretics, as well as glucocorticoids, inhibit granulation around cotton pellets implanted subcutaneously in rats. When drugs were given daily for 7 days, indomethacin, hydrocortisone, phenylbutazone, and aspirin, in descending order of potency, were effective (Winter, 1965). In Winter's experiment, 100 mg/kg daily of aspirin by mouth inhibited by about 20% granulation around a cotton pellet.

The inhibition of granulation was also seen in the experiment of Wilhelmi (1963) on wound healing in rats. In this experiment, pieces of skin 1.5 cm in diameter were excised and the lesion observed during healing. A daily oral dose of 300 mg/kg of salicylic acid or a twice daily application of 10% salicylic acid in Vaseline inhibited granulation and retarded the rate of healing.

B. Site of Anti-Inflammatory Action

Aspirin inhibits inflammation in such diverse sites as skin, limbs, body cavities, and subcutaneous tissue; it may therefore be supposed to act by influencing one or more of the systemic mechanisms that may regulate or mediate local responses to injury. There are several that might be involved—the central nervous system, the autonomic nervous system with the adrenal medulla, the adrenal cortex with the adrenocorticotropic cells of the anterior lobe of the pituitary body, the reticuloendothelial system, the widespread mechanisms that liberate histamine, kinins, and probably other mediators of inflammation locally at sites of injury, and the mechanism by which counterirritants inhibit an inflammatory response, if not one of the foregoing.

At this point, we may discuss whether aspirin exerts its antiphlogistic effect by influencing nerves or ductless glands. The influence of aspirin on the rest of the above mechanisms had best be discussed after other aspects of its anti-defensive activity have been scrutinized.

Although there are many reports of the effects of experimental nervous lesions or of anesthetic, hypnotic, tranquilizing, narcotic, analgetic, or ganglion-blocking drugs upon inflammation, studies on the effect of such lesions or drugs upon the anti-inflammatory activity of aspirin or its relatives have been rare and their results confusing. In some of the few experiments of this type that have been traced, Domenjoz (1955) and Domenjoz *et al.* (1957) showed that aprobarbital anesthesia inhibited the anti-inflammatory effect of sodium salicylate on formalin-induced edema of the rat paw, but did not inhibit the effect of phenylbutazone on the same response. Aprobarbital incompletely inhibited the effect of aspirin on dextran edema of the rat paw. Without thorough investigation of the effects of experimental lesions or of pharmacologic blockade of the nervous system upon the anti-inflammatory activity of aspirin, we cannot tell whether nervous influences play any important part in this.

The suggestion that aspirin inhibits inflammation by potentiating adrenocortical mechanisms has often been made and has recently been discussed in detail by Smith (1966b). This suggestion takes several forms, each of which may apply either to the adrenocorticotropic hormone of the pituitary gland or to the hormones of the adrenal cortex and medulla. Protagonists of this view have suggested that aspirin either causes more of one of these hormones to be liberated from its producing gland or from storage sites elsewhere, or that aspirin blocks the inactivation of the hormone after its release. For example, Maickel *et al.* (1965) and Brodie (1965) have suggested that nonsteroidal anti-inflammatory drugs act by liberating adrenocortical steroids from their binding with plasma protein.

A usual way of investigating the role of a ductless gland in the antiphlogistic action of aspirin has been to test whether the drug is effective after removal of the gland. There is general agreement that hypophysectomy does not lessen the effect of aspirin or sodium salicylate upon edema of the rat foot induced by egg white (Ungar *et al.*, 1952) or by formalin (Domenjoz, 1955, 1960) or hyaluronidase-induced bluing of rat skin (Mathies, 1958).

Experiments on the effect of adrenalectomy upon the antiphlogistic activity of salicylates have given conflicting results. Adrenalectomy did not reduce the inhibition by salicylate of the edema of rat foot induced by egg white (Ungar *et al.*, 1952). In early experiments with formalin-induced edema of the rat foot, adrenalectomy abolished the anti-inflammatory effect of aspirin (Bacchus and Bacchus, 1953; Domenjoz, 1955); but in later and more thorough studies with moderate doses of aspirin, adrenalectomy had no such effect (Domenjoz, 1960). Northover and Subramanian (1961a) found that adrenalectomy lessened, but did not abolish, the antagonism by salicylate of formalin-induced edema of the rat foot. Mathies (1958) found that adrenalectomy inhibited the antagonism by large doses of aspirin of bluing induced by hyaluronidase in rat skin. On the contrary, adrenalectomy did not lessen the inhibition by indomethacin of edema induced by carrageenin in the rat paw (Winter *et al.*, 1967). In anti-granulation tests in the rat, adrenalectomy did not significantly change the extent to which phenylbutazone, mefenamic acid, or meclofenamic acid inhibited granulation around an implanted cotton pellet (Winder *et al.*, 1962, 1965). Likewise, indomethacin lessened granulation in adrenalectomized as well as intact rats (Winter *et al.*, 1963).

In the hands of van Cauwenberge and his associates, adrenalectomy reduced the inhibitory effect of sodium salicylate upon experimental inflammation of skin, subcutaneous tissue, or foot in the rat (van Cauwenberge *et al.*, 1954, 1960; van Cauwenberge and Lecomte, 1957; Halkin and van Cauwenberge, 1960). Likewise, Kelemen and co-workers (Kelemen *et al.*, 1950, 1952; Tanos *et al.*, 1953) have concluded that, after adrenalectomy, sodium salicylate is a less effective anti-inflammatory agent in the rat.

The above results indicate that adrenalectomy in some circumstances reduces the anti-inflammatory activity of salicylates. This reduction might be attributed to the loss of glucocorticoids, of catecholamines, or of some other factor. There are three reasons for not attributing this effect of adrenalectomy to lack of glucocorticoids. First, adrenalectomy does not change the activity of phenylbutazone and fenamates against granulation in the rat, although granulation is very sensitive to glucocorticoids. Second, as Smith (1966b) concludes after thoroughly reviewing the published work, therapeutic doses of salicylate do not stimulate adrenocortical secretion in animals or man, although large toxic doses may do so. For example, neither aspirin nor sodium salicylate increased hydrocortisone secretion from the isolated perfused adrenal of the dog (Crampton *et al.*, 1962). Nor, again, did indomethacin increase the corticosterone level in the blood of rats *in vivo* (Winter *et al.*, 1967). Third, in their profiles of antiphlogistic activity, glucocorticoids differ from salicylates. For example, in the guinea pig, aspirin antagonizes skin erythema induced by UV-radiation, but glucocorticoids do not; whereas glucocorticoids inhibit the tuberculin reaction, but salicylates do not. Some of these facts also weaken the hypothesis that salicylates exert their antiphlogistic effect by liberating glucocorticoids from store or by inhibiting their destruction.

Since catecholamines have shown anti-inflammatory activity in several tests, there is a possibility that adrenalectomy, when it effectively depresses the action of salicylates, does so because these drugs act in part by releasing catecholamines from the adrenal glands. If so, we would expect the effect of adrenalectomy to be more obvious when tested with higher doses of salicylate. Kelemen *et al.* (1950) and Domenjoz (1960) report that this is so. Since, however, in several experiments, aspirin has been found effective in the absence of the adrenals, there seems good reason to suppose that release of catecholamines, if this occurs with high doses of drug, provides no more than a secondary reinforcement of its activity.

To summarize, aspirin can inhibit inflammation in many parts of the body and therefore it presumably acts upon a widely distributed mechanism. There is little or no evidence bearing on the proposition that aspirin may stimulate nerves that inhibit inflammation or inhibit nerves that stimulate it. The sum of existing evidence suggests that aspirin does not act mainly by increasing the availability of adrenal hormones, either by an effect on the anterior lobe of the pituitary, on the adrenal cortex or medulla, or on glucocorticoid storage sites. Other possible sites of its anti-inflammatory effect will be considered in the general analysis of its mode of action.

C. Aspirin and Clinical Inflammation

The laboratory analysis of the antiphlogistic property of aspirin shows that it is effective against some inflammations and not against others, although even where it is effective, inhibition is seldom or never complete. The other main useful antiphlogistic drugs, the glucocorticoids, show a different profile of activity in the laboratory. The choice of aspirin or other anti-inflammatory drug has therefore largely been established by clinical experience. Such experience stretches back into the last century; but from a scrutiny of inflammatory reactions, new uses of aspirin or other antiphlogistic drugs may yet emerge. For example, observation of the effect of aspirin in one individual suffering from dermographia, coupled with the seeming parallelism between dermographia and the skin erythema induced by ultraviolet radiation or thurfyl nicotinate led me to ask whether aspirin would inhibit dermographia. A controlled trial of this possibility is now being attempted (A. Herxheimer, personal communication); although Moore-Robinson and Warin (1967) did not report any diminution caused by aspirin in weal width in 10 patients with dermographia.

The question arises whether the clinical value of aspirin in rheumatoid arthritis depends upon its antiphlogistic or upon its analgetic effect. By using jeweller's rings, Boardman and Hart (1967) have shown that a large dose of aspirin (5.3 gm daily) significantly reduced joint size in this disease; but half this dose of aspirin or a large dose of paracetamol (6 gm daily) was ineffective. Since this dose of paracetamol and the smaller dose of aspirin may be expected to relieve pain, but are not adequate in treating rheumatism, we may conclude that the anti-inflammatory, distinct from the analgetic, effect of aspirin is useful in rheumatoid arthritis. This conclusion is confirmed by the experience that sodium salicylate is about as effective as aspirin in this disease, as it is against experimental inflammation of the foot or ankle (Table VIII), but not against nociception (Tables I and V).

V. Antagonism of Smooth Muscle Responses

We have seen that aspirin inhibits nociceptive responses induced by various physiologically important substances, such as acetylcholine, ATP, bradykinin, tryptamine, or potassium (Table V). In inhibiting these responses, aspirin is relatively more active against acetylcholine and less active against tryptamine or potassium, and its selectivity toward bradykinin is not particularly marked. In inhibiting the responses of smooth muscles to these substances, aspirin shows a different pattern of selectivity, at least in some preparations of the guinea pig (Table X).

A. Bronchoconstriction

Aspirin readily antagonized bronchoconstriction induced by bradykinin and other kinins in the Konzett-Rössler preparation of guinea-pig lungs *in vivo* (Collier *et al.*, 1959, 1960). In the same *in vivo* preparation, aspirin did not inhibit bronchoconstriction induced by acetylcholine, angiotensin, histamine, 5-hydroxytryptamine, substance P (Collier and Shorley, 1960; Bhoola *et al.*, 1962; Berry and Collier, 1964), or by eledoisin (Stürmer and Berde, 1963). Aspirin also antagonized bronchoconstriction induced by other kinins, such as wasp kinin and the decapeptide kallidin; but the substances antagonized were not only kinins, as was at first thought, but also SRS-A (Berry and Collier, 1964), ATP (Collier *et al.*, 1966), and impure arachidonic acid (Berry, 1966). Aspirin also antagonized that part of the bronchoconstrictor response to anaphylatoxin that antihistamines did not antagonize (Bodammer, 1968).[1] This effect of aspirin is therefore better described as selective toward certain substances, than as specific toward kinins.

In antagonizing kinins, SRS-A, or ATP, low doses of aspirin were effective and these could be surmounted by higher doses of bradykinin or of SRS-A. Higher doses of aspirin in turn reestablished the block; but the relationship broke down at massive doses of agonist and antagonist (Collier and Shorley, 1963). The antagonism of bradykinin occurred almost immediately after intravenous injection of aspirin and it persisted for several hours (Collier, 1963b). The antibradykinin effect was present after destruction of the brain and spinal cord and after adrenalectomy or β-adrenergic blockade (Collier *et al.*, 1965, 1966), as Fig. 2 shows.

Other antipyretics are also able to antagonize bronchoconstriction induced by bradykinin, SRS-A, or ATP in the guinea pig, but drugs of other groups tested, except those with adrenergic and/or bronchodilator effects, have so far

[1] B. B. Vargaftig, E. P. de Miranda, and B. Lacoume (1968, *Nature* **222**, 883) have reported that several antipyretics antagonized bronchoconstriction in the guinea pig induced by slow-reacting substance C (SRS-C) obtained by the action of cobra venom on egg yolk.

TABLE X
SELECTIVE ANTAGONISM BY ASPIRIN OF THE CONTRACTION OF SOME SMOOTH MUSCLES OF THE GUINEA PIG INDUCED BY CERTAIN CHALLENGE SUBSTANCES[a]

Response	Challenge substance	Effective dose of aspirin	Approx. relative potency of other antipyretics (aspirin = 1)	Challenge substances not antagonized	Reference
Bronchoconstriction *in vivo*	Bradykinin SRS-A	2 mg/kg i.v.	Am, 0.25–0.5; Fl, 2; In, 2; Me, 2; Pb, 0.5–2; Pm, 0.03–0.125; Sa, 0.03	Ach; An; El; Hi; 5-HT; SP	Collier and Shorley, (1960 1963); Stürmer and Berde (1963); Berry and Collier (1964)
	Kallidin				Bhoola *et al.* (1962)
	ATP				Collier *et al.* (1966)
	Arachidonic acid				Berry (1966)
Bronchoconstriction in isolated perfused lung	Bradykinin	1 μg/ml	Pb, 5	Hi, 5-HT	Greeff and Moog (1964)
Vasoconstriction in isolated perfused lung	Bradykinin	1 μg/ml	Pb, 5	5-HT	
Contraction of isolated ileum	Arachidonic acid	30 μg/ml	Am, 10; Pb, 3	Ach; $BaCl_2$	Jaques (1965)

[a] Key to abbreviations: Ach, acetylcholine; An, angiotensin; ATP, adenosine-5′-triphosphate; El, eledoisin; Hi, histamine; SRS-A, slow-reacting substance in anaphylaxis; SP, substance P (other abbreviations as in Tables I, II, V, and VIII).

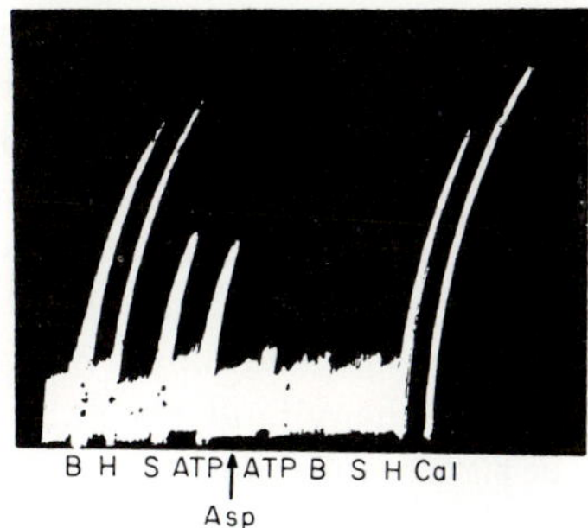

FIG. 2. Antagonism by aspirin of bronchoconstriction induced by bradykinin, by slow-reacting substance in anaphylaxis (SRS-A), and by adenosine triphosphate in the absence of the CNS and in the presence of β-adrenergic blockade. Air overflow volume during artificial ventilation is recorded by the method of Konzett and Rössler (1940), in a guinea pig of 350 gm, after destruction of the brain and spinal cord and pretreatment with pronethalol, 10 mg/kg intraperitoneally and 5 mg/kg intravenously. B, 1 μg of bradykinin; H, 0.25 μg of histamine; S, 0.2 mg of SRS-A; ATP, 0.6 mg of adenosine triphosphate; Asp, 4 mg/kg of sodium acetylsalicylate; all given intravenously. Cal, maximum air overflow volume; time, 30 sec. (Collier *et al.*, 1966.)

been ineffective (Collier and Shorley, 1960, 1963; Berry and Collier, 1964).[1] Among inactive drugs are glucocorticoids, narcotic analgetics, quinoline antimalarials, and antagonists of acetylcholine, histamine, and 5-HT.

Although this antagonism is very definite when kinins are administered intravenously to the guinea pig *in vivo*, the range of circumstances in which it operates has proved to be rather limited. Intravenous aspirin was ineffective against bradykinin dropped onto the pleural surface of the lung of the guinea pig *in vivo* (Bhoola *et al.*, 1962), but this failure is consistent with that of catecholamine aerosols to overcome bronchoconstrictors applied to the pleural surface of isolated guinea-pig lungs, reported by Dautrebande (1963). Again, when bradykinin was injected intravenously into the rabbit or rat, the resulting bronchoconstriction was not antagonized by aspirin (Bhoola *et al.*, 1962). In man, bronchoconstriction induced in chronic asthmatics by inhalation of bradykinin aerosol was slightly, but probably nonspecifically, reduced by aspirin, phenylbutazone, amidopyrine, flufenamic acid, mepyramine, or atropine (Stresemann, 1963). Antipyretic drugs did not antagonize bronchoconstriction induced in a few chronic asthmatics by inhalation of SRS-A aerosol (Herxheimer and Stresemann, 1966).

The antagonism of bradykinin-induced contraction of the bronchial muscle

[1] H. O. J. Collier, G. W. L. James and P. J. Piper (1968, *Brit. J. Pharmacol.* **34**, 76) have reported that phenelzine and mebanazine also weakly antagonized the bronchoconstrictor effect of bradykinin. Apart from these exceptions, this activity remains confined to the anti-inflammatory acids.

has been studied further *in vitro*. In the isolated heart-lung preparation of the guinea pig, bradykinin caused bronchoconstriction, which was readily suppressed by phenylbutazone; but in the cat this effect of phenylbutazone was slight or absent (Carpi *et al.*, 1962; Klupp and Konzett, 1965).

In the isolated lungs of the guinea pig perfused with Tyrode's solution via the pulmonary artery and artificially ventilated, bronchoconstriction can be elicited by acetylcholine, angiotensin, bradykinin, eledoisin, histamine, 5-HT, and kallidin. Aspirin (1 μg/ml) or phenylbutazone (0.2 μg/ml) antagonized this effect with a high degree of significance, but did not antagonize that of histamine or 5-HT (Greeff and Moog, 1964). Aarsen (1966), however, failed to obtain antagonism of bradykinin-induced bronchoconstriction with antipyretics in the isolated lungs of the guinea pig.

In the isolated trachea of the guinea pig, aspirin (100 μg/ml) antagonized SRS-A, but did not antagonize acetylcholine (Berry and Collier, 1964). In the same preparation, phenylbutazone (100 μg/ml) antagonized bradykinin more readily than it antagonized histamine (Bhoola *et al.*, 1962). The potency and selectiveness of aspirin or phenylbutazone against bradykinin or SRS-A in the isolated trachea, however, was less than in the isolated whole lungs perfused via the pulmonary artery (Greeff and Moog, 1964), in the heart-lung preparation (Klupp and Konzett, 1965) or in the whole animal (Collier and Shorley, 1960). If this difference were real, it would parallel the ineffectiveness of aspirin against bronchoconstriction induced by dropping bradykinin onto the pleural surface of the lung (Bhoola *et al.*, 1962), contrasting with its effectiveness against intravenous bradykinin.

Since the effectiveness of aspirin seems to depend upon the route by which bradykinin reaches the bronchial muscle and since aspirin antagonizes bronchoconstriction induced by substances such as bradykinin and SRS-A that appear to act at different receptors (Berry and Collier, 1964; Collier *et al.*, 1966), aspirin might be supposed to act in this situation by blocking some common route of these substances to or from their receptors. If the concept of bradykinin receptors on bronchial muscle of guinea pig that are blocked by antipyretic drugs ("A-receptors"), proposed some years ago (Collier, 1962), is retained, the A-receptors must be conceived as lying at some common point on the route by which kinins, SRS-A, ATP, and possibly other substances affect bronchoconstriction.

Gjuris *et al.* (1964a) have shown that, in lightly anesthetized, spontaneously breathing guinea pigs, relatively low intravenous doses of bradykinin induced tachypnea. Aspirin and other antipyretics readily antagonized this effect. Since this tachypnea could be abolished by isoprenaline or by cutting the vagi, Marquardt (1966) considers that it is a reflex response to bradykinin-induced bronchoconstriction. This conclusion is supported by the fact that the doses of bradykinin and kallidin that elicit tachypnea, and the absolute and relative doses of aspirin and other antipyretics that prevent it, correspond very closely with those inducing and antagonizing bronchoconstriction, respectively (Collier, 1965). Also, like bradykinin-induced bronchoconstriction, the tachypnea declines with repeated treatment.

That salicylates antagonize bronchoconstriction induced by bradykinin or by SRS-A in guinea-pig lung suggests that they might also reduce anaphylactic bronchoconstriction in that species; but early attempts to demonstrate this effect failed (Smith and Humphrey, 1949; Armitage *et al.*, 1952; Collier and Shorley, 1960). By suitable choice of the conditions of the experiment, however, aspirin could be shown to lessen anaphylactic bronchoconstriction quite effectively in the guinea pig (Collier *et al.*, 1963; Collier, 1965). In the rabbit, also, aspirin or phenylbutazone protected against anaphylactic shock, but large doses were needed (Campbell, 1948; Lepper *et al.*, 1950; Lecomte, 1960).

In anaphylactic shock in the guinea pig, SRS-A and kinins are liberated (Brocklehurst, 1956, 1960; Brocklehurst and Lahiri, 1962, 1963). The kinins and one component of SRS-A are bronchoconstrictors in that species (Collier *et al.*, 1960; Berry and Collier, 1964). The antagonism by aspirin of both these bronchoconstrictors is potent enough to account for its reduction of anaphylactic bronchoconstriction (Collier and James, 1966, 1967), but inhibition of histamine release in anaphylaxis (Trethewie, 1951; Mongar and Schild, 1957) or antagonism of other so far unidentified mediators could also be involved.

The failure in preliminary experiments of aspirin and other antipyretics to antagonize bronchoconstriction induced in chronic asthmatics by inhaling aerosols of bradykinin or of SRS-A suggests that these drugs are less effective in antagonizing kinins and SRS-A in man than in the guinea pig. There is evidence, however, that aspirin is sometimes efficacious in this disease. Thus, Cook (1947) wrote that aspirin is "curiously effective in an occasional asthmatic patient" and Pearson (1963) found that, of 1205 asthmatics, 6 had their symptoms "relieved or prevented by taking aspirin."[1] The fact that, also in Pearson's series, 24 hypersensitive patients had asthmatic attacks precipitated by aspirin explains why it is not more commonly used in this disease. The possibility remains that in suitable conditions, patients, doses, or combinations with other agents, some anti-inflammatory acids may yet show more widely useful antiasthmatic activity in man.

B. Other Muscles

In certain preparations of blood vessels, many physiologically active endogenous substances, including bradykinin, induce a contraction of the smooth muscle. In the guinea pig and rabbit, antipyretics antagonize the contraction induced by bradykinin or eledoisin, respectively, but there is doubt whether this antagonism is selective.

[1] C. A. Clarke (1969, *Brit. med. J.* **i**, 256) has recently confirmed the antiasthmatic effect of aspirin.

According to Konzett and his co-workers (Klupp and Konzett, 1965; Konzett and Bauer, 1966), in the anesthetized guinea pig, bradykinin or adrenaline induced a rise of pressure in the pulmonary artery. Flufenamic acid, mefenamic acid, and phenylbutazone (1–10 mg/kg) antagonized the rise due to bradykinin, but not that due to adrenaline. Similar results were obtained in the heart-lung preparation of the guinea pig *in vitro* and in isolated strips of guinea-pig pulmonary artery. In preparations of either the whole rabbit or of isolated pulmonary artery, eledoisin induced a rise in pulmonary blood pressure, or a contraction of the isolated smooth muscle, that antipyretics antagonized. Antipyretics did not, however, antagonize comparable responses to 5-HT, acetylcholine, or adrenaline. In the cat, in contrast with the guinea pig, phenylbutazone did not antagonize the increase in pulmonary arterial pressure induced by bradykinin.

In the isolated lungs of the guinea pig (Greeff and Moog, 1964) or of the rabbit (Lecomte and Troquet, 1960), but not in those of the cat (Greeff and Moog, 1964) or dog (Waaler, 1961), bradykinin contracted the pulmonary blood vessels. In the guinea pig, aspirin or phenylbutazone antagonized this effect without reducing a comparable effect of 5-HT, although the antipyretics somewhat lessened the effect of histamine (Greeff and Moog, 1964). In the rabbit, phenylbutazone inhibited the comparable action of bradykinin (Lecomte and Troquet, 1960).

Although the above workers found some degree of selectivity in the antagonism by antipyretics of the constriction of blood vessels in whole isolated lungs induced by bradykinin or other agents, Hauge *et al.* (1966) and Starr and West (1966) observed no selectivity of phenylbutazone or other antipyretics toward bradykinin in isolated strips of guinea-pig or rabbit pulmonary artery. Both these groups of workers, however, appeared to use higher doses of antipyretics than did Greeff and Moog (1964). In blood vessels of the rat or guinea pig, isolated from other sites than lung, antipyretic drugs antagonized non-specifically the contractions induced by several endogenous substances (Starr and West, 1966; Northover, 1967).

In contrast to its effect on the pulmonary circulation, bradykinin causes a sharp fall in systemic blood pressure. In the guinea pig, aspirin (4 mg/kg i.v.) lessened the duration, but not the depth, of this hypotensive response (Collier and Shorley, 1960; Collier *et al.*, 1968b). It did not, however, curtail the comparable response to prostaglandin E_1. In the rabbit also, quite small doses of aspirin and other antipyretics shortened the duration of the blood pressure fall induced by bradykinin (Türker and Kiran, 1964; Vargaftig, 1966).[1]

[1] B. B. Vargaftig, E. P. de Miranda, and B. Lacoume (1969, *Nature* **222**, 883) have recently reported that several anti-inflammatory acids lessened hypotension induced by crude SRS-C in the rabbit.

In the dog, intravenous infusion of aspirin (45 mg/kg) blocked the fall in systemic blood pressure and the rise in portal venous pressure induced by *Escherichia coli* endotoxin (Hinshaw *et al.*, 1967). Indomethacin had a similar effect on the systemic hypotensive response to endotoxin, and phenylbutazone curtailed it without lessening its depth (Erdös *et al.*, 1967).

Aspirin or phenylbutazone, at a concentration of 100 μg/ml did not inhibit the contraction of guinea-pig isolated ileum induced by acetylcholine, barium chloride, bradykinin, or histamine (Collier and Shorley, 1960; Jaques, 1965). On the contrary, aspirin (30 μg/ml) and phenylbutazone (3 μg/ml) inhibited the response of ileum to arachidonic acid peroxide (Jaques, 1965). Whereas morphine failed to antagonize bradykinin-induced bronchoconstriction (Collier and Shorley, 1960), morphine and other narcotic analgetics shared with aspirin and phenylbutazone the ability to antagonize selectively the contraction of isolated ileum induced by arachidonic acid peroxide (Jaques, 1965). At present this observation remains as another example of the diversity of the patterns of selectivity that aspirin displays.

C. Character of the Antagonism

Aspirin and other antipyretics sometimes potently antagonize the responses of some smooth muscles to certain endogenous substances. The antagonism by aspirin of bronchoconstriction induced by bradykinin in the guinea pig shows several features of receptor blockade: (1) It occurs in the absence of the CNS or of the adrenal glands; (2) it is surmountable by higher doses of bradykinin, which can in turn be overcome by higher doses of aspirin; (3) its onset is rapid; and (4) aspirin does not antagonize bronchoconstriction induced by acetylcholine, histamine, or 5-HT. For the following reasons, however, this antagonism by aspirin cannot be compared with that by antihistamine drugs of histamine-induced responses nor with the similar specific antagonism by atropine of the muscarinic effects of acetylcholine.

First, the pattern of selectiveness varies. Thus, in the guinea pig, aspirin antagonizes bronchoconstriction induced by bradykinin or arachidonic acid, but not that induced by acetylcholine or histamine, whereas, on pulmonary blood pressure, aspirin antagonizes bradykinin and histamine, but not 5-HT, and, on isolated ileum, it antagonizes arachidonic acid peroxide, but not bradykinin or acetylcholine. Again, aspirin not only antagonizes bronchoconstriction in the guinea pig, induced by bradykinin, but also that induced by SRS-A, arachidonic acid or ATP, although some or all of these probably act at different receptors.

A second difference between the antagonism by aspirin of certain endogenous substances and the receptor blocking action of antihistamines or of atropine is that the former is confined to certain species and organs. Thus, aspirin antagonizes bronchoconstriction induced by bradykinin in the guinea pig, but not in the rabbit or cat. Again, aspirin antagonizes the rise in pulmonary blood pressure induced by bradykinin in the guinea pig, but not the immediate fall in systemic blood pressure induced by the same challenge substance in the same species, although it lessens the duration of the fall.

A third feature that distinguishes aspirin from conventional receptor blocking agents is that, in the same organ system, antagonism by aspirin is more apparent in some circumstances than in others. For example, aspirin readily antagonizes bradykinin-induced bronchoconstriction in the guinea pig when the agonist is given intravenously, but not when it is dropped onto the pleural surface of the lung. Again, aspirin is more selective *in vivo* than in isolated trachea. These observations suggest that the effect of aspirin depends on the route by which it reaches the tissues.

These conclusions are puzzling, but the patterns of activity that aspirin shows against induced responses of smooth musculе agree at least in their variety with the patterns already noted in antinociception and anti-inflammation. They suggest that aspirin and other antipyretics act, not by blocking only one type of receptor for a particular mediator, such as the A-receptors for bradykinin (Collier, 1962), but rather by inhibiting some underlying cellular mechanism that takes part to different extents in different responses mediated by different endogenous substances.

VI. Antihemostasis

In the last century, both Balette and Binz considered that sodium salicylate might cause untoward bleeding in man (Gross and Greenberg, 1948). Since then, several authors, beginning with Fischer (1905), have suggested that large doses of aspirin might also have this effect. In animals, an antihemostatic effect seems first to have been reported by Link *et al.* (1943), who observed that salicylate delayed blood clotting in the rat. A single intravenous dose of 5 mg of sodium salicylate or an oral dose of 10 mg of salicylic acid per rat detectably increased prothrombin time, the peak effect being at about 12–24 hours after treatment. Feeding vitamin K prevented, and injecting prothrombin overcame the effect. In shed blood, addition of salicylate did not increase prothrombin time.

Soon afterward, several workers confirmed and extended the observations of Link and co-workers. Field (1945) showed that aspirin acted like salicylic acid and that it prolonged prothrombin time in suckling rats when fed to their mother. Rapoport *et al.* (1943) reported that rabbits, too, were susceptible to this effect of salicylates, although dogs were not. Meyer and Howard (1943) found that salicylate also diminished the prothrombin content of human blood.

In normal people, an oral dose of about 6 gm of aspirin was needed to produce a significant prolongation of prothrombin time (Quick and Clescari, 1960). The largeness of the dose lessens the likelihood of this particular antihemostatic effect being either useful or dangerous clinically.

Aspirin also inhibits other events in hemostasis. Thus, in healthy volunteers, 0.65 to 3.0 gm of aspirin by mouth prolonged the bleeding time (Gast, 1964; Quick, 1966; Weiss and Aledort, 1967). In similar doses, aspirin also decreased the aggregation of platelets in blood withdrawn after treatment (Beaumont *et al.*, 1955; Gast, 1964; Morris, 1967; Weiss and Aledort, 1967; Zucker and Peterson, 1968). O'Brien (1968a) found that a single oral dose of 150 mg of aspirin was enough to inhibit platelet aggregation induced by adrenaline or collagen in blood subsequently shed, whereas 2 gm of sodium salicylate was ineffective. The inhibition of platelet aggregation after one dose of aspirin lasted several days. Although phenylbutazone and indomethacin were slightly more active than aspirin, their effect was much briefer (O'Brien, 1968b). In rabbits, a comparable effect has been observed (Evans *et al.*, 1967). Salicylate and other anti-inflammatory drugs also inhibited aggregation of human blood platelets *in vitro* (Morris, 1967; Mustard *et al.*, 1967). O'Brien (1968b) found meclofenamate the most potent of such drugs.

Since hemostasis is one of the local reactions to injury, its inhibition may be regarded as an expression of the antidefensive activity of aspirin. Unlike some of its other antidefensive effects, the delay of hemostasis has not become the basis of a clinical use of aspirin; but Morris (1967) and O'Brien (1968a) suggested that this inhibition of platelet aggregation might be useful. Whether the antihemostatic effects of aspirin can be exploited clinically or not, they may well accentuate gastric bleeding, which is one of its main toxic hazards (Honigsberger, 1943).

VII. Lowering Some Raised Constituents of Blood

Fasting or exposure to cold raises the level of free fatty acids (FFA) in the blood (Paoletti *et al.*, 1963). Hormones, such as adrenaline, adrenocorticotropin, and glucagon, and drugs, such as amphetamine, chlorpromazine, and ethanol, also raise plasma FFA (Paoletti *et al.*, 1963; Steinberg, 1963). The mobilization of FFA from fat stores has been seen as a homeostatic mechanism to provide supplies of nutriment for energy.

In the rat, intraperitoneal doses of 25–300 mg/kg of sodium salicylate prevented the rise in FFA induced by fasting, by cold, or by injecting corticotropin, noradrenaline, amphetamine, or chlorpromazine (Bizzi *et al.*, 1965). At an intraperitoneal dose of 300 mg/kg, acetylsalicylic and benzoic acid were also effective, but salicylamide and *p*-aminobenzoic acid were not. Bizzi and coworkers used a technique for measuring plasma FFA that was unaffected by salicylate. Using the same technique, Carlson and Östman (1961) showed that large oral doses of aspirin lowered plasma FFA, both in normal human subjects and, more markedly, in diabetics, in whom the FFA level is raised.

Whereas large doses of salicylates may cause hyperglycemia in people with normal blood glucose levels, there is much evidence that salicylates reduce the glucose concentration of the blood and urine in patients with diabetes mellitus (Ebstein, 1876; Gross and Greenberg, 1948; Hecht and Goldner, 1959; Stowers, 1963; Smith, 1966a). In rats made diabetic by injuring the islets of Langerhans, the reduction of the levels of glucose in the blood and urine by aspirin (Ingle, 1950; Bornstein *et al.*, 1952; Ingle and Meeks, 1952) or by sodium salicylate (Smith *et al.*, 1952) can readily be reproduced in the laboratory. In the experiments of Ingle and Meeks (1952), treatment for 3 weeks with subcutaneous doses of aspirin, rising from 40–160 mg daily per rat, lowered both blood and urinary glucose. Unlike insulin, however, aspirin did not at the same time lower urinary nonprotein nitrogen. Although salicylates have been used in diabetes, much more satisfactory remedies are now available. Little seems to be known about any effect that salicylates may exert upon the hyperglycemia and glycosuria induced by burns or by surgery (Evans and Butterfield, 1951; Johnston, 1964, 1968), but the ability of salicylates to lower plasma FFA raised by cold, starvation, or diabetes suggests that these drugs might also lower the hyperglycemia of trauma.

Salicylates lower blood cholesterol, where this is elevated in myxedema, xanthomatosis, and coronary artery disease (Austen *et al.*, 1958; Macdougall and Alexander, 1963). Macdougall and Alexander (1963) and Smith (1966b), who have reviewed the literature on the hypercholesteremic effects of salicylates, do not report experiments on laboratory animals in which the blood cholesterol had been artificially raised. More recently, Wooles *et al.* (1967) failed to lower blood cholesterol with daily doses of 300 mg/kg sodium salicylate in rats made hypercholesteremic by dietary excess of cholesterol and cholic acid.

Salicylates are well known to lessen blood urate and to increase uric acid excretion in gout (Gutman, 1966). Attempts to mimic in laboratory animals this therapeutic effect of salicylates have failed. Salicylates do not greatly influence uric acid excretion in normal animals and there seems no satisfactory model of gout in laboratory animals (Gutman, 1966).

VIII. Damage to Epithelia

A. Gastric Mucosa

In his paper introducing aspirin, Dreser (1899) stated that the drug irritated and abraded the mucous membrane of the stomach, though he showed that it damaged the transparent fins of small fish less than did salicylic acid. Likewise, Manasse (1900) found that, when each was applied for 3 days to human skin, salicylic acid had greater keratolytic and inflammatory effects than had acetylsalicylic acid. Nonetheless, by 1948, when Gross and Greenberg drew up a list of fatal cases of aspirin poisoning, hemorrhage from the gastric mucosa had been noted in many. At that time, however, the fact that aspirin, in therapeutic doses, can damage the gastric mucosa was little appreciated, although Gregerson (1916), Douthwaite and Lintott (1938), and Hurst and Lintott (1939) had produced good evidence that this was so. So successfully had Wolf and Wolff (1943), Paul (1943), and Caravati and Cosgrove (1946) argued that aspirin caused negligible gastric damage that, in 1948, Gross and Greenberg concluded: "Bleeding from the gastrointestinal tract may occur in exceptional cases after small doses of salicylate and is probably due to abnormal sensitivity. Bleeding, frequently observed after toxic doses of salicylate, is due solely to a systemic action of salicylates" (p. 98).

Ignorance of the ability of aspirin to elicit bleeding remained so widespread that Modell and Patterson (1951) were able to describe a patient with chronic bleeding from the gut and with consequent anemia, who had been investigated in three different medical centers during 8 years, without discovery that the condition was due to chronic consumption of aspirin. When this drug, of which the patient was taking about 3 gm daily, was withdrawn, blood disappeared from the stools within a day and the blood hemoglobin doubled within 2 months.

The observation that aspirin erodes the mucous membrane of the stomach and causes gastric bleeding in experimental animals preceded by several years the same finding in man. In 1909, Chistoni and Lapresa reported that oral doses of acetylsalicylic acid induced hyperemia and ulceration in dogs and edema and hemorrhage in rabbits.

Experiments on gastric damage caused by aspirin in laboratory animals concern the following questions. What is the nature of the damage induced by aspirin? In what species is it seen? What is the effective dose by oral and parenteral routes? What is the time course of the effect? How is it affected by repeated dosage? Can the effect be lessened by changing the pharmaceutical formulation of aspirin? What is the potency of aspirin compared with other drugs having comparable therapeutic effects? What is the mechanism of its action? From many experiments in animals, some, but not all, of these questions have been answered.

Aspirin causes desquamation of epithelium, hyperemia, local ulceration, and/or hemorrhage in the stomach of guinea pig, rat, dog, man, and other species. The effective dose varies with the species and route. In the guinea pig, for example, Anderson (1964a) found that a single dose of 10 mg/kg by mouth was effective in most animals. An oral dose of 100 mg/kg of aspirin produced damage within a quarter of an hour in the stomach of one animal and within an hour in all animals treated.

Parenterally, doses up to 500 mg/kg of aspirin produced no gastric lesions in guinea pigs (Anderson, 1964a); but, in rats, Barbour and Dickerson (1938) obtained stomach ulcers by repeated subcutaneous or oral doses of 300 mg/kg daily. In dogs, oral doses of about 80–200 mg/kg of aspirin were effective (Chistoni and Lapresa, 1909; Hurley and Crandall, 1964). Hurley and Crandall did not obtain ulceration with intravenous sodium salicylate, but Dodd *et al.* (1937) found this effective in the dog. Hurley and Crandall also found that, during continued treatment of dogs with aspirin, ulcers tended to heal; but if treatment was stopped for more than 2 days and then started again, ulcers again appeared. In the dog there thus develops refractoriness to the ulcerogenic effect of aspirin; but the refractory period is short.

The short period of refractoriness to aspirin ulceration observed by Hurley and Crandall (1964) in dogs may be paralleled by a finding of Wilhelmi (1963). Oral treatment with sodium salicylate, in doses too small to induce ulceration, for 2 days before challenge with an ulcerogenic dose of 5-hydroxytryptamine, lessened the intensity of the resulting ulceration. A possible cross-refractoriness between the ulcerogenic activities of salicylates and 5-hydroxytryptamine is suggested.

In man, there has been a wealth of studies on the gastric damage induced by aspirin, in which gastroscopy, gastrectomy, and tests for blood in the feces have been used to assess the effect. These studies show that a single oral dose of aspirin caused gastric erosion in up to 20% of subjects (Muir and Cossar, 1955, 1961; Weiss *et al.*, 1961). On continued treatment with aspirin, most people lost >2 ml of blood daily in the feces and about 5% of patients lost >15 ml (Pierson *et al.*, 1961; Stubbé *et al.*, 1962; Wood *et al.*, 1962; Croft and Wood, 1967). In man, aspirin is seldom given other than by the oral route; but Grossman *et al.* (1961) found that relatively large intravenous doses of aspirin caused a slight fecal blood loss.

Because of its pharmaceutical importance, the possibility that certain formulations of aspirin might lessen gastric damage has been widely investigated. Anderson (1963) reported that aspirin tablets, whether plain acetylsalicylic acid, soluble aspirin, buffered aspirin, calcium aspirin urea, or aspirin glycine, each induced ulceration at about the same dose in the guinea pig. In man, the earlier claim that soluble aspirin was less likely than plain aspirin to damage the gastric mucosa (Muir and Cossar, 1955, 1961) was not supported by later observations (Stubbé *et al.*, 1962; Wood *et al.*, 1962). Dispersal of aspirin or soluble aspirin in water before swallowing did not lessen gastric damage (Wood, 1963), but giving the drug with sodium bicarbonate or other powerful antacid, or dissolving effervescent aspirin in water, which gives an alkaline solution, protected the mucosa in guinea pig (Anderson, 1963, 1964b), rat (Barbour and Dickerson, 1938), dog (Hurley and Crandall, 1964), and man (Wood, 1963; Stubbé, 1963). Occasionally, however, effervescent aspirin also caused bleeding (Stubbé, 1963).

Although Grossman *et al.* (1961) found that enteric-coated aspirin tablets caused bleeding, the view of Wood (1963)—that they were less active in this respect than ordinary tablets—is consistent with the finding that aspirin was less damaging to the gastrointestinal tract when given with alkali.

Contrary to the opinion of Dreser (1899), aspirin appeared to be more damaging to the stomach than was salicylic acid or sodium salicylate in guinea pig (Anderson, 1963), dog (Hurley and Crandall, 1964), or man (Wood, 1963). Mefenamic acid was also less toxic to human gastric epithelium than was aspirin (Lane *et al.*, 1964; Skyring and Bhanthumnavin, 1967). Anderson (1963) found phenylbutazone to be about as destructive as sodium salicylate in the guinea pig. In man, phenylbutazone (Mauer, 1955) and indomethacin (Croft, 1966) each caused gastric damage. Paracetamol, however, appeared to be relatively free of gastric toxicity (Wood *et al.*, 1962; Goulston and Skyring, 1964). Tudhope (1967) found that flufenamic acid was not more toxic to the gastric mucosa than was paracetamol.

Since the gastric lesions are reduced by administering enough alkali with aspirin to neutralize gastric acidity, the contention of Wood (1963) that nonionized acetylsalicylic acid causes the injury seems justified. His argument that the lesions are not caused by the acidity of aspirin is also acceptable, since salicylic acid is more acidic and less toxic to the mucosa.

Domenjoz (1966b) has suggested that antirheumatic drugs erode the epithelium of the digestive tract by inhibiting the cell division that occurs very frequently in the epithelial cells. Supporting this suggestion, Domenjoz quotes the finding of Karzel (1967) that aspirin (30–340 μg/ml) and other antirheumatic drugs inhibited the division of mouse fibroblasts and of Ehrlich ascites tumor cells in culture. Roth and Valdes-Dapena (1963) observed that aspirin coagulated the gastric mucosa of the cat. Menguy and Masters (1965) found that aspirin inhibited gastric mucous secretion in rats and dogs and they obtained some evidence that the quality of the mucus was altered. Menguy and Desbaillets (1967) found that phenylbutazone had similar effects in dogs. These authors suggested that such effects play a part in causing the gastric erosion induced by the anti-inflammatory drugs.

B. Renal Tubular Epithelium

The toxic effect of a drug on the epithelium of the human kidney tubule may be assessed by counting the number of renal tubular cells in the urine. When 0.65, 1.3, or 2.7 gm of aspirin was given by mouth to volunteers, the number of renal tubular cells in the urine rose sharply, the count being directly related to the dose (Scott *et al.*, 1963). When treatment with aspirin was continued daily, the cellular count returned to normal within $2\frac{1}{2}$–$3\frac{1}{2}$ weeks. In 2 patients, Scott *et al.* (1963) tested whether sodium bicarbonate, in large enough doses to bring the urine to a pH of 8–9, inhibited this nephrotoxic effect. A single dose of aspirin, however, still elicited a sharp rise in the count of urinary cells, and although this rise was a little less than sometimes occurred without bicarbonate, the difference was not significant.

Sodium salicylate was about as effective as aspirin in exfoliating the renal tubular epithelium (Scott *et al.*, 1963). Other drugs often taken as analgetics, alone or in mixtures, were also effective (Prescott, 1966a). The counts of renal tubular cells in groups of volunteers taking large doses of analgetic drugs daily, made by Prescott (1966a), show that paracetamol had a just detectable nephrotoxic effect, caffeine and phenacetin were slightly more toxic than paracetamol, and aspirin was much more toxic, judged by the urinary cell count (Table XI).

TABLE XI

EFFECT OF ASPIRIN AND OTHER ANTIPYRETICS ON RENAL TUBULAR CELL COUNT IN HEALTHY VOLUNTEERS[a]

Drug	Daily dose (gm)	No. of subjects	Mean total control count[b] (thousands)	Mean total treatment count[b] (thousands)	Percent increase	*P*
Placebo	—	10	5,814	6,153	6	N.S.[c]
Paracetamol	3.6	21	5,645	6,286	11	<0.05
Caffeine citrate	2.4	10	6,308	8,660	37	<0.01
Phenacetin	3.6	10	6,064	10,494	73	<0.05
A.P.C.[d]	4.8	10	6,012	11,435	90	<0.01
Aspirin	3.6	10	6,065	57,294	945	<0.01

[a] Prescott (1966a).

[b] The urinary renal tubular cells were counted for a 5-day control period followed by a 5-day treatment period.

[c] N.S., not significant.

[d] A.P.C. consisted of aspirin (1.8 gm), phenacetin (1.8 gm) and caffeine citrate (1.2 gm).

Because the exfoliative response to aspirin became refractory to repeated doses, Scott *et al.* (1963) argued that "it is doubtful if any serious damage is done to the kidney by salicylates in therapeutic dosage, even after long periods". The refractoriness of the response, however, may only be due to exhaustion of the supply of cells liable to exfoliate.

There are several reasons why the nephrotoxicity of aspirin may be more serious than Scott *et al.* (1963) supposed. First, an increase of red blood corpuscles accompanied that of renal tubular cells in the urine during aspirin treatment (Prescott, 1966a). Second, patients with rheumatoid arthritis showed an unexpectedly high incidence of renal papillary necrosis and of interstitial nephritis (Clausen and Pedersen, 1961; Brun *et al.*, 1965). Third, Clausen (1964) has shown that rabbits, receiving either aspirin or phenacetin (1–2 gm daily 5 days a week) for about a year, developed histologically evident kidney lesions, especially in the distal part of the nephron. These findings suggest that persistent consumption of aspirin, as well as that of phenacetin, should be suspected as a cause of kidney damage.

C. Conclusions

Experiments in which aspirin was applied directly to visible sites, for example, fish fins (Dreser, 1899), human skin (Manasse, 1900), and human lip (Roth *et al.*, 1963), show that it damages dry or moist epithelia. In the therapeutic use of aspirin such damage is most likely to occur in the stomach, where the concentration of aspirin in contact with epithelial cells is highest and where the acidic environment leads to more acetylsalicylic acid being present in nonionized form.

In the lumen of the kidney tubule the situation is less clear. After an oral dose of aspirin, little acetylsalicylic acid is likely to be present in the tubule, but salicylate may be expected there, its ionization depending on the pH of the urine. The renal tubular toxicity of aspirin may thus rather be due to salicylic acid or even a derivative of it than to aspirin itself. This conclusion is in line with the finding of Scott *et al.* (1963) that sodium salicylate appears to cause as much kidney damage as does aspirin.

The mechanism is unknown whereby aspirin and other salicylates damage epithelia in general and the moist linings of the stomach and of kidney tubules in particular. Nonetheless, this toxic property seems to conform with the character of aspirin as an antidefensive drug, since these epithelia, however internal, may be regarded as boundaries between the body and the outside world.

IX. The Mechanism of Aspirin Action

In the last analysis, a drug may be supposed to act upon living material by influencing some active macromolecule that operates an important biochemical process. Macromolecules that might react to a drug include genes and enzymes and some less well-defined entities, such as the storage sites, the carriers across living boundaries, and the receptors of living cells that take up and react to hormones and metabolites. If a drug interferes with a macromolecule that handles a hormone or metabolite, we think of the drug as antagonizing the substance to which the macromolecule reacts. Substances thus supposed to be antagonized are normally of small molecular weight. If they mediate local reactions they may well be liberated locally and hence may be called local hormones or humoral mediators.

Within the general concept that a drug acts by interfering with the working of a macromolecule, the particular possibilities are many, since the living body is a complex system of such operating macromolecules. The defensive reactions that aspirin inhibits are several, and so we might expect the drug to interfere with the operation of several different types of macromolecules; but the alternative exists that a single type of macromolecule of widespread occurrence taking part in several defensive reactions is involved. Since we should aim, on principle, to explain as much as possible with as few hypotheses as possible, this alternative will be kept in mind. If aspirin acts by affecting only one process, however, this cannot be central, as of the C.N.S. or a ductless gland, because the potency of aspirin relative to sodium salicylate differs between tests (Tables I and VI).

In each of the main reactions to experimental challenge that aspirin inhibits —fever, pain, inflammation, movement of smooth muscle, or hemostasis—the drug might act in one (or both) of two possible ways. It might depress a mechanism that promotes the reaction, or it might strengthen a mechanism that inhibits it. We should therefore consider the natural mechanisms by which defensive reactions are brought about and those by which they are moderated; and we should sift the evidence that aspirin depresses mechanisms of the one type or potentiates those of the other.

To interpret an effect of aspirin in terms of the antagonism or potentiation of a particular endogenous factor, evidence of three kinds is desirable. First, in an appropriate biologic preparation, aspirin should antagonize the mediator or potentiate the natural inhibitor more readily than it does other factors. Second, chemical relatives of aspirin should show effects upon the mediator or the inhibitor, corresponding to those they exert upon the induced response. Third, aspirin should antagonize the mediator or mimic the inhibitor over a range of biologic responses.

A. Depression of Defensive Reactions

1. *Effect on Nervous or Humoral Mechanisms*

The way in which the body effects defensive reactions are not always well understood, but they may be supposed to be either humoral or both nervous and humoral. Thus, the clotting of shed blood must depend upon a purely humoral mechanism, whereas flight in response to noxious stimulation of a nerve fiber is mainly nervous, but would at least involve some humoral transmission at nerve endings.

Both pain and fever involve nervous pathways, in which humoral mechanisms might be limited to junctions between nerves or to sites at the ends of efferent nerve fibers. There is good evidence, however, that in at least some forms of fever and pain, humoral mechanisms also operate on the afferent side.

Thus, fever induced by bacterial toxins is thought to be mediated by endogenous pyrogen released from leukocytes and pain associated with inflammation may be mediated by the release of endogenous pain substance.

The extent to which nerves are involved in the induction of inflammation is probably slight. For example, in the experiments of Fearn *et al.* (1965) in the rat, summarized in Table XII, inflammatory responses to such common noxae as xylol, dextran, or heat did not depend on the integrity of the central nervous system. The response to xylol probably involves an axon reflex, since it was abolished by degeneration of the femoral and sciatic nerves or by cocaine, but responses to dextran or mild heat were not abolished by either procedure and presumably depend on humoral mechanisms.

TABLE XII

EFFECTS OF EXPERIMENTAL NERVE LESIONS ON INFLAMMATORY RESPONSES TO NOXAE IN THE RAT[a]

Lesion	Response to noxa		
	Dextran[b]	Heat[c]	Xylol[d]
Chronic denervation[e]	P[f]	P	A[g]
Cocaine, 5 mg/kg s.c.	P	P	A
Decerebration[h]	P	P	P
Destruction of spinal cord[h]	P	P	P
Transection of spinal cord[h]	P	P	P
Adrenalectomy[i]	P	P	P

[a] Fearn *et al.* (1965).
[b] Dextran (180 mg/kg) injected intravenously.
[c] Hind paw immersed in water at 45°C for 30 minutes.
[d] Xylol applied to skin of hind paw.
[e] Femoral and sciatic nerves cut 3 weeks before challenge.
[f] P, inflammation present.
[g] A, inflammation absent.
[h] Carried out 3 hours before challenge.
[i] Bilateral adrenalectomy 4 days before challenge.

The view that aspirin acts by inhibiting the nervous mechanisms of fever, pain, and so on is widely held and is stated, for example, in the third edition of "The Pharmacological Basis of Therapeutics," edited by Goodman and Gilman (Woodbury, 1965). Although some of the toxic effects of aspirin may be brought about by a direct action on nerve cells, the view that its therapeutic effects are so mediated is becoming untenable. The evidence against this view has been discussed above, but a few points are worth restating.

With antipyretic doses of aspirin, very little of this drug could be found in the brain (Lim *et al.*, 1967a); but when sodium salicylate was injected into a cerebral ventricle it stimulated respiration and heat production (Cameron, 1968). Furthermore, therapeutic doses of sodium salicylate, injected intravenously, lessened fever induced by endogenous pyrogen prepared from leukocytes, when this was also injected intravenously, but not when the pyrogen was injected into a cerebral ventricle (Cooper *et al.*, 1968). Again, in inhibiting nociceptive responses, aspirin was effective when these were elicited by injection of an irritant substance into the peritoneal cavity or into an artery, but not when the skin was subjected to noxious stimulation (Table V), although the nervous mechanisms in the two responses may be comparable.

The same picture emerges from studies of the effect of aspirin against the bronchoconstrictor responses of the guinea pig to intravenous injection of endogenous substances. Thus, even after destruction of the external nerve supply of the lungs, aspirin blocked the response to bradykinin or SRS-A (Collier *et al.*, 1966). That neither atropine nor propranolol blocked the response to bradykinin or SRS-A, and that aspirin did not stop the lungs responding to acetylcholine, shows that this effect of aspirin is not likely to be due to an influence on autonomic nerve cells. Furthermore, aspirin exhibits some of its antidefensive effects in situations where there are no nerve cells at all, as in preparations of blood platelets or of leukocytes *in vitro*. These and other observations, cited in earlier sections of this review, combine to suggest that, if aspirin acts by inhibiting natural defensive mechanisms, rather than by potentiating a system that controls them, it does so by depressing a humoral process involved, rather than by affecting nerve cells directly.

If aspirin depresses some local humoral process in a natural defensive reaction it may do so in various possible ways. One way would be to interfere with the development of the means to react, such as the synthesis of the precursor of some humoral mediator or the formation of antibody, as certain corticoid and noncorticoid immune suppressants may be supposed to act. Although immune-suppressant drugs of the antimetabolite type inhibited inflammatory responses of limbs and subcutaneous tissue (Page *et al.*, 1962; Rosenthale and Nagra, 1967; Trnavsky, 1967), they differed from aspirin in both profile of activity and time course of action. For example, in profile, 6-mercaptopurine suppressed both allergic encephalomyelitis and adjuvant arthritis in rats, whereas aspirin was only effective against the latter (Rosenthale and Nagra, 1967). In time course, immune-suppressants must be given daily over some days (Page *et al.*, 1962), whereas aspirin and similar drugs need only be given in a single dose near the time of challenge. Thus, sodium salicylate began to lessen fever in man 5 minutes after its intravenous administration (Cranston and Rosendorff, 1968).

Aspirin seems more likely therefore to interfere with the humoral mediation of the defensive reaction, either by directly antagonizing the mediator, by inhibiting its release, or by hastening its destruction. Some effects of aspirin and related drugs upon substances that may mediate defensive reactions, or upon the enzymes that liberate these substances are therefore discussed below.

2. *Amines*

As the clinical efficacy of antihistamine drugs finally established, histamine is involved in some forms or phases of pathologic inflammation. The possibility that salicylates act by antagonizing histamine has been tested in several preparations. In guinea-pig lungs *in vivo*, large intravenous doses of aspirin did not antagonize histamine-induced bronchoconstriction (Collier and Shorley, 1960). On the contrary, in the skin of guinea pig, rat and rabbit, large systemic doses of salicylates detectably lessened the increase in capillary permeability induced by intradermal histamine (Swyer, 1948; Smith and Humphrey, 1949; Spector and Willoughby, 1959; Marks *et al.*, 1961; Starr and West, 1967). When sodium salicylate was mixed directly with histamine, however, and both were injected intradermally in the rabbit or rat, capillary permeability was not reduced (Smith and Humphrey, 1949; Willoughby *et al.*, 1965; Starr and West, 1967), although salicylate effectively reduced permeability when it was injected mixed with kallikrein, globulin permeability factor, or lymph node permeability factor (Willoughby *et al.*, 1965).

Histamine is stored in inactive form in the body, particularly in mast cells, and released from store by noxae. The possibility has therefore been studied whether salicylates act by inhibiting the release of histamine, rather than by directly antagonizing its action on cells. Salicylates inhibited histamine release during anaphylaxis of isolated guinea-pig lung (Trethewie, 1951; Ungar and Damgaard, 1955; Mongar and Schild, 1957), but high concentrations of salicylate were needed. This inhibition, therefore, seems unlikely to account for the antagonism by salicylates of defensive reactions *in vivo*.

Another amine suspected of mediating fever, pain, and inflammation is 5-hydroxytryptamine (5-HT). As with histamine, however, antagonism by salicylates of 5-HT is either absent, weak, or nonspecific. Thus, in guinea-pig lung, *in vivo* or *in vitro*, aspirin antagonized neither bronchoconstriction nor vasoconstriction induced by 5-HT (Collier and Shorley, 1960; Greeff and Moog, 1964). In rat skin, large systemic doses of sodium salicylate lessened the increase of permeability induced by intradermal injection of 5-HT, as they did the like response to histamine (Spector and Willoughby, 1959; Starr and West, 1967). Intradermal injection of salicylate, mixed with 5-HT, lessened, but did not abolish the increase of blood vessel permeability induced by this amine. In the experiments of Winter (1965), aspirin was less effective against the edema of rat foot elicited by 5-HT than against that elicited by six other noxae (Fig. 1). Since aspirin does not appreciably lower normal body temperature, it is unlikely to act as an antipyretic by antagonizing 5-HT in the hypothalamus in those species in which this amine induces fever.

The above findings suggest that, if 5-HT is involved in any of the defensive reactions considered, aspirin is unlikely to act by antagonizing it. That aspirin might inhibit the mechanism by which 5-HT is released remains a possibility about which experimental evidence has not been traced.

A third amine that should be considered is acetylcholine. This is certainly a mediator of the transmission of some nervous messages and might perhaps be involved in eliciting pain after injury. Whereas large doses of aspirin failed to antagonize bronchoconstriction induced by acetylcholine in guinea-pig lungs *in vivo* (Collier and Shorley, 1960), aspirin was more effective against nociception induced by acetylcholine than it was against that induced by bradykinin in the mouse (Collier *et al.*, 1964, 1968a) and probably also in the dog (Guzman *et al.*, 1964).

3. *Peptides*

The evidence is strong that kinins mediate some phase of anaphylactic bronchoconstriction in the guinea pig (Collier and James, 1966, 1967; Collier, 1968) and of edema induced by mild heat in the rat paw (Starr and West, 1967). Experiments cited in previous sections of this review have shown that aspirin antagonizes kinins to extents that vary with the test preparation used, but no preparation in which the antagonism is completely specific has yet come to light.

In guinea-pig lungs, the antagonism by aspirin of chemically induced bronchoconstriction was selective toward a small group of agents, including kinins and SRS-A, leaving others, such as acetylcholine and histamine, unaffected (Collier and Shorley, 1960; Berry and Collier, 1964; Collier *et al.*, 1966). This antagonism was also potent, in that parenteral doses of 1–10 mg/kg were effective, and was of short latency, in that the effect was seen very soon after injecting aspirin intravenously and lasted several hours (Collier, 1963b).

In antagonizing nociceptive responses to bradykinin, aspirin was less selective, less potent, and less quick in onset than it was against bronchoconstriction. In the mouse, aspirin was less effective against nociception induced by intraperitoneal bradykinin than by acetylcholine (Collier *et al.*, 1964, 1966, 1968a) and, in the guinea pig, it was completely ineffective against intradermal bradykinin (Collier and Lee, 1963). Aspirin also failed to suppress nociception elicited by bradykinin in human skin (Lewis, 1963). In the dog, the latency of onset of the inhibition of nociception after intravenous aspirin was about 19 minutes (Guzman *et al.*, 1964).

Salicylates also lessened the duration, but not the intensity, of the hypotension induced by bradykinin (Türker and Kiran, 1964; Vargaftig, 1966; Collier *et al.*, 1968b). Such a curtailment was not seen when hypotension was induced by prostaglandin E_1 (Collier *et al.*, 1968b). In some other effects of kinins, such as the induction of local edema, antagonism by aspirin is weak or absent and selectivity is correspondingly low. In rat skin, for example, sodium salicylate did not inhibit whealing due to bradykinin when both were injected intradermally (Table XIII).

TABLE XIII
ACCUMULATION OF TRYPAN BLUE IN RAT SKIN AFTER INTRADERMAL INJECTION OF VARIOUS PERMEABILITY FACTORS AND ITS INHIBITION BY SODIUM SALICYLATE OR GUINEA-PIG PLASMA[a]

	Inhibitor[b]		
Permeability factor	None	Salicylate (2.5 mg/ml)	Guinea-pig plasma (50%)
Bradykinin	6.2[c]	6.1	0.5
Histamine	6.5	6.3	6.4
5-HT	6.4	3.2	6.1
Substance P	6.4	6.0	5.9
Kallikrein[d]	7.3	1.0	7.1
Globulin PF	7.0	0.5	0.5
Lymph node PF	7.1	1.0	0.5

[a] Willoughby *et al.* (1965).
[b] Inhibitors were injected admixed with permeability factors.
[c] Values are micrograms of trypan blue extracted from skin weals at appropriate times after intradermal injection of permeability factors (PF).
[d] The kallikrein was from saliva.

Substance P is another peptide that may be involved in some defensive reactions. In guinea-pig lungs *in vivo* (Bhoola *et al.*, 1962) and in rat skin (Table XIII) salicylate did not antagonize substance P.

4. *Other Mediators*

The prostaglandins form another group of local hormones that might be involved in some defensive reactions, but their relationship to aspirin remains to be worked out.[1]

Although aspirin does not antagonize, specifically and in most of its actions, any humoral mediator of defensive reactions that has been chemically characterized, the possibility remains that it may so antagonize some humoral factor of uncertain chemical type. The slow-reacting substances form one group of

[1] Although anti-inflammatory acids did not antagonize bronchoconstriction induced by prostaglandin $F_{2\alpha}$ in the guinea pig *in vivo* (Berry and Collier, 1964; G. W. L. James, 1969, *J. Pharm. Pharmacol.* **21**, 379), they were surprisingly effective in antagonizing the contraction of human isolated bronchial muscle induced by that prostaglandin (H. O. J. Collier and W. J. F. Sweatman, 1968, *Nature* **219**, 864).

such factors, and aspirin did antagonize the bronchoconstriction induced by one component of SRS-A in the guinea pig (Berry and Collier, 1964). The biologic effects of this type of SRS-A are rather limited and it has not yet been purified. We therefore do not yet know whether aspirin selectively antagonizes any of its other effects.

Another mediator of unknown structure, whose relationship to aspirin may explain an important therapeutic effect of the drug, is endogenous pyrogen. Recent work suggests that salicylates act by preventing either the release of endogenous pyrogen from leukocytes (Gander *et al.*, 1967) or its entry into the brain (Cooper *et al.*, 1968), but which of these mechanisms is more important is not yet settled.

5. *Enzymes*

An alternative to the possibility that aspirin antagonizes a small molecular mediator of defensive responses is that it inhibits an enzyme concerned in these responses. Many workers have tried to explain the anti-inflammatory effect of aspirin and related drugs as the inhibition of an enzyme concerned in metabolism. These attempts have been reviewed by Smith (1963, 1966c) and by Whitehouse (1965). Whitehouse has supported the suggestion of Adams and Cobb (1958) that the ability of such drugs to uncouple oxidative phosphorylation accounts for their suppression of inflammation; but Smith (1966c) believes that "an uncoupling action may either have no anti-inflammatory significance or merely play a supporting role to other sites of interaction" (p. 223).

If aspirin does indeed inhibit inflammation by uncoupling oxidative phosphorylation, its antipyretic activity must be attributed to a quite different mechanism from the anti-inflammatory. Also, if salicylates act therapeutically by uncoupling oxidative phosphorylation, we would expect 2,4-dinitrophenol to have potent anti-inflammatory and correlated activity, which it does not (Adams and Cobb, 1958; Winder *et al.*, 1958; Marks *et al.*, 1961; Collier *et al.*, 1966; Goldstein *et al.*, 1968). Smith (1963) has suggested, however, that uncoupling is more likely to account for the stimulation of metabolism by high doses of aspirin than for its anti-inflammatory effect.

The mucopolysaccharides of the body include chondroitin sulfate, heparin, hyaluronidate, and keratosulfate. The mucopolysaccharides, which may exist as complexes with peptides, influence the structure, rigidity, and other properties of the supporting tissue of the body. The metabolic turnover of the mucopolysaccharides is fairly fast and is susceptible to hormonal influences. Thus their half-life is prolonged when the thyroid is inhibited with propylthiouracil, and their synthesis is depressed by corticosteroids.

Aspirin (30 μg/ml) and other antirheumatic drugs, including fenamates, indomethacin, phenylbutazone, chloroquine, hydrocortisone, and prednisone, inhibited the synthesis of mucopolysaccharides by cultures of mouse fibroblasts

(Karzel, 1967). Moderate concentrations of sodium salicylate and many other antirheumatic drugs also inhibited the incorporation of radioactive glucose, acetate, or sulfate into the mucopolysaccharide sulfates of ox cartilage slices *in vitro* (Whitehouse, 1962, 1963, 1965). Potency in this respect did not, however, seem to correspond altogether with antirheumatic potency in man. Thus, Kodicek and Loewi (1955) found 2,4-dinitrophenol more effective than aspirin or sodium salicylate, and cortisone ineffective, in inhibiting the incorporation of radioactive sulfur into regenerating tendons of guinea pig *in vitro*. Again, drugs not used as antirheumatics, such as estrogens and chlorpromazine, also inhibited mucopolysaccharide biosynthesis.

In rat rib cartilage *in vivo*, sodium salicylate, phenylbutazone, flufenamic acid, and hydrocortisone inhibited the biosynthesis of mucopolysaccharide sulfate (Boström *et al.*, 1964). In these experiments, drugs, such as flufenamic acid and phenylbutazone, seemed no more potent than sodium salicylate, but 2,4-dinitrophenol seemed to be so. Thus, although sodium salicylate and other antirheumatic drugs inhibit the biosynthesis of mucopolysaccharides, there appears to be little correlation between this effect and therapeutic activity against rheumatism.

The possibility has also been entertained that aspirin acts against inflammation by inhibiting a mechanism by which histamine is formed. Skidmore and Whitehouse (1966) have reported that sodium salicylate or phenylbutazone inhibited a histidine decarboxylase from rat fetus. Another possibility is that aspirin may inhibit the enzyme concerned in the release of a mediator of a defensive reaction. Such an enzyme is kallikrein, which liberates kinins.

Experiments on whether salicylates inhibit kallikrein have given seemingly contradictory results in the hands of different workers; but the contradictions may partly arise through differences in the circumstances of the tests used. Table XIII shows that a high concentration of sodium salicylate inhibited exudation of fluid from blood vessels induced by intradermal injection of human salivary kallikrein in the rat. Intravenous indomethacin (10 mg/kg) had the same effect (Walters and Willoughby, 1965b). Northover and Subramanian (1961b) found that aspirin, sodium salicylate, and related drugs inhibited the hypotensive effect in the dog of diluted human saliva, used as a source of salivary kallikrein. Their figure also shows (although they do not comment on this) that salicylate lessens the duration, but not the intensity, of the hypotensive response to bradykinin in the dog, as Vargaftig (1966) later demonstrated in the rabbit. Northover and Subramanian (1961b) reported that aspirin and related drugs also delayed the onset of exudation induced by intradermal injection of human salivary kallikrein in the rabbit, but Lewis (1963) was unable to obtain such an effect of aspirin.

Northover and Subramanian (1961b) also claimed that kallikrein was inhibited by incubation with salicylates *in vitro*. Other authors (Lewis, 1963;

Hebborn and Shaw, 1963; Davies *et al.*, 1966) were unable to confirm that moderate concentrations of salicylates inhibit kallidin formation by kallikrein *in vitro*. The balance of evidence at present therefore seems to indicate that large doses of salicylates may inhibit some effects of salivary kallikrein *in vivo*, but that this inhibition is slight or absent *in vitro*.

Instead of inhibiting the enzymatic action of kallikrein, aspirin might conceivably act by preventing the formation of this enzyme or of its substrate (kininogen) or by potentiating a peptidase that destroys kinins. Smith (1966c) has discussed these possibilities, but no experimental evidence as yet exists to support or to oppose them. The question of whether aspirin potentiates natural inhibitors of kallikrein will be discussed below.

Yet another enzyme that may be involved in inflammation is the lymph node permeability factor (LNPF) of Willoughby *et al.* (1962). This factor has been extracted from lymph nodes and many other mammalian tissues. Injected intradermally, it induced exudation of fluid and emigration of leukocytes from blood vessels and the deposition of fibrinoid (Willoughby and Spector, 1964; Walters and Willoughby, 1965a). LNPF has been distinguished by pharmacologic tests from other suspected mediators of inflammation (Willoughby *et al.*, 1963; Willoughby and Walters, 1965).

Table XIII shows that a high concentration of sodium salicylate inhibited exudation induced by intradermal LNPF in the rat. Indomethacin (10 mg/kg intravenously) also inhibited the exudation, but reduced neither the leukocyte emigration nor the deposition of fibrinoid induced by LNPF (Walters and Willoughby, 1965b). Thus, as with nociception and with the responses of smooth muscles, antipyretic drugs may inhibit one, but not another, response to the same endogenous substance.

Hyaluronidase is another enzyme that has been proposed as the target of salicylate inhibition. Smith (1953, 1966c) has reviewed the reasons why the mechanism of action of aspirin cannot be interpreted as an inhibition of hyaluronidase.

Glucocorticoids and chloroquine have been supposed to inhibit inflammation by stabilizing lysosomes and thus preventing the release of enzymes inducing inflammation. Drugs of the aspirin group, however, do not seem to stabilize lysosomes (Weissmann, 1964).

6. *Conclusions*

Although we cannot be sure that aspirin acts by depressing at some point or points the mechanisms of defensive responses, rather than by potentiating their natural inhibitors, aspirin does block several endogenous substances suspected of mediating the responses it antagonizes. Exactly how this occurs we do not yet know; but everywhere the same picture emerges. Aspirin antagonizes one effect of an endogenous substance, but not another effect. Likewise it antagonizes a few such substances, but it does not antagonize others. In different responses, the pattern of selectivity of aspirin toward a range of substances differs. Such findings have led to the suggestion that "aspirin and like-acting drugs block a route leading to or from the specific receptors for the agonists rather than blocking those receptors themselves" (Collier *et al.*, 1966).

Quastel (1963) has expressed an alternative point of view in these words "The potent effects of salicylates in changing the rates of transport of substances in and out of cells, brought about primarily by diminution of cell ATP, may be directly associated with some of its therapeutic effects." The connection with ATP is particularly interesting, because aspirin was later found to block bronchoconstriction induced by ATP in the guinea pig, and, moreover, tachyphylaxis of this preparation induced to ATP also produced insensitivity to SRS-A (Collier *et al.*, 1966).

What might be the nature of the route blocked by aspirin? One possibility would seem to be that, in situations where they are inhibited by aspirin, humoral mediators require an intermediate mechanism to enable them to reach their target, and that this mechanism is inhibited by aspirin. Such a mechanism might be envisaged as one transferring mediators across cellular or other boundaries; alternatively the release of an intermediary substance might be susceptible to aspirin blockade.[1] Since bradykinin elicits a response from bronchial muscle within 6 seconds of intravenous injection and since aspirin blocks this effect if injected just before the bradykinin, both the intermediate mechanism and its blockade would have to act rapidly, at least in some situations. That aspirin was ineffective when injected after the bradykinin suggests that it might act at an early stage of the intermediate mechanism.

B. Potentiation of Natural Inhibitory Mechanisms

An alternative to the proposition that aspirin acts by depressing a humoral mechanism mediating a defensive response is that it acts by potentiating a natural inhibitory mechanism of such responses. Various mechanisms that moderate defensive responses are well known, although how they are mediated or the relative contribution of humoral or nervous factors to their performance may not be fully understood.

Many observations have shown that central nervous processes can counteract pain (Beecher, 1957; Gardner *et al.*, 1960; Lim, 1966). To what extent other defensive reactions are susceptible to central inhibition is unknown; but in so far as release of glucocorticoids or of catecholamines can be activated by

[1] P. J. Piper and J. R. Vane (1969, *Nature* **223**, 29) have recently reported that bradykinin, SRS-A or antigen released from guinea pig isolated lungs an unidentified bronchoconstrictor substance and that this release was blocked by aspirin, mefenamate, or indomethacin.

nerves, other defensive reactions are also likely to be modifiable by the central nervous system. The reasons for thinking that aspirin does not depress defensive reactions by an effect on nerve cells apply also against the possibility that it might potentiate inhibitory mechanisms in such a way.

1. *Counterirritation*

Another mechanism known to inhibit defensive reactions is counter-irritation. Table XIV illustrates the efficacy of hydrocortisone, noradrenaline, and counterirritants to lessen the edema of rat paw induced by several noxae. For reference, indomethacin and oxyphenbutazone have also been used.

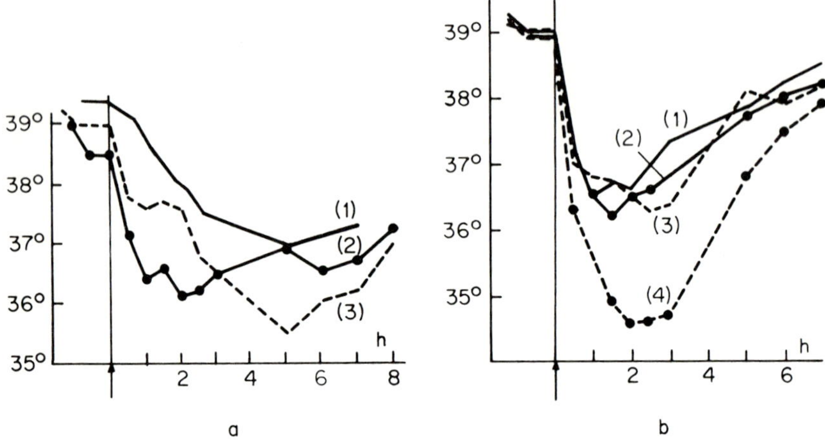

FIG. 3. Antipyretic effect of counterirritants in the rat. Fever was induced with yeast; test materials were injected intraperitoneally. A: (1) 100 mg/kg of phenylbutazone; (2) 40 mg/kg of sodium hydroxide; (3) 200 mg/kg of hydrogen peroxide. B: (1) 100 and (2) 200 mg/kg of kaolin; (3) 100 and (4) 200 mg/kg of talc. (Büch and Wagner-Jauregg, 1960.)

In situations in which it has been tested experimentally, application of a chemical irritant may reduce fever, nociception, or inflammation. In the instance of fever, Büch and Wagner-Jauregg (1960) found that hydrogen peroxide, caustic soda, talc, or kaolin, injected intraperitoneally, lowered fever induced by yeast in the rat (Fig. 3). In the instance of nociception, Winter and Flataker (1965) found that formalin injected into a foot or phenylquinone injected intraperitoneally, raised the threshold tail pressure needed to elicit a squeak from the rat. Again, Hitchens *et al.* (1967) reported that kaolin, formalin, or croton oil inhibited nociception both in the mouse and rat. In the instance of inflammation, intraperitoneal injection of acetic acid or formalin reduced the edema of the rat foot elicited by subplantar injection of carrageenin, compound 48/80, dextran, 5-hydroxytryptamine, kaolin, or yeast

TABLE XIV

COUNTERACTION BY INDOMETHACIN, OXYPHENBUTAZONE, HYDROCORTISONE, NORADRENALINE, OR ACETIC ACID OF FOOT EDEMA INDUCED BY VARIOUS NOXAE IN THE RAT[a]

Noxa	Indomethacin (10 mg p.o.)[b]	Oxyphenbutazone (100 mg p.o.)	Noradrenaline (1 mg s.c.)	Hydrocortisone (15 mg p.o.)	Acetic acid, 0.6% (10 ml i.p.)	
					Intact	Adrenalectomized[c]
Carrageenin	142[d]	65	14 (N.S.)[e]	60	82	76
Yeast	27	49	46	30	46	55
Kaolin	105	48	45	34 (N.S.)	50	—
Dextran	94	47 (N.S.)	68	42	100	62
Compound 48/80	92	52	94	43	77	50
5-HT	59	8 (N.S.)	+2 (N.S.)	66	45	48

[a] Garattini *et al.* (1965).

[b] Doses are per kilogram; routes of administration are abbreviated as in Table I.

[c] Rats were adrenalectomized 3 days before challenge.

[d] Results are expressed as the sums of the percentage inhibition of the edema, compared with controls, at three different times, between 0.5 and 6 hours, after challenge.

[e] N.S., not significant.

(Table XIV). Conversely, injection of silver nitrate into a foot joint of the rat lessened the volume of exudate induced by injecting an irritant into the pleural cavity (Laden *et al.*, 1958). Counterirritation may be effective quite quickly, as when intraperitoneal injection of 5-hydroxytryptamine inhibited the swelling of the rat foot induced by simultaneous injection of bradykinin, which reached a peak within 30 minutes (Horáková and Muratová, 1965).

Noxae are effective as counterirritants to different degrees according to the route by which they are given. Thus Benitz and Hall (1963) failed to inhibit with oral carrageenin or diatomaceous earth, inflammation induced in rats by subcutaneous injection of the same substance, although intraperitoneal injection of either irritant exerted a clear counterirritant effect. Some noxae, however, are effective by mouth as well as by other routes. For instance, croton oil inhibited inflammatory or nociceptive responses in the rat or mouse when given by the oral, intraperitoneal, or subcutaneous routes (Goldstein *et al.*, 1967; Hitchens *et al.*, 1967).

Various workers have investigated whether adrenalectomy, hypophysectomy, or cutting the sciatic nerve eliminates counterirritant inhibition of inflammatory responses. In no experiment in which these procedures have been tested did they abolish the counterirritant effect (Laden *et al.*, 1958; Garattini *et al.*, 1965; Horáková and Muratová, 1965; Goldstein *et al.*, 1967). That counterirritant inhibition of inflammation can be due to a humoral factor is suggested by the experiments of Goldstein *et al.* (1967), who showed that counterirritant suppression of inflammation in one rat is echoed in a parabiotic with linked circulation. In parabiotic rats, however, counterirritant suppression of a nociceptive response in one animal was not echoed in the other member of the pair (Hitchens *et al.*, 1967).

There is little evidence about the relationship between salicylates and counterirritation, but what evidence there is suggests that they antagonize rather than reinforce one another. Thus, in the experiments of Bowman *et al.* (1961), the swelling of one foot induced by injection of silver nitrate into the ankle joint of a rat was lessened by injecting the same noxa into the opposite ankle 15 hours previously. If sodium salicylate was given before silver nitrate, it lessened the swelling of the ankle, but it abolished the inhibitory effect of that silver nitrate injection upon a second injection 15 hours later into the other ankle. Although this experiment implies that salicylates do not act by potentiating counterirritation, salicylates might themselves be sufficiently irritant to exert some effect of this type. This seems unlikely, however, because aspirin, injected along with an irritant into the peritoneal cavity of the mouse, reduced the incidence of nociceptive responses (Collier *et al.*, 1968a).

2. *Adrenocortical Mechanisms*

An alternative to the proposition that aspirin acts by eliciting or potentiating counterirritation is that it potentiates corticosteroid mechanisms. There are two good reasons for rejecting corticosteroid potentiation as a major factor in aspirin action. First, in the absence of pituitary or adrenal glands, aspirin or other antipyretic drugs can effectively suppress several induced defensive responses. Second, the pattern of the inhibitory activity of aspirin toward a variety of induced responses is quite different from that of glucocorticoids. For example, in the guinea pig, aspirin antagonizes skin erythema induced by UV-radiation or bronchoconstriction induced by bradykinin, but glucocorticoids do not. Again, in this species, glucocorticoids inhibit the tuberculin reaction, but salicylates do not. Other differences between salicylates and corticoids are also apparent. For example, salicylates increase the rate of metabolism, but corticoids do not (Smith, 1966b). Again, cortisone increases and salicylate decreases deposits of glycogen in the liver (Hailman, 1952; Smith, 1966a), and salicylates even antagonize steroid-induced glycogen deposition (Smith, 1952; Winters and Morrill, 1955). Although many effects of salicylates and glucocorticoids are similar, the above list of exceptions could be lengthened.

3. *Catecholamines*

Catecholamines form a third kind of natural inhibitor of induced responses of the type antagonized by aspirin. The extent to which liberation of catecholamines might contribute to the antiphlogistic effects of aspirin should be further explored since, as already discussed, adrenalectomy has sometimes been found to reduce some of these effects. Supporting such exploration is the report of Smith (1955) that adrenal demedullation lessened and total adrenalectomy reversed the hyperglycemic response to sodium salicylate in rats.[1]

In the instance of bradykinin-induced bronchoconstriction, the contribution of a release of catecholamines elicited by aspirin must be negligible, since aspirin was effective after adrenalectomy or β-adrenergic receptor blockade with pronethalol (Collier *et al.*, 1965). Moreover, adrenaline inhibited the bronchoconstrictor response to histamine, but aspirin did not (Collier *et al.*, 1960). The question whether catecholamine release by aspirin plays a part in its antinociceptive or anti-inflammatory activity might best be answered by determining the effect of adrenergic blockade upon the activity of aspirin.

In some species, such as the cat (Feldberg and Myers, 1963; Feldberg, 1965), adrenaline, injected into a cerebral ventricle, lowered body temperature. Aspirin might therefore be thought to act as an antipyretic by potentiating the effect of noradrenaline in the hypothalamus. This seems unlikely for two

[1] L. Riesterer and R. Jaques (1969, *Helv. Physiol. Pharmacol. Acta* **26**, 287) have recently reported that drugs blocking β-receptors for adrenaline impaired the ability of sodium salicylate to lessen pleurisy induced by turpentine in the rat; but, their potency in this effect did not parallel that in blockading β-receptors.

reasons: First, aspirin does not appreciably lower normal body temperature; and second, in the rabbit, in which aspirin is as effective as in the cat (Table I), intraventricular noradrenaline did not raise, but lowered body temperature (Cooper *et al.*, 1965).

Some of the above observations suggest that salicylates probably do not act by releasing catecholamines. The finding that aspirin and catecholamines can have opposite effects, for example, on the level of free fatty acids in the plasma (Bizzi *et al.*, 1965), strengthens this suggestion.

4. *Enzyme inhibitors*

We have considered some of the systemic mechanisms by which defensive reactions are naturally restrained; but there remain also some other controlling factors that might be involved. For example, mammalian serum contains two α-globulins that are specific inhibitors of the enzyme kallikrein (Trautschold *et al.*, 1966). The possibility therefore exists that aspirin or related drugs liberate from store or otherwise activate an inhibitor of kallikrein or of some other factor that mediates one or more defensive reactions.

Table XIII compares the effects of sodium salicylate with those of an inhibitor present in guinea-pig plasma upon several endogenous factors that may mediate inflammation. This table, from the paper of Willoughby *et al.* (1965), shows that sodium salicylate and the plasma inhibitor had slightly different patterns of activity. Although the possibility remains open that aspirin antagonizes induced responses by potentiating a natural enzyme inhibitor, the evidence for this is not convincing.

5. *Conclusion*

Although many efforts have been made to show that aspirin inhibits defensive reactions by influencing nerve cells or by potentiating the natural mechanisms that moderate such reactions, the balance of evidence now lies in favor of the view that aspirin acts mainly by interfering with one or more of the humoral mechanisms that mediate defensive reactions.

C. General Conclusions

When Gross and Greenberg (1948) published their critical bibliographic review of the salicylates, they cited more than four thousand references. The modern successor of this book, with the same title (Smith and Smith, 1966), cites only about one quarter of that number of references. Nonetheless, by now the total of original publications on aspirin and other salicylates probably runs into five figures. This review has tried to discern and discuss some threads, running through these observations and making a coherent pattern in the biologic effects of aspirin. In attempting this, the chapter expands a view, advanced some years ago (Collier, 1963a), that aspirin may be characterized as an antidefensive drug, and that its main therapeutic value derives from its ability to counteract such defensive reactions as fever, pain, and the inflammatory responses of blood vessels, when these become excessive. Not only the therapeutic, but some of the main toxic effects of aspirin—such as its ability to prolong bleeding and to damage gastric epithelium—might be included in the anti-defensive category.

In the last analysis, the antagonism by aspirin of defensive reactions may be attributable to a direct action upon macromolecules that operate one or more important biochemical processes. Such a macromolecule could be the receptor site of the carrier for a small mediator molecule or it could be some enzyme involved in defensive processes. No such macromolecule has yet been identified, although, in the opinion of the author of this review, the most likely candidate is a hypothetical macromolecule concerned in the transport of certain messenger substances (of which kinin may be one) between their sites of liberation and of taking effect. Attempts to account for the main therapeutic effects of aspirin through the inhibition of enzymes have succeeded, however, in explaining some of its unwanted effects such as the increased consumption of oxygen, with resulting fever and acidosis (Smith, 1963).

The slow progress of our understanding of the mode of therapeutic action of aspirin calls attention to a paradox in its pharmacology that must be faced if further advances are to be made. The paradox is that, according to the dosage, the state of the biologic preparation, and possibly other circumstances, aspirin may have opposite effects. Thus, in fever, it is antipyretic, yet aspirin intoxication sometimes produces fever. In gout, aspirin is uricosuric; but in normal animals it may have the opposite effect (Gutman, 1966). In diabetes of man or animals, aspirin is hypoglycemic; yet in normal animals large doses can be hyperglycemic (Gross and Greenberg, 1948; Ingle, 1950; Bornstein *et al.*, 1952; Ingle and Meeks, 1952; Smith, 1966a). In rare cases of asthma, aspirin has a beneficial effect; yet it can induce a severe asthmatic attack in sensitive individuals (Cook, 1947; Pearson, 1963).

A part of this paradox resides in the fact that the toxic effects of high doses of aspirin may be very different from, and even opposite to, the therapeutic effects of lower doses. To explain what remains of the paradox, we might suppose that, in disease, a process (or processes) is set in motion, upon which some of the symptoms depend, and that aspirin readily affects this process. Whether or not this process is operating, aspirin may also be supposed to act directly in other ways on healthy tissues. If this line of approach is correct, a clue to the mode of therapeutic action of aspirin should continue to be sought, not in normal animals or their parts, but in those in an injured or unhealthy state, where the process with which aspirin may be supposed to interfere is in operation.

Explaining the mechanism by which a drug acts is a continuing process, in which understanding becomes better as a succession of questions is answered. To characterize aspirin as an antidefensive drug gives some insight into its therapeutic activity. To conclude that it exerts these antidefensive effects locally, rather than through an influence on the central or autonomic nervous system, or on the pituitary or adrenal glands, adds further to our understanding. To say that aspirin antagonizes some humoral mediators that induce defensive responses adds something more. To conclude that aspirin does not block these mediators as antihistamines block histamine, by a receptor antagonism, but rather that it inhibits some underlying mechanism coming between the mediator and its effect, is to increase our understanding by another step. To demonstrate what mechanism aspirin inhibits, and how it affects this inhibition, would bring us to a new level of insight into its mode of action.

REFERENCES

Aarsen, P. N. (1966). *Brit. J. Pharmacol.* **27**, 196.

Adams, S. S. (1960). *J. Pharm. Pharmacol.* **12**, 251.

Adams, S. S., and Cobb, R. (1958). *Nature* **181**, 773.

Adams, S. S., and Cobb, R. (1963). *In* "Salicylates: An International Symposium" (A. St. J. Dixon, B. K. Martin, M. J. H. Smith, and P. H. N. Wood, eds.), p. 127. Churchill, London.

Anderson, K. W. (1963). *In* "Salicylates: An International Symposium" (A. St. J. Dixon, B. K. Martin, M. J. H. Smith, and P. H. N. Wood, eds.), p. 217. Churchill, London.

Anderson, K. W. (1964a). *Arch. Intern. Pharmacodyn.* **152**, 379.

Anderson, K. W. (1964b). *Arch. Intern. Pharmacodyn.* **152**, 392.

Andersson, B., Jobin, M., and Olsson, K. (1966). *Acta Physiol. scand.* **67**, 50.

Antweiler, H. (1957). *Klin. Wochschr.* **35**, 1087.

Armitage, P., Herxheimer, H., and Rosa, L. (1952). *Brit. J. Pharmacol.* **7**, 625.

Atkins, E. (1960). *Physiol. Rev.* **40**, 580.

Austen, F. K., Rubini, M. E., Meroney, W. H., and Wolff, J. (1958). *J. Clin. Invest.* **37**, 1131.

Bacchus, H., and Bacchus, A. (1953). *Federation Proc.* **12**, 7.

Balme, H. W. (1967). *Practitioner* **198**, 769

Barbour, H. G. (1919). *Arch. Internal Med.* **24**, 624.

Barbour, H. G., and Dickerson, V. C. (1938). *Arch. Intern. Pharmacodyn.* **58**, 78.

Batterman, R. C., and Grossman, A. J. (1955). *J. Am. Med. Assoc.* **159**, 1619.

Bavin, E. M., Macrae, F. J., Seymour, D. E., and Waterhouse, P. D. (1952). *J. Pharm. Pharmacol.* **4**, 872.

Beaumont, J. L., Willie, A., and Lenègre, J. (1955). *Bull. Soc. Med. Hop. Paris* **71**, 1077.

Beecher, H. K. (1957). *Pharmacol. Rev.* **9**, 59.

Beecher, H. K., Keats, A. S., Mosteller, F., and Lasagna, L. (1953). *J. Pharmacol. Exptl. Therap.* **109**, 393.

Benitz, K.-F. and Hall, L. M. (1963). *Arch. Intern. Pharmacodyn.* **144**, 185.

Benjamin, F. B. (1958). *Science* **128**, 303.

Bennett, I. L., and Beeson, P. B. (1953a). *J. Exptl. Med.* **98**, 477.

Bennett, I. L., and Beeson, P. B. (1953b). *J. Exptl. Med.* **98**, 493.

Berry, P. A. (1966). Ph.D. Thesis, Council for National Academic Awards, London.
Berry, P. A., and Collier, H. O. J. (1964). *Brit. J. Pharmacol.* **23**, 201.
Bertagnini, C. (1856). *Ann. Chem. Liebigs* **97**, 248.
Bhoola, K. D., Collier, H. O. J., Schachter, M., and Shorley, P. G. (1962). *Brit. J. Pharmacol.* **19**, 190.
Bianchi, C., Lumachi, B., and Pegrassi, L. (1967). *Arzneimittel-Forsch.* **17**, 246.
Bizzi, A., Garattini, S., and Veneroni, E. (1965). *Brit. J. Pharmacol.* **25**, 187.
Blane, G. F. (1967). *J. Pharm. Pharmacol.* **19**, 367.
Bligh, J. (1966). *J. Physiol.* (*London*) **185**, 46P.
Boardman, P. L., and Hart, F. D. (1967). *Brit. Med. J.* **4**, 264.
Bodammer, G. (1968). *Arch. Exptl. Pathol. Pharmakol.* **260**, 16.
Bondi, S., and Katz, H. (1911). *Z. Klin. Med.* **72**, 177.
Bonnycastle, D. D., and Leonard, C. S. (1950). *J. Pharmacol. Exptl. Therap.* **100**, 141.
Bornstein, J., Meade, B. W., and Smith, M. J. H. (1952). *Nature* **169**, 115.
Boström, H., Berntsen, K., and Whitehouse, M. W. (1964). *Biochem. Pharmacol.* **13**, 413.
Bowman, D. C., Doemling, D. B., and Harris, S. C. (1961). *Proc. Soc. Exptl. Biol. Med.* **108**, 432.
British Pharmaceutical Codex (1963). p. 610. Pharmaceutical Press, London.
Brittain, R. T., and Spencer, P. S. J. (1965). *J. Pharm. Pharmcol.* **17**, 389.
Brocklehurst, W. E. (1956). *In* "Histamine" (G. E. W. Wolstenholme and C. M. O'Connor, eds.), p. 175. Churchill, London.
Brocklehurst, W. E. (1960). *J. Physiol.* (*London*) **151**, 416.
Brocklehurst, W. E., and Lahiri, S. C. (1962). *J. Physiol.* (*London*) **160**, 15P.
Brocklehurst, W. E., and Lahiri, S. C. (1963). *J. Physiol.* (*London*) **165**, 39P.
Brodie, B. B. (1965). *Proc. Roy. Soc. Med.* **58**, 946.
Brown, D. M., and Robson, R. D. (1964). *Nature* **202**, 812.
Brownlee, G. (1937). *Quart. J. Pharm. Pharmacol.* **10**, 609.
Brownlee, G., and Gaddum, J. H. (1939). *Quart. J. Pharm. Pharmacol.* **12**, 45.
Brun, C., Olsen, S. T., Raeschou, F., and Sørensen, A. W. S. (1965). *Nephron* **2**, 65.
Büch, O., and Wagner-Jauregg, T. (1960). *Arzneimittel-Forsch.* **10**, 834.
Buller, R. H., Miya, T. S., and Carr, C. J. (1957). *J. Pharm. Pharmacol.* **9**, 128.
Buss, C. E. (1875). *Zentr. Med. Wiss.* **13**, 276.
Cameron, I. R. (1968). *Brit. J. Pharmacol.* **32**, 438P.
Campbell, B. (1948). *Science* **108**, 478.
Caravati, C. M., and Cosgrove, E. F. (1946). *Ann. Internal Med.* **24**, 638.
Carlson, L. A., and Östman, J. (1961). *Metab. Clin. Exptl.* **10**, 781.
Carpi, A., Klupp, H., and Konzett, H. (1962). *Arch. Exptl. Pathol. Pharmakol.* **243**, 356.
Chistoni, A., and Lapresa, F. (1909). *Arch. Farmacol. Sper.* **8**, 63.
Clausen, E. (1964). *Lancet* **ii**, 123.
Clausen, E., and Pederson, J. (1961). *Acta Med. Scand.* **170**, 631.
Climenko, D. R. (1936). *Proc. Soc. Exptl. Biol. Med.* **34**, 807.
Coffman, J. D. (1964). *Federation Proc.* **23**, 252.
Collier, H. O. J. (1962). *Biochem. Pharmacol.* **10**, 47.
Collier, H. O. J. (1963a). *Sci. Am.* **209**, 96.
Collier, H. O. J. (1963b). *In* "Salicylates: An International Symposium" (A. St. J. Dixon, B. K. Martin, M. J. H. Smith, and P. H. N. Wood, eds.), p. 120. Churchill, London.
Collier, H. O. J. (1964). *In* "Evaluation of Drug Activities: Pharmacometrics" (D. R. Laurence, and A. L. Bacharach, eds.), Vol. 1, p. 183. Academic Press, New York.
Collier, H. O. J. (1965). *In* "Non-Steroidal Anti-Inflammatory Drugs" (S. Garattini, and M. N. G. Dukes, eds.), p. 139. Excerpta Med. Found., Amsterdam.

Collier, H. O. J. (1968). *Sci. Basis Med., Ann. Rev.* p. 308.
Collier, H. O. J., and Chesher, G. B. (1956). *Brit. J. Pharmacol.* **11**, 20.
Collier, H. O. J., and James, G. W. L. (1966). *J. Physiol.* (*London*) **185**, 71P.
Collier, H. O. J., and James, G. W. L. (1967). *Brit. J. Pharmacol.* **30**, 283.
Collier, H. O. J., and Lee, I. R. (1963). *Brit. J. Pharmacol.* **21**, 155.
Collier, H. O. J., and Shorley, P. G. (1960). *Brit. J. Pharmacol.* **15**, 601.
Collier, H. O. J., and Shorley, P. G. (1963). *Brit. J. Pharmacol.* **20**, 345.
Collier, H. O. J., Holgate, J. A., Schachter, M., and Shorley, P. G. (1959). *J. Physiol.* (*London*) **149**, 54P.
Collier, H. O. J., Holgate, J. A., Schachter, M., and Shorley, P.G. (1960). *Brit. J. Pharmacol.* **15**, 290.
Collier, H. O. J., Warner, B. T., and Skerry, R. J. (1961). *Brit. J. Pharmacol.* **17**, 28.
Collier, H. O. J., Hammond, A. R., and Whiteley, B. (1963). *Nature* **200**, 176.
Collier, H. O. J., Hammond, A. R., Horwood-Barrett, S., and Schneider, C. (1964). *Nature* **204**, 1316.
Collier, H. O. J., James, G. W. L., and Piper, P. J. (1965). *J. Physiol.* (*London*) **180**, 13P.
Collier, H. O. J., James, G. W. L., and Schneider, C. (1966). *Nature* **212**, 411.
Collier, H. O. J., Dinneen, L. C., Johnson, C. A., and Schneider, C. (1968a). *Brit. J. Pharmacol.* **32**, 295.
Collier, H. O. J., Dinneen, L. C., Perkins, A. C., and Piper, P. J. (1968b). *Arch. Exptl. Pathol. Pharmakol.* **259**, 159.
Comby, M. (1900). *Bull. Soc. Med. Hop. Paris, 3rd Ser.* **17**, 997.
Cook, R. A. (1947). "Allergy in Theory and Practice", p. 161. Saunders, Philadelphia, Pennsylvania.
Cooper, K. E. (1965). *Proc. Roy. Soc. Med.* **58**, 740.
Cooper, K. E., Cranston, W. I., and Honour, A. J. (1965). *J. Physiol.* (*London*) **181**, 852.
Cooper, K. E., Cranston, W. I., and Honour, A. J. (1967). *J. Physiol.* (*London*) **191**, 325.
Cooper, K. E., Grundman, M. J., and Honour, A. J. (1968). *J. Physiol.* (*London*) **196**, 56P.
Courvoisier, S., Fournel, J., Ducrot, R., Kolsky, M., and Koetschet, P. (1953). *Arch. Intern. Pharmacodyn.* **92**, 305.
Crampton, R. S., Black, W. C., Verdesca, A. S., Nedeljkovic, R. I., and Hilton, J. G. (1962). *Nature* **194**, 295.
Cranston, W. I., and Rosendorff, C. (1968). *Brit. J. Pharmacol.* **32**, 436P.
Croft, D. N. (1966). *J. Pharm. Pharmacol.* **18**, 354.
Croft, D. N., and Wood, P. H. N. (1967). *Brit. Med. J.* **i**, 137.
Dautrebande, L. (1963). *In* "The Regulation of Human Respiration" (D. J. C. Cunningham, and B. B. Lloyd, eds.), p. 143. Blackwell, Oxford.
Davies, G. W., Holman, G., Johnston, T. P., and Lowe, J. S. (1966). *Brit. J. Pharmacol.* **28**, 212.
Decourt, P., Brunaud, M., and Brunaud, S. (1953). *Compt. Rend. Soc. Biol.* **147**, 1605.
Deffenu, G., Pegrassi, L., and Lumachi, B. (1966). *J. Pharm. Pharmacol.* **18**, 135.
Deneau, G. H., Waud, R. A., and Gowdey, C. W. (1953). *Can. J. Med. Sci.* **31**, 387.
Dickerson, G. D., Engle, R. J., Guzman, F., Rodgers, D. W., and Lim, R. K. S. (1965). *Federation Proc.* **24**, 677.
Dodd, K., Minot, A. S., and Arena, J. M. (1937). *Am. J. Diseases Children* **53**, 1435.
Domenjoz, R. (1955). *Arch. Exptl. Pathol. Pharmakol.* **225**, 14.
Domenjoz, R. (1960). *Ann. N.Y. Acad. Sci.* **86**, 263.
Domenjoz, R. (1966a). *Advan. Pharmacol.* **4**, 143.
Domenjoz, R. (1966b). *Med. Pharmacol. Exptl.* **14**, 321.

Domenjoz, R., and Morsdorf, K. (1965). *In* "Non-steroidal Anti-inflammatory Drugs" (S. Garattini, and M. N. G. Dukes, eds.), p. 162. Excerpta Med. Found., Amsterdam.

Domenjoz, R., Morsdorf, K., Stenger, E. G., and Theobald, W. (1957). *Arch. Exptl. Pathol. Pharmakol.* **230**, 325.

Douthwaite, A. H., and Lintott, G. A. M. (1938). *Lancet* **ii**, 1222.

Dreser, H. (1899). *Arch. Ges. Physiol. Pfluegers* **76**, 306.

Ebstein, W. (1876). *Berlin. Klin. Wochschr.* **13**, 337.

Emele, J. F., and Shanaman, J. (1963). *Proc. Soc. Exptl. Biol. Med.* **114**, 680.

Erdös, E. G., Hinshaw, L. B., and Gill, C. C. (1967). *Proc. Soc. Exptl. Biol. Med.* **125**, 916.

Evans, E. I., and Butterfield, W. J. H. (1951). *Ann. Surg.* **134**, 588.

Evans, G., Packham, M. A., Nishizawa, E. E., and Mustard, J. F. (1967). *J. Clin. Invest.* **46**, 1053.

Fearn, H. J., Karady, S., and West, G. B. (1965). *J. Pharm. Pharmacol.* **17**, 761.

Feldberg, W. (1965). *Proc. Roy. Soc. Med.* **58**, 395.

Feldberg, W., and Lotti, V. J. (1967). *Brit. J. Pharmacol.* **31**, 152.

Feldberg, W., and Myers, R. D. (1963). *Nature* **200**, 1325.

Feldberg, W., and Myers, R. D. (1964). *J. Physiol.* (*London*) **173**, 226.

Feldberg, W., and Myers, R. D. (1965). *J. Physiol.* (*London*) **177**, 239.

Feldberg, W., Hellon, R. F., and Myers, R. D. (1966). *J. Physiol.* (*London*) **186**, 410.

Feldberg, W., Hellon, R. F., and Lotti, V. J. (1967). *J. Physiol.* (*London*) **191**, 501.

Fessler, J. H., Cooper, K. E., Cranston, W. I., and Vollum, R. L. (1961). *J. Exptl. Med.* **113**, 1127.

Field, J. B. (1945). *Am. J. Physiol.* **143**, 238.

Findlay, J. D., and Robertshaw, D. (1967). *J. Physiol.* (*London*) **189**, 329.

Fischer, E. (1905). *Arch. Intern. Laryngol.* **20**, 136.

Floersheim, G. L. (1965). *In* "Non-steroidal Anti-inflammatory Drugs" (S. Garattini, and M. N. G. Dukes, eds.), p. 232. Excerpta Med. Found., Amsterdam.

Fürbringer, P. (1875). *Zentr. Med. Wiss.* **18**, 273.

Gander, G. W., Chaffee, J., and Goodale, F. (1967). *Proc. Soc. Exptl. Biol. Med.* **126**, 205.

Garattini, S., and Dukes, M. N. G., eds. (1965). "Non-steroidal Anti-inflammatory Drugs". Excerpta Med. Found., Amsterdam.

Garattini, S., Jori, A., Bernardi, D., Carrara, C., Paglialunga, S., and Segre, D. (1965). *In* "Non-steroidal Anti-inflammatory Drugs" (S. Garattini and M. N. G. Dukes, eds.), p. 151. Excerpta Med. Found., Amsterdam.

Gardner, W. J., Licklider, J. C. R., and Weisz, A. Z. (1960). *Science* **132**, 32.

Gast, L. F. (1964). *Ann. Rheumatic. Diseases* **23**, 500.

Geschikter, C. F., O'Malley, W. E., and Roubacky, E. P. (1960). *Am. J. Clin. Pathol.* **34**, 1.

Gibson, R. D., Miya, T. S., and Edwards, L. D. (1955). *J. Am. Pharm. Assoc. Sci. Ed.* **44**, 605.

Gilfoil, T. M., Klavins, I., and Grumbach, L. (1963). *J. Pharmacol. Exptl. Therap.* **142**, 1.

Gilfoil, T. M., Klavins, I., and Dunn, J. T. (1964). *Federation Proc.* **23**, 285.

Gjuris, V., Heicke, B., and Westermann, E. (1964a). *Arch. Exptl. Pathol. Pharmakol.* **247**, 429.

Gjuris, V., Heicke, B., and Westermann, E. (1964b). *Arch. Exptl. Pathol. Pharmakol.* **248**, 540.

Goldstein, S., Demeo, R., and Shemano, I. (1968). *Proc. Soc. Exptl. Biol. Med.* **128**, 980.

Goldstein, S., Shemano, I., Demeo, R., and Beiller, J. M. (1967). *Arch. Intern. Pharmacodyn.* **167**, 39.

Goulston, K., and Skyring, A. (1964). *Gut* **5**, 463.

Grant, R., and Whalen, W. J. (1953). *Am. J. Physiol.* **173**, 47.

Greeff, K., and Moog, E. (1964). *Arch. Exptl. Pathol. Pharmakol.* **248**, 204.
Gregerson, J. P. (1916). *Ugeskrift Laeger* **78**, 697; *J. Am. Med. Ass.* **67**, 84.
Gross, M., and Greenberg, L. A. (1948). "The Salicylates: A Critical Bibliographic Review". Hillhouse Press, New Haven, Connecticut.
Grossman, M. I., Matsumoto, K. K., and Lichter, R. J. (1961). *Gastroenterology* **40**, 383.
Guerra, F. (1944). *J. Pharmacol. Exptl. Therap.* **82**, 103.
Guerra, F., and Barbour, H. G. (1943). *J. Pharmacol. Exptl. Therap.* **79**, 55.
Guerra, F., and Brobeck, J. R. (1944). *J. Pharmacol. Exptl. Therap.* **80**, 209.
Gutman, A. B. (1966). *Advan. Pharmacol.* **4**, 91.
Guzman, F., Braun, C., and Lim, R. K. S. (1962). *Arch. Intern. Pharmacodyn.* **136**, 353.
Guzman, F., Braun, C., Lim, R. K. S., Potter, G. D., and Rodgers, D. W. (1964). *Arch. Intern. Pharmacodyn.* **149**, 571.
Hagebush, O. E., and Kinsella, R. A. (1930). *Proc. Soc. Exptl. Biol. Med.* **27**, 922.
Hailman, H. F. (1952). *J. Clin. Endocrinol. Metab.* **12**, 454.
Haining, C. G. (1963). *Brit. J. Pharmacol.* **21**, 104.
Hajnal, J., Sharp, J., and Popert, A. J. (1959). *Ann. Rheumatic. Diseases* **18**, 189.
Halkin, F., and van Cauwenberge, H. V. (1960). *Compt. Rend. Soc. Biol.* **154**, 1668.
Hardy, J. D. (1961). *Physiol. Rev.* **41**, 521.
Harris, S., and Harris, T. N. (1950). *Proc. Soc. Exptl. Biol. Med.* **74**, 186.
Harris, S. C., and Fosdick, L. S. (1952). *Northwest. Univ. Bull. Dental Res. Graduate Studies* **53**, 6.
Hart, E. R. (1947). *J. Pharmacol. Exptl. Therap.* **89**, 205.
Hauge, A., Lunde, P. K. M., and Waaler, B. A. (1966). *Acta Physiol. Scand.* **66**, 269.
Hebborn, P., and Shaw, B. (1963). *Brit. J. Pharmacol.* **20**, 254.
Hecht, A., and Goldner, M. G. (1959). *Metab. Clin. Exptl.* **8**, 418.
Hendershot, L. C., and Forsaith, J. L. (1959). *J. Pharmacol. Exptl. Therap.* **125**, 237.
Herxheimer, H., and Stresemann, E. (1966). *J. Physiol. (London)* **165**, 78P.
Hesse, E., Roesler, G., and Buhler, F. (1930). *Arch. Exptl. Pathol. Pharmakol.* **169**, 453.
Hinshaw, L. B., Solomon, L. A., Erdös, E. G., Rains, D. A., and Gunter, B. J. (1967). *J. Pharmacol. Exptl. Therap.* **157**, 665.
Hitchens, J. T., Goldstein, S., Shemano, L., and Beiler, J. M. (1967). *Arch. Intern. Pharmacodyn.* **169**, 384.
Honigsberger, M. (1943). *Brit. Med. J.* **ii**, 57.
Hook, G. (1966). *Therapiewoche* **16**, 1066.
Horáková, Z., and Muratová, J. (1965). *In* "Non-steroidal Anti-inflammatory Drugs" (S. Garattini, and M. N. G. Dukes, eds.), p. 237. Excerpta Med. Found., Amsterdam.
Houde, R. W., and Wallenstein, S. L. (1953). *Federation Proc.* **12**, 332.
Humphrey, J. H. (1951). *Brit. J. Exptl. Pathol.* **32**, 274.
Hurley, J. W., and Crandall, L. A. (1964). *Gastroenterology* **46**, 36.
Hurst, A., and Lintott, G. A. M. (1939). *Guy's Hosp. Rept.* **89**, 173.
Ingle, D. J. (1950). *Proc. Soc. Exptl. Biol. Med.* **75**, 673.
Ingle, D. J., and Meeks, R. C. (1952). *Am. J. Physiol.* **171**, 600.
Jacob, J. (1967). *In* "Methods of Drug Evaluation" (S. Mantegazza and F. Picini, eds.), p. 278. North-Holland Publ., Amsterdam.
Jacob, J., and Szerb, J. (1951). *Arch. Intern. Pharmacodyn.* **87**, 251.
Jacob, J., and Szerb, J. (1952). *Arch. Intern. Pharmacodyn.* **90**, 301.
Jaques, R. (1965). *Helv. Physiol. Pharmacacol. Acta* **23**, 156.
Johnston, I. D. A. (1964). *Ann. Roy. Coll. Surgeons Engl.* **35**, 270.
Johnston, I. D. A. (1968). *Sci. Basis Med., Ann. Rev.* p. 224.
Jori, A., and Bernardi, D. (1966). *Med. Pharmacol. Exptl.* **14**, 500.

Karzel, K. (1967). *Arch. Intern. Pharmacodyn.* **169**, 70.

Keith, E. F. (1960). *Am. J. Pharm.* **132**, 202.

Kelemen, E., Majoros, M., Ivanyi, J., and Kovacs, K. (1950). *Experientia* **6**, 435.

Kelemen, E., Majoros, M., Soltesz, R., and Tanos, B. (1952). *Deut. Med. Wochschr.* **77**, 1317.

Kellett, D. N. (1965). *In* "Non-steroidal Anti-inflammatory Drugs" (S. Garattini and M. N. G. Dukes, eds.), p. 203, Excerpta Med. Found., Amsterdam.

King, M. K., and Wood, W. B. (1958). *J. Exptl. Med.* **107**, 305.

Klupp, H., and Konzett, H. (1965). *Arch. Exptl. Pathol. Pharmakol.* **249**, 479.

Kodicek, E., and Loewi, G. (1955). *Proc. Roy. Soc.* (*London*) **B144**, 100.

Kolbe, H. (1874). *Z. Prakt. Chem.* **10**, 89.

Konzett, H., and Bauer, G. (1966). *In* "Hypotensive Peptides" (E. G. Erdös, N. Back, and F. Sicuteri, eds.), p. 375. Springer, New York.

Konzett, H., and Rössler, R. (1940). *Arch. Exptl. Pathol. Pharmakol.* **195**, 71.

Koster, R., Anderson, M., and de Beer, E. J. (1959). *Federation Proc.* **18**, 412.

Laden, C., Blackwell, R. A., and Fosdick, L. S. (1958). *Am. J. Physiol.* **195**, 712.

Lane, A. Z., Holmes, E. L., and Moyer, C. E. (1964). *J. New Drugs* **4**, 333.

Lecomte, J. (1960). *Compt. Rend. Soc. Biol.* **154**, 1118.

Lecomte, J., and Troquet, J. (1960). *Compt. Rend. Soc. Biol.* **154**, 1115.

Lepper, M. H., Caldwell, E. R., Smith, P. K., and Miller, B. F. (1950). *Proc. Soc. Exptl. Biol. Med.* **74**, 254.

Lester, D., Lolli, G., and Greenberg, L. A. (1946). *J. Pharmacol. Exptl. Therap.* **87**, 329.

Lewis, G. P. (1963). *In* "Salicylates: An International Symposium" (A. St. J. Dixon, B. K. Martin, M. J. H. Smith, and P. H. N. Wood, eds.), p. 134. Churchill, London.

Lim, R. K. S. (1966). *In* "The Salicylates, A Critical Bibliographic Review" (M. J. H. Smith and P. K. Smith, eds.), p. 155. Wiley, New York.

Lim. R. K. S., Guzman, F., Rodgers, D. W., Goto, K., Braun, C., Dickerson, C. D., and Engle, R. J. (1964). *Arch. Intern. Pharmacodyn.* **152**, 25.

Lim, R. K. S., Leung, P. M., and Guy, J. L. (1967a). *Federation Proc.* **26**, 619.

Lim, R. K. S., Miller, D. G., Guzman, F., Rodgers, D. W., Rogers, W., Wang, S. K., Chao, P. Y., and Shih, T. Y. (1967b). *Clin. Pharmacol. Therap.* **8**, 521.

Link, K. P., Overman, R. S., Sullivan, W. R., Huebner, C. F., and Scheel, L. D. (1943). *J. Biol. Chem.* **147**, 463.

Lish, P. M., and McKinney, G. R. (1963). *J. Lab. Clin. Med.* **61**, 1015.

Lisin, N., and Leclerq, R. (1963). *Compt. Rend. Soc. Biol.* **157**, 1536.

Long, D. A. (1955). *Intern. Arch. Allergy Appl. Immunol.* **6**, 337.

Long, D. A., and Miles, A. A. (1950). *Lancet* **i**, 492.

Macdougall, A. I., and Alexander, W. D. (1963). *In* "Salicylates: An International Symposium" (A. St. J. Dixon, B. K. Martin, M. J. H. Smith, and P. H. N. Wood, eds.), p. 92. Churchill, London.

Maclagan, T. (1876). *Lancet* **i**, 342, 383.

Maickel, R. P., Miller, F. P., and Brodie, B. B. (1965). *Pharmacologist* **7**, 182.

Manasse, K. (1900). Therapeutisches uber Aspirin. Wurzburg Thesis. Quoted in Gross and Greenberg (1948), p. 122.

Margolin, S. (1965). *In* "Non-steroidal Anti-inflammatory drugs" (S. Garattini, and M. N. G. Dukes, eds.), p. 214. Excerpta Med. Found., Amsterdam.

Marks, V., Smith, M. J. H., and Cunliffe, A. C. (1961). *J. Pharm. Pharmacol.* **13**, 218.

Marquardt, H. (1966). *Arch. Exptl. Pathol. Pharmakol.* **253**, 207.

Martelli, E. A. (1967). *J. Pharm. Pharmacol.* **19**, 617.

Mathies, H. (1958). *Arzneimittel-Forsch.* **8**, 233.

Mauer, E. F. (1955). *New Engl. J. Med.* **253**, 404.
Menguy, R., and Desbaillets, L. (1967). *Proc. Soc. Exptl. Biol. Med.* **125**, 1108.
Menguy, R., and Masters, Y. F. (1965). *Surg. Gynecol. Obstet.* **120**, 92.
Meyer, O. O., and Howard, B. (1943). *Proc. Soc. Exptl. Biol. Med.* **53**, 234.
Modell, W., and Patterson, R. (1951). *J. Am. Med. Assoc.* **147**, 124.
Mongar, J. L., and Schild, H. O. (1957). *J. Physiol.* (*London*) **135**, 301.
Moore-Robinson, M., and Warin, R. P. (1967). *Brit. Med. J.* **4**, 262.
Morris, C. D. W. (1967). *Lancet* **i**, 279.
Muir, A., and Cossar, I. A. (1955). *Brit. Med. J.* **ii**, 7.
Muir, A., and Cossar, I. A. (1961). *Am. J. Digest. Diseases* **6**, 1115.
Mustard, J. F., Glynn, M. F., Nishizawa, E. E., and Packham, M. A. (1967). *Federation Proc.* **26**, 106.
Newbould, B. B. (1963). *Brit. J. Pharmacol.* **21**, 127.
Niemegeers, C. J. E., Verbruggen, F. J., and Janssen, P. A. J. (1964). *J. Pharm. Pharmacol.* **16**, 810.
Nilsen, P. L. (1961). *Acta Pharmacol. Toxicol.* **18**, 10.
Northover, B. J. (1963). *J. Pathol. Bacteriol.* **85**, 361.
Northover, B. J. (1967). *Brit. J. Pharmacol.* **31**, 483.
Northover, B. J., and Subramanian, G. (1961a). *Brit. J. Pharmacol.* **16**, 163.
Northover, B. J., and Subramanian, G. (1961b). *Brit. J. Pharmacol.* **17**, 107.
Northover, B. J., and Subramanian, G. (1962). *Brit. J. Pharmacol.* **18**, 346.
O'Brien, J. R. (1968a). *Lancet* **i**, 779.
O'Brien, J. R. (1968b). *Lancet* **i**, 894.
Page, A. R., Condie, R. M., and Good, R. A. (1962). *Am. J. Pathol.* **40**, 519.
Paoletti, R., Maickel, R. P., Smith, R. L., and Brodie, B. B. (1963). *Proc. 1st Intern. Pharmacol. Meeting, Stockholm,* 1961 **2**, 29.
Pardo, E. G., and Rodriguez, R. (1966). *Life Sci.* **5**, 775.
Paul, W. D. (1943). *J. Iowa State Med. Soc.* **33**, 155.
Pearson, R. S. B. (1963). *In* "Salicylates: An International Symposium" (A. St. J. Dixon, B. K. Martin, M. J. H. Smith, and P. H. N. Wood, eds.), p. 170. Churchill, London.
Perese, D. M. (1961). *J. Am. Med. Assoc.* **175**, 75.
Pierson, R. N., Holt, P. R., Watson, R. M., and Keating, R. P. (1961). *Am. J. Med.* **31**, 259.
Prescott, L. F. (1966a). *J. Pharm. Pharmacol.* **18**, 331.
Prescott, L. F. (1966b). *Lancet* **ii**, 1143.
Quastel, J. H. (1963). *Appl. Therap.* **5**, 252.
Quick, A. J. (1966). *Am. J. Med. Sci.* **252**, 265.
Quick, A. J., and Clescari, L. (1960). *J. Pharmacol. Exptl. Therap.* **128**, 95.
Randall, L. O. (1963). *In* "Physiological Pharmacology. The Nervous System" (W. S. Root, and F. G. Hofman, eds.), Vol. 1, Pt. A, p. 313. Academic Press, New York.
Randall, L. O., and Selitto, J. J. (1957). *Arch. Intern. Pharmacodyn.* **111**, 409.
Rapoport, S., Wing, M., and Guest, G. M. (1943). *Proc. Soc. Exptl. Biol. Med.* **53**, 40.
Rénon, L. (1900). *Bull. Soc. Med. Hop. Paris,* 3rd *Ser.* **17**, 993.
Rodgers, D. W. (1964). *Pharmacologist* **6**, 182.
Rosenthale, M. E., and Nagra, C. L. (1967). *Proc. Soc. Exptl. Biol. Med.* **125**, 149.
Roth, J. L. A., and Valdes-Dapena, A. (1963). *In* "Salicylates: An International Symposium" (A. St. J. Dixon, B. K. Martin, M. J. H. Smith, and P. H. N. Wood, eds.), p. 224, Churchill, London.
Roth, J. L. A., Valdes-Dapena, A., Pieses, P., and Buchman, E. (1963). *Gastroenterology* **44**, 146.
Sancilio, L. P., and Rodriguez, R. (1965). *Federation Proc.* **24**, 677.

Sancilio, L. P., and Rodriguez, R. (1966). *Proc. Soc. Exptl. Biol. Med.* **123**, 707.
Schmidt, J. (1963). *Acta Biol. Med. Ger.* **10**, 194.
Scott, J. T., Denman, A. M., and Dorling, J. (1963). *Lancet* **i**, 344.
Seed, J. C. (1965). *Clin. Pharmacol. Therap.* **6**, 354.
Sheth, U. K., and Borison, H. L. (1960). *J. Pharmacol. Exptl. Therap.* **130**, 411.
Shwartzman, G., and Schneierson, S. S. (1953). *Ann. N.Y. Acad. Sci.* **56**, 733.
Shwartzman, G., Schneierson, S. S., and Soffer, L. J. (1950). *Proc. Soc. Exptl. Biol. Med.* **75**, 175.
Siegmund, E., Cadmus, R., and Lu, G. (1957). *Proc. Soc. Exptl. Biol. Med.* **95**, 729.
Silvestrini, B. (1965). *In* "Non-steroidal Anti-inflammatory Drugs" (S. Garattini and M. N. G. Dukes, eds.), p. 180. Excerpta Med. Found., Amsterdam.
Silvestrini, B., Garau, A., Pozzatti, C., and Cioli, V. (1966). *Arzneimittel-Forsch.* **16**, 59.
Sim, M. F. (1965). *In* "Non-steroidal Anti-inflammatory Drugs" (S. Garattini and M. N. G. Dukes, eds.), p. 207. Excerpta Med. Found., Amsterdam.
Skidmore, I. F., and Whitehouse, M. W. (1966). *Biochem. J.* **99**, 5P.
Skyring, A., and Bhanthumnavin, K. (1967). *Med. J. Australia* **1**, 601.
Smith, A. E. W., Frommel, E., and Radouco-Thomas, S. (1963). *Arzneimittel-Forsch.* **13**, 338.
Smith, D. L., D'Amour, M. C., and D'Amour, F. F. (1943). *J. Pharmacol. Exptl. Therap.* **77**, 184.
Smith, M. J. H. (1951). *J. Pharm. Pharmacol.* **3**, 409.
Smith, M. J. H. (1952). *Biochem. J.* **52**, 649.
Smith, M. J. H. (1953). *J. Pharm. Pharmacol.* **5**, 81.
Smith, M. J. H. (1955). *Brit. J. Pharmacol.* **10**, 110.
Smith, M. J. H. (1963). *In* "Salicylates: An International Symposium" (A. St. J. Dixon, B. K. Martin, M. J. H. Smith, and P. H. N. Wood, eds.), p. 47. Churchill, London.
Smith, M. J. H. (1966a). *In* "The Salicylates: A critical Bibliographic Review" (M. J. H. Smith and P. K. Smith, eds.), p. 49. Wiley, New York.
Smith, M. J. H. (1966b). *In* "The Salicylates: A critical Bibliographic Review" (M. J. H. Smith and P. K. Smith, eds.), p. 107. Wiley, New York.
Smith, M. J. H. (1966c). *In* "The Salicylates: A critical Bibliographic Review" (M. J. H. Smith and P. K. Smith, eds.), p. 203. Wiley, New York.
Smith, M. J. H., and Smith, P. K., eds. (1966). "The Salicylates: A Critical Bibliographic Review." Wiley, New York.
Smith, M. J. H., Meade, B. W., and Bornstein, J. (1952). *Biochem. J.* **51**, 18.
Smith, P. K. (1960). *Ann. N.Y. Acad. Sci.* **86**, 38.
Smith, P. K., Gleason, H. L., Stoll, C. B., and Orgorzalek, S. (1946). *J. Pharmacol. Exptl. Therap.* **87**, 237.
Smith, W., and Humphrey, J. H. (1949). *Brit. J. Exptl. Pathol.* **30**, 560.
Spector, W. G., and Willoughby, D. A. (1959). *J. Pathol. Bacteriol.* **77**, 1.
Starr, M. S., and West, G. B. (1966). *J. Pharm. Pharmacol.* **18**, 838.
Starr, M. S., and West, G. B. (1967). *Brit. J. Pharmacol.* **31**, 178.
Steinberg, D. (1963). *In* "The Control of Lipid Metabolism" (J. K. Grant, ed.), Biochem. Soc. Symp. No. 24, p. 111. Academic Press, New York.
Stone, E. (1763). *Phil. Trans. Roy. Soc. London* **53**, 195.
Stowers, J. M. (1963). *In* "Salicylates: An International Symposium" (A. St. J. Dixon, B. K. Martin, M. J. H. Smith, and P. H. N. Wood, eds.), p. 65. Churchill, London.
Stresemann, E. (1963). *Acta allergol.* **18**, 235.
Stubbé, L. Th. F. L. (1963). *In* "Salicylates: An International Symposium" (A. St. J. Dixon, B. K. Martin, M. J. H. Smith, and P. H. N. Wood, eds.), p. 236. Churchill, London.

Stubbé, L. Th. F. L., Pietersen, J. H., and van Heulen, C. (1962). *Brit. Med. J.* **1**, 675.
Stürmer, E., and Berde, B. (1963). *J. Pharmacol. Exptl. Therap.* **140**, 349.
Swyer, G. I. M. (1948). *Biochem. J.* **42**, 28.
Tanos, B., Kelemen, E., and Soltesz, R. (1953). *Acta Med. Acad. Sci. Hung.* **4**, 419.
Theobald, W., and Domenjoz, R. (1958). *Arzneimittel-Forsch.* **8**, 18.
Thiersch, C. (1875). *Samml. Klin. Vortr.* **84/85**, 637.
Trautschold, I., Fritz, H., and Werle, E. (1966). *In* "Hypotensive Peptides" (E. G. Erdös, N. Back, and F. Sicuteri, eds.), p. 221. Springer, New York.
Trethewie, E. R. (1951). *Australian J. Exptl. Biol. Med. Sci.* **29**, 443.
Trnavsky, K. (1967). *Acta Rheumatol. Balneol. Pistiniana* **3**, 66.
Truelove, L. H., and Duthie, J. J. R. (1959). *Ann. Rheumatic Diseases* **18**, 137.
Tudhope, G. R. (1967). *Ann. Phys. Med., Suppl.*, 58.
Türker, K., and Kiran, B. K. (1964). *Arzneimittel-Forsch.* **14**, 1318.
Ungar, G., and Damgaard, E. (1955). *J. Exptl. Med.* **101**, 1.
Ungar, G., Damgaard, E., and Hummel, F. P. (1952). *Am. J. Physiol.* **171**, 545.
Ungar, G., Kobrin, S., and Sezesny, B. R. (1959). *Arch. Intern. Pharmacodyn.* **123**, 71.
van Cauwenberge, H. V., and Lecomte, J. (1952). *Experientia* **8**, 469.
van Cauwenberge, H. V., and Lecomte, J. (1957). *Compt. Rend. Soc. Biol.* **151**, 405.
van Cauwenberge, H. V. Lecomte, J., and Goblet, J. (1954). *Experientia* **10**, 30.
van Cauwenberge, H. V., Lapière, C. M., and Lecomte, J. (1960). *Compt. Rend. Soc. Biol.* **154**, 440.
Vander Wende, C., and Margolin, S. (1956). *Federation Proc.* **15**, 494.
Vargaftig, B. (1966). *Experientia* **22**, 182.
Villablanca, J., and Myers, R. D. (1965). *Am. J. Physiol.* **208**, 703.
Vogin, E. E., and Rossi, G. V. (1963). *Arch. Intern. Pharmacodyn.* **144**, 151.
von Euler, C. (1961). *Pharmacol. Rev.* **13**, 361.
von Rechenberg, H. K. (1962). "Phenylbutazone", p. 147. Arnold, London.
Waaler, B. A. (1961). *J. Physiol. (London)* **157**, 475.
Wallenstein, S. L., and Houde, R. W. (1954). *Federation Proc.* **13**, 414.
Walters, M. N. I., and Willoughby, D. A. (1965a). *J. Pathol. Bacteriol.* **89**, 255.
Walters, M. N. I., and Willoughby, D. A. (1965b). *J. Pathol. Bacteriol.* **90**, 641.
Ward, J. R., and Cloud, R. S. (1966). *J. Pharmacol. Exptl. Therap.* **152**, 116.
Warren, M. R., and Werner, H. W. (1946). *J. Am. Pharm. Assoc., Sci. Ed.* **35**, 257.
Weis, J. (1963). *Med. Exptl.* **8**, 1.
Weiss, A., Pitman, E. R., and Graham, E. C. (1961). *Am. J. Med.* **31**, 266.
Weiss, B., and Laties, V. G. (1961). *J. Pharmacol. Exptl. Therap.* **131**, 120.
Weiss, H. J., and Aledort, L. M. (1967). *Lancet* **ii**, 495.
Weissmann, G. (1964). *Blood* **24**, 594.
Whitehouse, M. W. (1962). *Nature* **194**, 984.
Whitehouse, M. W. (1963). *In* "Salicylates: An International Symposium" (A. St. J. Dixon, B. K. Martin, M. J. H. Smith, and P. H. N. Wood, eds.), p. 55. Churchill, London.
Whitehouse, M. W. (1965). *Prog. Drug. Res.* **8**, 321.
Whittle, B. A. (1964). *Brit. J. Pharmacol.* **22**, 246.
Wiesinger, D. (1965). *In* "Non-steroidal Anti-inflammatory Drugs" (S. Garattini and M. N. G. Dukes, eds.), p. 221. Excerpta Med. Found., Amsterdam.
Wilhelmi, G. (1949). *Schweiz. Med. Wochschr.* **79**, 577.
Wilhelmi, G. (1963). *In* "Salicylates: An International Symposium" (A. St. J. Dixon, B. K. Martin, M. J. H. Smith, and P. H. N. Wood, eds.), p. 176. Churchill, London.
Wilhelmi, G. (1965). *In* "Non-steroidal Anti-inflammatory Drugs" (S. Garattini and M. N. G. Dukes, eds.), p. 174. Excerpta Med. Found., Amsterdam.

Wilhelmi, G., and Domenjoz, R. (1951). *Arch. Intern. Pharmacodyn.* **85**, 129.
Williams, M. W. (1959). *Toxicol. Appl. Pharmacol.* **1**, 590.
Williams, M. W., Williams, C. S., and Kartchner, M. J. (1965). *Toxicol. Appl. Pharmacol.* **7**, 45.
Willoughby, D. A., and Spector, W. G. (1964). *J. Pathol. Bacteriol.* **88**, 557.
Willoughby, D. A., and Walters, M. N. I. (1965). *J. Pathol. Bacteriol.* **90**, 193.
Willoughby, D. A., Boughton, B., Spector, W. G., and Schild, H. O. (1962). *Life Sci.* **7**, 347.
Willoughby, D. A., Boughton, B., and Schild, H. O. (1963). *Immunology* **6**, 484.
Willoughby, D. A., Walters, M. N. I., and Spector, W. G. (1965). *Immunology* **8**, 578.
Wilson, C. W. M. (1965). *Proc. Roy. Soc. Med.* **58**, 405.
Winder, C. V. (1947). *Arch. Intern. Pharmacodyn.* **74**, 219.
Winder, C. V. (1959). *Nature* **184**, 494.
Winder, C. V., Sarber, R. W., Hemans, M., Wax, J., and Bratton, A. C. (1957). *Arch. Intern. Pharmacodyn.* **112**, 212.
Winder, C. V., Wax, J., Burr, V., Been, M., and Rosiere, C. E. (1958). *Arch. Intern. Pharmacodyn.* **116**, 261.
Winder, C. V., Wax, J., Scotti, L., Scherrer, R. A., Jones, E. M., and Short, F. W. (1962). *J. Pharmacol. Exptl. Therap.* **138**, 405.
Winder, C. V., Wax, J., Serrano, B., Jones, E. M., and McPhee, M. C. (1963). *Arthritis Rheumat.* **6**, 36.
Winder, C. V., Wax, J., and Welford, M. (1965). *J. Pharmacol. Exptl. Therap.* **148**, 422.
Winter, C. A. (1965). *In* "Non-Steroidal Anti-inflammatory Drugs" (S. Garattini and M. N. G. Dukes, eds.), p. 190. Excerpta Med. Found., Amsterdam.
Winter, C. A., and Flataker, L. (1965). *J. Pharmacol. Exptl. Therap.* **148**, 373.
Winter, C. A., and Nuss, G. W. (1963). *Toxicol. Appl. Pharmacol.* **5**, 247.
Winter, C. A., Risley, E. A., and Nuss, G. W. (1962). *Proc. Soc. Exptl. Biol. Med.* **111**, 544.
Winter, C. A., Risley, E. A., and Nuss, G. W. (1963). *J. Pharmacol. Exptl. Therap.* **141**, 369.
Winter, C. A., Risley, E. A., and Silber, R. H. (1967). *Federation Proc.* **26**, 620.
Winter, J. E., and Barbour, H. G. (1928). *Proc. Soc. Exptl. Biol. Med.* **25**, 587.
Winters, R. W., and Morrill, M. F. (1955). *Proc. Soc. Exptl. Biol. Med.* **88**, 409.
Witthauer, R. (1900). *Therap. Monatsch.* **14**, 534.
Wolf, S., and Wolff, H. G. (1943). "Human Gastric Function" p. 165. Oxford Univ. Press, London and New York.
Wood, P. H. N. (1963). *In* "Salicylates: An International Symposium" (A. St. J. Dixon, B. K. Martin, M. J. H. Smith, and P. H. N. Wood, eds.), p. 194. Churchill, London.
Wood, P. H. N., Harvey-Smith, E. A., and Dixon, A. St. J. (1962). *Brit. Med. J.* **1**, 669.
Wood, W. B. (1958). *Lancet* **ii**, 53.
Woodbury, D. M. (1965). *In* "The Pharmacological Basis of Therapeutics" (L. S. Goodman, and A. Gilman, eds.), 3rd Ed., p. 312. Collier-Macmillan, London.
Wooles, W. R., Borzelleca, J. F., and Branham, G. W. (1967). *Toxicol. Appl. Pharmacol.* **10**, 1.
Zimmermann (1875). *Arch. Exptl. Pathol. Pharmakol.* **4**, 248.
Zucker, M. B., and Peterson, J. (1968). *Proc. Soc. Exptl. Biol. Med.* **127**, 547.

Author Index

Numbers in parentheses are reference numbers and indicate that an author's work is referred to, although his name is not cited in the text. Numbers in italics show the page on which the complete reference is listed.

C

D

E

F

G

H

I

J

K

L

M

N

O

T

U

V

X

Y

Z

Subject Index

D

E

F

Q

R

S

T

U

V

W